Of a Demon in My View

Jean M. Porro

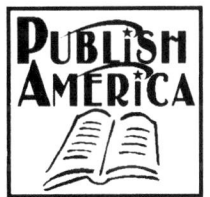

PublishAmerica
Baltimore

© 2002 by Jean M. Porro.
All rights reserved. No part of this book may be reproduced in any form without written permission from the publishers, except by a reviewer who may quote brief passages in a review to be printed in a newspaper or magazine.

First printing

This is a work of fiction. Names, characters, places, and incidents are either the product of the author's imagination or are used fictitiously, and any resemblance to actual persons, living or dead, business establishments, events or locales is entirely coincidental.

ISBN: 1-59129-748-6
PUBLISHED BY PUBLISHAMERICA BOOK PUBLISHERS
www.publishamerica.com
Baltimore

Printed in the United States of America

To Mom and Dad
To Danny

"Alone"
By Edgar Allen Poe, 1829

From childhood's hour I have not been
As others were—I have not seen
As others saw—I could not bring
My passions from a common spring—
From the same source I have not taken
My sorrow—I could not awaken
My heart to joy at the same tone—
And all I lov'd—I lov'd alone—
Then—in my childhood—in the dawn
Of a most stormy life—was drawn
From ev'ry depth of good and ill
The mystery which binds me still—
From the torrent, or the fountain—
From the red cliff of the mountain—
From the sun that' round me roll'd
In the autumn tint of gold—
From the lightening in the sky
As it pass'd me flying by—
From the thunder, and the storm—
And the cloud that took the form
(When the rest of Heaven was blue)
Of a demon in my view.

—From *The Unabridged Edgar Allen Poe*

PROLOGUE

The bureau sat in the corner of the room, a dusty memorial to her sister. On top of the large dresser lay Nina's comb, brush, perfumes and a framed photograph of the two girls. Millie Giannetti sat Indian style on the floor and carefully placed her dead sister's personal items into a small box. Each piece of clothing represented a piece of Nina, her favorite white sweater with the Angora collar. The short blue nightgown that she wore on hot summer nights.

When she pulled open the bottom drawer she saw her sister's journals. The diaries that Nina had been writing in since she was a little girl. Millie smiled as she thumbed through a few pages.

> *It was a nice day. The whole family was here, even Tommy came with his wife and Peter brought the new baby. We sat around and talked and ate all day. I even had fun with Suzy. Then Millie and I went for a walk along the tracks.*

They were wonderful moments and Millie was enchanted with the fact that she was able to share the same recollections. She felt a sudden sense of her sister's spirit when she read the familiar stories.

> *One night Poppa decided he was going to help some one. He bought a Christmas tree from a little boy who was working to support his family.*
>
> *"I made him so happy," Poppa bragged. "He had a big smile on his face."*
>
> *But the tree was crooked and the top branch where we hung the angel tilted toward the wall. It was so comical to see the angel flopping downward that when my father turned on the tree lights, Momma couldn't resist commenting,*
>
> *"That angel, she put on a few pounds since last year."*

Millie giggled at Nina's entries about Tommy and his temper tantrums, or Paul with his obnoxious ability to constantly taunt. She read over and over her sister's descriptions of the times they spent together. How they walked along the railroad tracks. Spent summer days and warm nights outside. Through her sister's words Millie was able to capture what it was like to sit and watch the neighborhood women gossip while the children played baseball or pleaded for pennies to give to the ice cream man on his nightly visit.

Nina loved to read and write so it was no surprise to Millie that her sister had kept track of everything she had ever read. The girl had filled one journal with titles, and authors, sorted by reading dates. She even highlighted notes about her favorite books.

>   (*Wuthering Heights*) *Did Emily Bronte know a real Heathcliffe?*

But as the young girl continued to read she began to see a dark side to some of Nina's writings.

>   *Please God, do not let him near my little sister. Promise me you won't let him touch her.*

At first she didn't understand but as Millie continued to read, her sister's sentences took on a bizarre strangeness and it soon became apparent that something horrible had happened to her sister.

>   *May 21, 1948*
>
>   Dear Momma:
>   *It was as an eleven-year-old girl that I first became caught up in the beauty of a tree. The tree of Heaven it was called.*
>   *It took me a long time to realize that I didn't have to be present each time he came to me and attacked my senses. I was grateful that I was able to leave this world to be transported out of myself and into the worlds that surround me.*
>   *I learned to leave my body and escape into the magic of words. Every time he violated me, my mind would whisk me away to some imaginary place in order to remove me from the devil that stirred around in my body.*
>   *To him it felt normal and right, that's what he told me, Momma.*

Millie, her eyes filling with tears, continued to read.

> *I pleaded with him each time but he would just smile and say it is alright. "You understand that's why I came to you, because you and I are just alike. We love deeper," he told me. Then he placed his hand under my blouse and his fingers grasped at my breast. I could feel the beat of his heart and face wet against me. Then he groped my thighs with sweaty hands and pushed my legs apart. He said he loved me, Momma, should I believe him?*
>
> *I wish I could tell you. I'm not sure what to say anymore. But if this is really what love is about why do I feel so sick, Momma?*
>
> *At first I believed him, now I just want it to end.*

She pressed the book closed and cried. It was horrible and unspeakable and her sister's revelations were devastating. She felt a terrible sadness. Nina wasn't just her older sister. They were best friends. She thought they had shared everything. But their closeness didn't include this secret. And Millie began to realize that her sister's only true confidante was herself and the words lost between the pages of her book.

Across the room was her sister's empty bed. The brown and white stuffed dog with the large ears, Nina's since she was a little girl, lay across the blue chenille bedspread.

Millie caught her breath as a quick breeze floated through the room. She began to fold the rest of her sister's clothes. She tied the box and placed it in a corner of the room. But not the journals; instead she placed them in the top drawer of her bureau. When Nina died Millie was left with a deep void. Today she felt a different sense of loss. She knew that what she had read would haunt her for a lifetime.

CHAPTER ONE

Once upon a time when the air was clean and the days were marked with innocence, Norwich seemed like a perfect world. A world with quiet, lazy streets and pretty neighborhoods lined with trees and smiling familiar faces.

In the early 1950s each house had a yard with a garden and a clothesline filled with white sheets that fluttered against soft breezes. Even the ominous dead end was nothing more than a deserted old railroad track that lured you to faraway places made up of summer dreams and inner simplicity. But within one short season the world would change and the essence of youth would trickle through adulthood and leave behind years of vulnerability, innocence and the ultimate sacrifice of naivete.

What happened in the small town of Norwich would change the dream of an ideal lifestyle forever with such devastating consequences that it would literally shake the tiny ethnic neighborhood out of existence.

For some the nightmare will never end. It still remains in the cemetery that overlooks the sober little town; where granite marks the grave of a young girl named Nina Giannetti. Whose death remains shrouded in mystery, and the horror of that time continues to hold her within its icy grasp.

It was the end of another innocent summer in 1952; but the busy citizens of Norwich didn't realize that their world was about to be shattered.

It started with a concern from a rash of sexual pranks that plagued young females. Though no one had been seriously hurt the parents of the teenage girls felt frightened and angered that the police had not been able to apprehend the attackers.

The pretty dark-haired girl lowered her head. "It's Maria," she said. "Marie Iatolla."

"I'm sorry, Marie," the police chief said. "This will only take a few minutes."

Mrs. Iatolla sat next to her daughter. "It's all right," she said, "this man needs to know everything."

"I know it was late, but I only live three blocks down from the Gershons. I didn't remember the street light was out until I reached the corner."

The old woman shook her head. "When they gonna fix that light?"

"That's when I heard the footsteps. So I turned around," the young girl began to cry. "Then that bag was shoved over my head."

Her eyes dropped to the floor. "His hands were under my blouse," she whispered. "I tried to fight, but he held the bag so tight against my neck I couldn't breathe. Then he forced me to the ground."

"It's all right," her mother said handing the girl a tissue. "You tell the police man what happened next."

"I lay still for a few minutes. I didn't know what to do. Then I heard footsteps again and the bag felt loose around my neck. That's when I pulled the sack off my head and threw up. Afterwards I ran home."

"You never saw anyone," the police chief asked.

"No sir. I didn't see anything."

"Well," Mrs. Iatolla said, "she tell the same story just like the other girls. How you gonna catch him, if no one ever sees him?"

"We will catch him, Mrs. Iatolla, I promise you."

Marty looked at the young girl. "Thank you, Maria."

The girl had given him nothing new to go on. Still there was little doubt in Marty's mind that this was some young kid acting out his sexual fantasies. Although he was concerned and wanted to wring the kid's neck he didn't believe that these events would escalate beyond some little shit trying to grab the breast of a few young girls. At least that's what he hoped.

In order to visualize the mood of a small town in Massachusetts during the post war years one must dig deep into the recesses of his or her memory or imagination. Lower Norwich was a haven for the ethnic cultures of Italian, Irish and Polish, immigrants who settled in the modest town after the war looking for a better way and the promises of tomorrow for their families.

In the years that followed the aftermath of World War II, the country seemed destined to grow up quickly. Most areas had gone from clusters of neighborhoods to main streets where schools, recreation facilities and churches were all being designed and built to carry the influx of new people and the bulging communities.

By 1950 the average yearly income was somewhere between $8,000 and $12,000. The purchase of a modest house with a new kitchen and a shiny new car could be had for less than fifteen thousand dollars.

Still with the explosion of post war pride, modular neighborhoods, and new technology there were left behind a few small towns that existed for years because of the local mill and other homebred industries. Norwich was one of them. With a policy of hire residents first and its ability to instill a sense of community drenched in tradition and loyalty it maintained a high ratio of citizenship. Diversified cultures lived side by side with the same moral and social qualities that hadn't changed since the Victorian era.

Lower Norwich or Ethnic Village, as it was often called, was made up of blue-collar workers, and immigrant families. People shared neat rows of double-decker houses each with its own front porch, where young mothers in stained aprons gossiped and carefully eyed their kids.

These cultural neighborhoods remained generation after generation. Neighbors watched their children grow up together, attend the same schools, football games and church dances. Next door romances blossomed into couples who married and continued the same familiar cycle. Yet the small community evaporates as one moves further into town.

The village is set apart by a large park that acts as a centerpiece for the town. A huge gazebo sits right in the middle of the park surrounded by pathways. In one section is a memorial dedicated to the veterans of World War I. All year long the common reflects the different seasons; alive with colorful flowers in summer or Christmas lights, the common is the focal point of the town.

At one end is the old brick building that houses the civic offices, the fire station and the police station. Along the sides of the common are wood benches shaded by large oak trees and filled with local gentry. The men gather in conversation and smoke their pipes or cigars, oblivious to the hustle and bustle of the locally-owned businesses that surround them, such as Pearson's Hardware and Edna Kelly's Bridal Shop.

On the other end of the park is St. Bartholomew's Catholic Church with its conspicuous cement, stone structure and steeple. The tower stares down at the town and maintains a constant vigil that overlooks its congregation.

The expanding population in Lower Norwich is no way a part of mainstream society. In fact with the small neighborhood's many cultural markets and brand new bank it is totally separate and dependent of the village or town center.

The main square, however, is dedicated to the needs of the residents who live in the traditional part of town. The doctors, bankers and businessmen tuck their families into large homes with front foyers and picture windows.

Their children play in quiet groups separated by white fences and private schools. As young adults the children attend out of state colleges and marry strangers; eventually they move away to unfamiliar places.

Yet with all the differences there is one common denominator that brings these two contrary communities together. Each Sunday, as the bells toll from the steeple of St. Bart's Church, the Catholic population from both sides of town comes together to listen to the Monsignor give his Sunday sermon.

On a warm weekend in August the unsuspected churchgoers kneeled and prayed together in harmony. They had no idea that their carefree lifestyle would soon be destroyed by an enigma that would crawl along the streets and eventually blanket the whole town, in a consuming plague.

CHAPTER TWO

He slid his knees behind Dorothy Miller's legs and forced her down. He knew the woman was drowning in terror. In his hand was a heavy statue. The attacker lifted the bronze figure and looked into the eyes of the pretty dark-haired woman. Swiftly and devoid of emotion he smashed it against the side of her head and watched as the blood oozed down her right cheek. Then he thrust himself into the nearly unconscious woman over and over again until he reached his own perverted climax.

The victim, barely alive, moaned. Pulling her limp body off the couch he placed it against the back wall. In his hand he cupped the woman's chin and stared at her lifeless image. With a sudden detached coldness he took her head and smashed it against the painted wall again and again.

When he was finished, he surveyed the room. The attacker picked up the woman's scattered clothes and began to fold them. First her skirt, then her blouse, and his hand brushing the collar of the white blouse. After he folded the underwear and placed it on top of the pile, he smoothed the wrinkles away with his hand.

The attacker stepped onto the couch and then lifted himself out the window. His shadowy form disappeared into the night.

Martin Sacco had been the police chief in Norwich for five years. Tonight he stood in the apartment of a woman who had just been brutally murdered.

"The Miller woman was probably dead before this guy decided to use her head as a hammer," the medical examiner told him. He had in his hand a bronze statue splattered with blood. "My guess is she was hit pretty hard with this first."

Marty reached his hand into the pocket of his shirt for that long absent pack of cigarettes. *Norwich hadn't dealt with anything this serious since the Roache disappearance ten years ago*, he thought. *A petty thief or belligerent drunk didn't account for any real trouble. This, this was different. This looked like rape and murder.*

He had been there for almost forty minutes and was about to head out the door. "What do you make of this?" a young detective called to him.

Marty knelt down. He pulled a pencil from his pocket and picked up a pair of silk panties that sat on top of a pile of neatly folded clothes.

"I don't know yet."

The chief dropped the underwear and placed the pencil back in his pocket. "But I'm sure I'll find out," he said.

Dorothy Miller's apartment was one flight up in the old brick building. Marty walked down the stairs and out of the front door. He looked up at the broken street light. It was cool and the night air felt crisp as he gathered his jacket around him. He would rather walk back to the office—but instead he slipped into the front seat of the police car.

"Tell me again what you saw, Mr. Benchek?" He heard Taylor ask the elderly man when he walked through the station door. The detective was taking notes while an elderly gentleman spoke. Both men sat on the bench just outside Marty's office.

"My wife and I have dinner at Tango's. Then we walk to Common Street. That's where we live. When we are less than one block from the house I notice that damn streetlight is out. It's very dark on that corner," he said. "My wife—she's called the town three times but nobody fix the light."

"Yes Mr. Benchek," Jim said. "Then what happened?"

The old man smiled at the detective. "I'm sorry," he said. "We walk by the apartment house and I hear a noise. When I look this man jump from the window and run. 'Hey, what you doing there?' I yell to him."

"Was there anything about him you recognized?" Taylor asked.

"No."

"How about his clothes?"

"All I see was a dark figure run across the street and down by the field where the old railroad tracks go. Then I don't see him no more. My wife, she run to somebody's house and asked them to call the police."

Sacco walked up to the old man and bent down. "Would you excuse us for one minute?"

Taking Jim aside he asked, "Who's that?"

"Mr. Benechek. It was his wife that called the police."

"Did he see anything?"

"No, just a shadow running across the street." Taylor pulled a cigarette out of his pocket. "This one is pretty brutal," he remarked. He placed the cigarette in his mouth. "The killer could be an ex or a new boyfriend. Maybe she pissed one of them off. But you can be sure of one thing," he said with a mouth full of smoke. "It's not our kid who's been copping a feel under a potato sack."

Sacco looked away from Taylor. His eyes focused on the old man who was still on the bench. "I'm not sure this murder is that simple," he said. "There's no evidence of an argument. Nothing appears out of place." He shook his head then looked back towards Taylor. "My guess is if this isn't a jealousy thing. Then we've got one mad son-of-a-bitch on our hands. And he isn't gonna stop with Dorothy Miller."

It was unusual for the chief of police to investigate a case. Even one this outrageous. But Marty wanted this case. "I'm on this one," he told Taylor. "I'm working this case with you."

"Just like the old days." Taylor smiled.

"Yeah, just like the old days."

CHAPTER THREE

Driving through Ethnic Village one can see that fundamentally it does still exist, but without the closeness and intimacy of its earlier heritage. The community where Millie Giannetti lived, as a young girl was once drenched in tradition with cultures that thrived on togetherness, a lifestyle so basic during the forties and fifties.

The houses like their owners appear haggard and distressed. The pampered backyards with nurtured vegetable gardens are now gone. And in their place stand large plastic swing sets that move idly in the sun. Neighbors no longer chat on street corners; instead they bury their faces and rush past one another.

The Kerchak house is gone and in its place stands a dingy brick building with a crooked sign that flashes lights over the entrance. "We cash checks. No identification needed" is printed in black on the dirty window. Every once in a while a middle-aged man, tall with gaunt features, paces the sidewalk. His eyes dart back and forth and a cigarette hangs loosely from his lips. Millie catches a quick glance and for a moment his face seems familiar.

The Giannetti house is still there but the huge white structure with its two big porches and dozen of lighted windows is now dark and empty.

Millie eases the car into the empty driveway of what once was her home. It seems like forever since she has been back. But it doesn't matter because the memories are still there, especially the ones about her sister.

Every day Nina would take her book and walk to the shed. Even now for Millie that memory was alive. She could still see her pretty sister with that soft smile and long black hair.

She stood in the doorway of what was once Nina's private reading place. It hadn't changed much. There was still that familiar groan when you opened the door.

Despite the coats of paint the smell of death still seeped through the walls. Similar, she thought, to the way her sister's death haunts her mind. That night was filled with so much chaos and horror. And suddenly it is all back. The sounds of the whining police cars in the driveway, the metal shininess visible under the white sheet when her sister's body is lifted onto the hearse. The whispers of neighbors gathered collectively in corners.

Nauseous and overwhelmed she runs outside. The fresh air feels good on her face. And she leans against the shed. A strong breeze takes hold of the door and slams it into the wind. Millie takes one last look into the cold cement building and then turns the knob. She twists the lock into place and walks away.

It was so long ago. And the sounds of confusion and the sense of drama can linger only in the memories. But the sadness of what happened will forever remain, because in reality she is left with the grief of an undeniable loss.

Millie walked back to her car. She took one last look at the back stairway. How strange it all seemed now, her past as she once lived it. Certainly there was nothing special about her family or her neighborhood. But it was real and secure and boringly consistent. And that was all she knew.

She drove to the end of the street and stopped the car. The railroad tracks lay right ahead. Her eyes scanned across the field. This too was once a secret garden, a place where young girls talked and laughed. Each day as they made their way home from school they would test their balance on the wooden tracks, or pick wildflowers. Sometimes Millie and Nina would sit on the old stone wall and share a secret or gossip about a new boy.

But that had changed too. The field was ravaged with litter. Instead of patches of wild flowers it was trash infested and overgrown with weeds.

Millie knew her sister's death was devastating. But Nina's death reached beyond the family. The grief carried through the neighborhood and into the town. People lost their sense of fellowship. The security and trust that was once a part of life was over. The open doors suddenly closed after the murder. And the people hid behind fear and ugly rumors. Nina Giannetti's death became the prelude for what would become the loss of Main Street innocence.

As youngsters the Giannetti girls lived in a house full of restrained love, noisy emotions and with such a large family, the necessary guidelines.

"Hey," Momma would say. "Have some hot bread." She would tear a piece from a fresh loaf, drizzle it with olive oil, stuff the soft center with fresh basil and her pudgy fingers would push the two ends together.

The house was actually a three family structure. On the first floor lived John and Elsie Provenz. The couple had lived there for as long as Millie could remember.

But the Giannettis took over the second and third floor. Her father expanded the house each time the family grew. Eventually the small third floor apartment became three bedrooms to accommodate all eight children.

By the time Millie came along Momma and Poppa were tired. And the older siblings were forced to take over the duties of their parents. The girls would bathe Millie, read her stories and listen to her prayers at night. Tommy helped with school projects. And Peter walked her to school for the first few years.

Tommy and Peter, in their late twenties, were married and had left home by the time Millie turned ten. "Peter and Domenic were the smart ones," Momma reminded everybody, "'cause they always busy." Eventually Peter graduated from college with a degree in accounting, married Audrey Dellacorte and moved out of state.

Tommy worked as a mechanic and eventually opened his own garage. Eventually he opened his own garage. Poppa always bragged about his sons. Anytime something needed to be fixed, it was Tommy he called. "There is nothing he can't fix."

"Except his temper," Momma would answer back.

Tommy was known for his quick emotional outbursts. He would get so angry banging his fist, turning red and then two minutes later it was as if his fury never happened and he was calm. Whenever he would get mad Millie would leave the room. Once he got so mad she thought the veins in the top of his head were going to explode.

The older sister, Rose, married Frank Curly and left her job to live in South Boston. Momma, who believed that not being Italian was a sin, could never say Rose's name without making the sign of the cross. "That poor girl, now she live with all the Irish."

Finally there was Poppa's favorite, Susan or Susie, with her statuesque figure and stylishly short dark hair. The boys would fall all over themselves to get a date with her. "When your sister Susie married Joey DeNardo," Poppa told his two younger daughters, "all the young men in the town cried."

Joey married her the year she turned twenty-two and then moved Susie out of Norwich and into his hometown of Brockton.

Millie loved to listen to Poppa's stories; most times they were rich in color and full of imagination. But he wasn't wrong about Susie. Guys would line the sidewalk just to walk on the same side of the street with her.

Yet as a sibling Susie was hard to like. One day Millie watched her stroll across the bedroom, a book balanced on the top of her head and her body erect.

"Susie, will you teach me how to walk like that?"

"Not now," she answered in her typical style. "Walking straight takes a certain poise. Something I don't think you have."

If Susie exasperated Millie, it was their brother Paul, just barely older, who irritated Nina. He had rugged good looks and a highly warped sense of humor. If he wasn't torturing some poor dumb animal then it was Nina, especially if she had a boyfriend. He loved to bully her with his super show of macho power. And if Nina complained he would roll his eyes and say, "Hey, that's what a big brother does."

But his attitude went beyond the brother stuff. And Nina considered him more than an overzealous protector. He was also a troublemaker who never accepted blame. If he were involved in anything that Poppa didn't like it was the other person's fault. "I didn't start it, he did," was his automatic reply.

One time when he stole some cupcakes at the local market, he held his ground with his excuse.

"It wasn't my fault," Paul insisted. "It's Mr. Jansen's fault. He's the one who placed them on the counter."

His no-fault attitude was not exclusively his own either, when you considered his environment and the family discussions.

There were eight Giannetti siblings including their stepbrother, Domenic, Poppa's son from his first marriage. "His wife die of pneumonia," Momma told Millie one day. "There he was, a poppa at twenty-five taking care of a little boy.

"Then one day he sees me walking along the road near my house and he falls in love all over again."

Momma Giannetti was barely nineteen when she married Salvatore and took over the care of little Domenic.

"I never think anything of it," she said. "It was just like my own from the very first day."

And Momma was right. Millie didn't realize Domenic was her step-brother until she was ten years old.

By then he was a twenty-seven-year-old theology student who seemed pretty mysterious in those days, especially because he spent most of his time at the seminary. Which suited the prepubescent Nina and Millie just fine. When he would come home from school for the holidays, Poppa would insist that his young son needed peace and quiet. "So he can study."

Only his room was one flight up from theirs and that meant they couldn't play the radio. One day after Poppa told her to turn off the record player Nina became angry. "Why does he have to come home?" she said. "All he does is study anyway."

Being so much older gave Domenic an edge over the rest of the siblings. He was already a college graduate and he had a vision. But it wasn't just his age that separated him from the other brothers. He liked to study. And he preferred track to football. He wasn't interested in constant dates. The older boy rarely bullied anybody and he had decent manners. And from what Millie could see he was neater, not always sweaty and smelly like Paul.

There was one time when Millie was surprised by something her brother did. Her mother had told her to call Domenic to the table so she climbed the stairs to his room. She was just ready to speak when she saw him toss something on the bedroom floor. Whatever it was shattered into pieces. He stood there and looked down at all the broken shards of glass. After a few minutes he fell to his knees, scooped up the debris and tossed it in the trash bucket. Then he placed the bucket back under his desk.

Millie loved all her siblings but she admired Nina. It was the way her seventeen-year-old sister could put her emotions aside. Nina was elusive and often times distanced herself from the strains that existed within the household. She had a maturity that went way beyond seventeen and yet there was this innocence about her life. If she was angered she could look at you with visible detachment. Yet there was this emotional warmth that was always accessible.

It was these very qualities that Millie admired that irritated the other siblings, especially Paul. No matter what Nina did Paul managed to use it against her.

"Nina walked home alone from the library tonight, Poppa," Paul told his father.

"What did I tell you about that?" Poppa would say.

"It was still light outside, Poppa."

Whatever Paul's problem was, Nina found herself constantly on the defensive.

On occasion Momma would give her son a steely glance.

"Why you don't mind your own business?" she would say. Then in a dramatic grumble Paul would generally toss an arm in the air and yell, "You tell me to watch out for my sisters, but when I do you get angry."

And his claims of protection could sometimes border on cruelty. One time when Nina made a silly remark Paul slapped her across the face. Within seconds he knew he had gone too far. But when he tried to apologize she ran into the shed and locked the door.

Millie sat on the back steps and listened as he shouted through the shed door, "Nina, I'm sorry," But she wouldn't open the door until he left.

And she could remain so isolated from him that it would take weeks before she spoke to him again. Nina was different from all of the siblings. She had little interest in anything they did or talked about.

Nina retreated into her books. She could become so engrossed in a story that she would settle into the main character. While reading *A Tree Grows in Brooklyn*, she would become Francie and for days wore her hair in pigtails. When she read *Wuthering Heights*, she would refer to Paul as Heathcliffe.

Her choice of books was extraordinary as well as diverse. She had no favorite. She loved every author and every story. If she wasn't reading then she was writing in her journal. Millie never held a memory of her sister when she didn't have a book in her hand.

As a young girl Millie didn't always comprehend the reason her sister withdrew from the real world. Now it is easy to understand why her sister was surrounded by an essence of melancholy, a sadness that embraced her and made her vulnerable even when she smiled.

The Giannetti house was big and roomy, full of slamming doors and drafty hallways, and constantly full of people. Aunts and uncles shared Friday night fish, Sunday dinners and all the holidays.

"Momma, Auntie and Uncle are here," Millie would yell with excitement when Aunt Claire would arrive with her kids Angela and her obnoxious son Steven, a pimple-faced adolescent who loved to provoke trouble for the girls.

Once after he tried to kiss Millie she slugged him.

He had the nerve to yell to his mother, "Momma, Millie slapped me in the face."

"Millie," Auntie Claire asked. "What Steven do that you slap him in the face?"

"He tried to kiss me."

"That's 'cause he loves you," she said. "He's you cousin. Now go ahead, you kids, go and play."

Although Steven was annoying he was harmless. But his father was another story.

"Come give your uncle a kiss," he would request each time he visited. His mouth slobbered over the girl's cheeks. And he would stare at them. Mainly their breasts. If he asked one of them a question Uncle Ed would never look them in the eye. Instead he stared below their necks.

One time Nina mentioned it. "He just stares at my breasts," she said.

"That's your Uncle Ed. He's known you since you were a baby," Momma said. "Why you think like that?"

Every weekend was the same. He would paste a kiss on one cheek and pat the other one.

Still when Friday nights came and the group of adults gathered around the table to sip wine and rehashed their lives in the old country, the young cousins would gather in the den and play games or refurbish the family legends. It didn't matter about the little issues back then. Millie felt safe and secure. Her family loved and nurtured her and she took to heart her mother's words. "Remember, family is all there is."

But now so many years later in the shadow of her old house saddened by more than just the loss of those days, Millie realized that her mother's theory was as flawed as the old cement driveway she was standing on.

CHAPTER FOUR

Marty Sacco stood and stared out the window of the civic building, which overlooked the common. In the middle of the park was a display of pilgrims with musket rifles in their hands while they stared down a group of wooden Indians. It was almost Thanksgiving and six weeks after Dorothy Miller's murder Marty was no closer to her killer.

However, despite the ugliness of the incident the local gentry wanted the murders buried. This was, after all, the holiday season and the clever shop owners were determined to eradicate the gloom of the tiny area with a replacement of seasonal decorations. And so with only seven days left the cautious residents of Norwich began to settle into preparations for the regular turkey feast.

The crime had doubly affected the residents of Ethnic Village. Dorothy Miller lived there and the murderer had escaped from there, terrible in the eyes of everyone. Still it was almost forgotten, as the festivities of the coming holiday season made it easy to ignore.

That was true about the Giannettis and especially Millie's mother. Plump and aged beyond her years she spent her days in the house surrounded by her daily habits. It was her custom, once fall arrived, to begin preparations for the special days. One of her favorite pastimes was to wash all the lace tablecloths and napkins by hand. Once they were all ironed, folded and stored neatly away in the drawer of the shiny mahogany hutch, Momma would exclaim, "They smell so good. Now we are ready."

Despite the cold, and the arthritis that invaded her body, Momma enjoyed the coolness that came with the fall season. "The quiet sometimes reminds me of Naples."

She was a stubborn woman and insisted on doing certain things her own way with little help. At the end of those exhausting days she would sit with a cup of coffee and stare out at the neighborhood.

Momma loved to talk about how she met her husband. Many days Millie would plant herself in a chair with a cup of cocoa and listen to her mother retell the same story. Only every time she would add a new embellishment. It was within those quiet solitary moments of conversation that Millie learned the most.

"Everybody think Poppa's wife die from pneumonia," Momma whispered one day. "But that's not true. She really die from a sickness in here," she said and pointed to her head.

"What kind of sickness?"

"I don't know but she was very bad. Your poppa tell me she would sometimes scream for days. One day he come home and she was crying. She told Poppa Domenic was dead. Your father, he ran to the crib to find the blanket over the baby's head. That's when he called the doctor and they took her away."

"That is so sad," Millie said.

"I know." Then she placed her finger on her lips and said, "Don't tell Poppa I told you."

Millie promised and she never did tell anyone. Still she never forgot the vision of a young woman trying to smother her own baby.

Another time she asked, "What are you looking at, Momma?" when she saw her mother staring out the window.

"That house it is very sad."

"The Kerchak house. How can a house be sad?"

"Because of the people who live there. I think that poor Grace Kerchak is a very sad woman."

The Kerchak family lived across from the Giannettis separated by the driveway and a tiny shed. Momma didn't like George Kerchak and it was no secret to any of the family. She had witnessed his meanness more than once.

Normally it was unusual for the Kerchaks to join in the resident activities, yet late one summer afternoon they did. George and Grace stood and chatted among a group of neighbors.

Later that evening he said goodnight and headed towards his house. When he realized his wife wasn't with him. She was with a group of the neighborhood women. He walked up to her and grabbed her arm. "Did you not hear me say goodnight?" he snapped.

"Poor Grace, her face turned white. She looked at us and whispered, 'Goodnight.' But the expression on the son's face," Momma said. "Scare me more than the father."

She turned to her daughter. "In all the years your poppa and me are married he never lift his hand to me." Then she smiled and tossed her hand, "Ahh, maybe he wanted to. But he never did."

The sound of the old kitchen clock was hypnotic and Millie could barely keep awake. Her mother leaned back in her chair and yawned.

"Call your sister from the shed," she said. "You girls go to bed."

Momma's daily habit to sit and stare out the window was a familiar sight in the neighborhood. Every day when the two girls arrived home she would be there to wave them up the back stairs. One day when Millie and Nina got off the bus at the corner, Momma saw Josef Kerchak speak to them.

"What that boy want?" Momma asked when Millie and Nina walked into the house.

"He wanted to paint Nina's picture," Millie said.

"Like an artist."

"Yes, Momma."

"What did you say?"

"I told him no."

Momma looked at Nina. "You don't like him."

"No. Nobody does."

"The kids make fun of him all the time at school," Millie volunteered.

"You don't like him, Nina," she said.

"No, Momma."

Momma might not have understood but Millie knew why her sister didn't like Josef. She thought of him like a pest. He was always around her, watching everyone she talked to. When she stepped off the bus he was there. Like today. He wanted to know if Nina would pose for him for a drawing he needed for school.

"It's a-a project for art cl-class," he said.

"I'm not posing for you," she told him. "School project or not."

"He makes my skin crawl," Nina said when they walked away. Then she told Millie something that happened in school. "Josef was behind me in line and he pushed himself into me. Yuck," she continued. "I wanted to vomit."

By Thanksgiving Day, Millie had tucked the conversations somewhere in the back of her head. The house was in an uproar as the Giannettis began to prepare for the holiday. Momma had set the dining room table, baked her breads and had placed a 22-pound turkey in the oven. Family was everywhere. Uncle Ed and Poppa were in the living room with the cousins and grandchildren and all the females were busy in the kitchen. Auntie Claire folded the napkins, Rose mashed the potatoes and Susie was busy with the water glasses.

"When will the turkey be done?" Millie asked.

"Soon," her mother said. "Relax, every year we rush around like crazy. We cook, clean, so much work, fifteen minutes everybody eat everything and then what? We do dishes all day."

"I know," Aunt Claire agreed, "but you wouldn't change it for the world."

"Yeah, don't be too sure..." she said with a wink.

"Why what do you mean?"

"This year I do something a little different. This year I break tradition. I invite the neighbors to come and share dessert."

"What neighbors?" Millie asked.

"The Kerchaks."

"Why did you do that, Momma?" Nina asked.

"Because, I feel sorry for the wife."

"Does Poppa know?"

"What do you think? Of course, I tell your father."

That afternoon dinner at the Giannettis' was like a dining room assembly line. Hands were everywhere. First came the soup, then the lasagna and sausages. After that, the table was cleared for the turkey, potatoes, stuffing and of course the salad.

Then it was dessert and coffee.

"Happy Thanksgivin'," Poppa greeted the Kerchaks when they arrived at the door.

"Please come in," Momma said. Mr. Kerchak followed Poppa out of the room and into the parlor. Mrs. Kerchak and Josef joined the rest of the family in the dining room. Grace Kerchak carried something to the buffet.

Momma looked down at the dark crusted sugar-topped pastry. "Oh you bring some strudel," she said.

"Yes," the frail woman answered, "it's the only dessert my George will eat."

"That's too bad," Momma said, before she announced the coffee was ready. Within a few minutes the room filled as the family began to wander into the dining room to eat nut breads, Italian cookies, cannolis, pumpkin pie, and the family's favorite, Riccotta pie.

Suzy walked in the room and made some usual nasty comments. This time it was directed at Tommy.

"Could you fit anything else on that plate?"

"Hey, why don't you go and check your husband's plate."

Nina tried to disappear from the dining room but Momma spotted her and patted the chair. "Come sit next to me," she said. Millie sat at the opposite end of the table and watched everybody, especially Josef, who was watching Nina. Now Millie understood why her sister felt so uncomfortable around him, his eyes never left her. And Momma also noticed it. Her eyes darted back and forth from her daughter's face to Josef's. Momma whispered something in Nina's ear and she moved from her seat and left the room. Then Momma sat herself directly in Josef's view.

"So," she said, "my girls tell me you like to draw."

He lowered his eyes. "Yes," he said.

Nina walked back into the room and he became distracted. "I'm—I'm s-s-studying bodies."

"You like to draw people," she said. "Well, maybe you should try to do the houses. I know these archytecturers make a lot of money."

"You mean architects," Domenic said eavesdropping. He had just sliced himself some dessert. "Momma, your Riccotta pie," he said, "gets better every year."

"I'm glad you enjoy," she turned to Grace, "you know my son, Domenic."

Later that evening after everyone else had left Nina walked back into the dining room and took a seat next to her mother. "I think maybe," she said while she stroked her daughter's dark hair, "I make a mistake when I invite the Kerchaks here. I don't like that he looks at you that way."

"Don't worry, Momma," Nina said. "He doesn't bother me."

CHAPTER FIVE

As he ran he breathed in the cold air and suddenly he felt revitalized. Then came this incredible surge of release. His pace quickened and he rushed along the tracks. *Faster*, he told himself over and over. Faster, until I'm invisible and become part of the midnight wind.

Two days later the holiday atmosphere would come to a quick end, when Marty Sacco was summoned to 189 Charles Street, in Lower Norwich.

Marty and Detective Taylor stood next to a middle-aged man who was visibly upset. As they listened Taylor would write in his notebook.

"My wife and I got home about 10:30," John Meddick said. "We had been at my in-laws' in Andover for the Thanksgiving holiday. When we pulled into the driveway, Lois got out to open the garage door. Then she tells me she saw somebody in the backyard. I went to the shelf to get the flashlight. But I didn't see anybody," Mr. Meddick said.

"I decided to walk next door to see if the Robertsons heard anything suspicious. Their back door was open, so I knocked and then walked inside."

"Was it unusual for their back door to be open?" Taylor asked.

"No, Stanley is a night volunteer for the local fire station, and his wife Betty would wait up for him. She would be downstairs with the television on so she would leave the door open for him."

"Then what happened?"

"All the lights were on so I walked inside and called to her. It seemed strange she didn't answer. I walked towards the front of the house and that's when I saw her." His voice cracked and his eyes filled.

"Mr. Meddick, did you touch anything?"

"No," he said. "I ran home to call you guys."

"Thank you, sir," Taylor said. "One of the officers will take your statement."

Marty felt genuinely sorry for Meddick. He knew what it was like to walk into a grisly scene. The killer had added another victim to the scenario. The poor man would live with what he saw every day.

The police chief walked past a young officer and through the doorway. He stood in the front foyer. A woman's nude body, her head hung low sat in a puddle of blood, slumped against the wall. Her name was Betty Robertson. Marty could see that her head had been pummeled. He bent down to look closer at the lifeless body and then out of habit felt for a pulse.

Doctor Curran, the M.E. looked at the woman. "This guy likes to pound heads," he said.

Marty gently let go of her wrist and looked up at the M.E. "I'm gonna look around."

He walked into the living room. Nothing appeared to be touched. There was no sign of a struggle. A lifetime of memories sat on a dusty table, and not one appeared out of place.

In the kitchen he found a few dirty dishes and a coffee can full of cigarette butts. He heard the coroner's van arrive and the familiar sound of the metal dolly when it clanked against the floor in the front hall.

Forty-eight hours later he reviewed the coroner's report and then he called for a meeting. He could almost feel his hair turn gray as he peered out at the young men gathering.

"This is the coroner's report," he said. "It states Mrs. Robertson had massive head injuries. In other words she died the same way Dorothy Miller did. With her head being slammed against a hard surface."

Marty, seated on the corner of his desk, turned and tossed the file. "Based on what Dr. Curran found he is pretty sure she was raped after she sustained the injuries."

"Does that mean she was raped after she was dead?" somebody yelled.

"Or she could have been raped while she was dying," Detective Taylor answered.

"I don't have to tell you how important it is to get this sick bastard," he told his men. "Until we find him this guy is not gonna stop. That's it any problems see either Jim or me. Now go on get out of here," he said.

Marty looked at Taylor's solemn face. "What's wrong?" he asked.

"I know her husband. I volunteer with him down at the firehouse."

"I'm sorry, Jim. Why didn't you tell me? Do you want some time off?"

Taylor crushed his cigarette on the floor. "No," he answered. He walked over to the window and remained silent for a few minutes with his back towards Sacco.

"I see Robertson once a week for eight hours at the fire station. And all he ever talked about was his wife. This is gonna devastate that man."

When he turned back he smiled at his friend. "Do you remember when we worked our first case together."

"Yeah, the Jessup robbery. Hat's Polaski was chief." Sacco grinned. "That old man never went anywhere without his hat," Taylor said.

Then his expression turned dark. "This is a bad one. I think we got a real sick son-of-a-bitch on our hands."

"Your right," Marty said. "And I think he's right here all the time. Watching all of us."

Jim stuck another cigarette in his mouth. "But where? This isn't some big city that he can hide in. This is Norwich, for Christ's sake."

Marty sank further down in his chair behind the pea green metal desk. "Jesus," he said. His hand unconsciously searched for that invisible cigarette pack. *Two years and I still crave them.* "We have two victims and not a clue. And this guy scares me. I mean how many more victims is it gonna take before we catch this asshole."

CHAPTER SIX

It was two weeks to the day since the Robertson murder and not one lead. The chief knew the business community insisted on low publicity in order to try and keep a holiday mood. "After all we want to enjoy a prosperous season," the owner of Pearson's Hardware had quipped at the last town meeting.

"Yeah," Marty groaned when he heard a tap at the door.

The door opened and a man said, "I need a favor."

"Hey, what can I do for you, buddy?" he said when his friend Don walked in.

"Marge is a bit nervous about the wedding. I think she needs a diversion. So I came by to see if I could persuade you and Connie to have dinner with us tonight."

"Sounds good to me but you know I don't make the important decisions."

"I saw Connie at the hospital earlier and she said it was fine with her."

"Well, I guess we're all set then."

"Great. To be honest I'm more nervous than Marge about Stephanie getting married."

"Hey, don't be," Marty said, "Brad's a great guy."

"Oh I know that," Don agreed. "It's just this sense of something being wrong."

"Christ, now you sound like Marge."

"I know," he said. "But I can't shake it."

"Hey, why wouldn't you feel a bit strange, Stephanie is a beautiful young woman and you want to be sure your only child is secure." Marty placed his arm around Don's shoulder. "Still," he joked, "anyone who got hooked into spending as much as you should be worried."

"Oh that really makes me feel better."

"Get out of here," Marty said. "I got work to do."

Don held out his hand for his friend to shake. "Thanks," he said, "I owe you."

"Ha, Delahunt, you're gonna owe more than me after this wedding."

That evening when Marty and Connie rushed into their favorite local restaurant, they were greeted by the owner.

"Hey, Paolo, what's good tonight?"

"Here everything good. But tonight, Marie cooks something special for you. You see, Mr. Sacco."

The Delahunts and the Saccos shared affectionate hellos. And Connie was surprised to see that Stephanie and Brad had joined them for dinner. "I am so thrilled to see you both," she said.

"Dad convinced us to join you," Stephie said. "I hope we haven't spoiled your dinner plans."

"How could you spoil our plans?" Connie said. Then she reached over and embraced the young woman.

Connie took a seat near Marge. "And the mother of the bride," she asked. "How are you doing?"

"I'm excited and nervous and always on the verge of tears. Stephanie had her final fitting today," she said. "You should have seen how lovely she looked."

"You promised, Mom." The young woman frowned. "Every time she talks about it she starts to cry."

The evening was full of fun. Old memories and new stories were shared along with the wine and food. And before the dinner ended, Don had made several toasts. But there was one final toast he was determined to make before the night ended. He looked towards his friends and said, "I know how special Stephie is to you both. But what we want you both to know," he said and raised his glass, "is how special you both are to all of us."

Marty smiled at the young couple across from him. It was obvious how much in love they were. And Stephanie wasn't the only one who fell for Brad. All the Delahunts had fallen in love with Brad Pierson.

"I had fun tonight," Connie told Marty on the walk home.

"Me too."

"I can't imagine how bittersweet this must be for Marge."

The following Friday the Saccos returned home from a quick dinner. Marty had just poured a drink and turned on the television to watch his favorite show when the phone rang. With a look of bewilderment she handed him the phone. "It's Don."

"Marty," he yelled. "Please, can you come over here?" The next thing he heard was the phone crash to the floor.

"What the hell?" he said. He pulled his coat out of the closet and ran through the front door. "I don't know what's going on," he yelled to Connie.

The Delahunts and the Saccos had been friends for fifteen years. He had never heard such chaos in Don's voice before.

Marty ran past the four houses that separated the couples. He saw his friends on the couch through the picture window.

He rushed through the front door. "What's wrong?"

Marge sat mute, lifeless and pale. Her eyes were red and swollen. The expression on her husband's face terrified Marty.

"What's happened?" he asked.

Don's ashen face pointed in the direction of the kitchen. Marty hesitated. "What is it?" he asked again. But he was answered by a blank stare. The police chief cautiously made his way across the parlor to the kitchen door. He took a step into the normally neat room and felt the insides of his belly tighten. With a deep resigned sigh that erupted from the pit of his stomach he walked into the room.

In the back corner of the kitchen he saw the broom closet door open and there was something propped up against it. Marty's occupation had in no way prepared him for what he was about to see.

"Oh, dear Jesus," he cried. His knees buckled and he fell to the floor. There squat against the door was the nude body of Stephanie Delahunt.

The lovely young blonde was in the same haunting position as the last two victims. Her pretty blonde hair was matted with a layer of dried blood. It was obvious that she had been raped.

"Fuck," Marty whispered and turned away, the saliva sticking in his throat. He took a handkerchief out of his pocket and picked up the telephone.

"This is Chief Sacco," he said to the night clerk at the station house. "Get someone over to the Delahunts' house right away."

He walked back to Stephanie's body. There it was, the eerie ritual of neatly folded clothes. Composed he bent down and took a pencil out of his pocket and gently lifted the small pair of underwear that lay on top of her pink flannel nightgown.

"Now we have three," he murmered. When he was finished he walked outside and placed his hand against the cold clapboards and vomited. He walked to the front of the house, stood on the lawn and waited until he heard the echoed sounds of the police sirens in the distance.

"Call the coroner," he told Detective Taylor, "then tape the area." He slid behind the front seat of Taylor's vehicle and pressed the radio button.

"It's Sacco," he told the dispatcher, "get my wife."

It wouldn't matter how he told her, he could never prepare Connie for such horrific news.

"Oh my God."

"Honey, Marge and Don are going to need us tonight."

"I know," she said with a sob. "Just give me a few minutes."

"I'll have an officer take them over. I'm sorry I can't be with you right now," he told her. "Are you sure you're up to this?"

"No," she said. "But I'll be okay."

Behind him were the headlights of the coroner's van with the boys from the lab.

"Wait," Marty told them on their way up the pathway. "Just give me a few minutes." He knew it was important to take their statement. But he just couldn't put them threw that right now. "To Hell with regulations," he whispered.

He walked over to his friend. "Connie and I want you and Marge to stay with us tonight. There's nothing you can do here." Don rubbed the top of his forehead.

"My men will be here all night," Marty said. "You don't want Marge to watch this."

"C'mon, honey," Don said and put his arm around his wife's waist. She backed away from him and cried. "No, I can't leave my little girl."

"She's gone," he said. "It's better if we leave."

It was obvious that Margaret Delahunt had come to the end of her joy. It was evident in her tear-stained face that she knew there was little more she could do than shake her head and stare at the mirror image photograph of her lovely daughter. She took the framed picture and held it to her breast. After she was seated inside the police car Marty walked over to Don. The devastated father collapsed in his arms. "What will we do now?" he cried.

He gently helped his friend into the police car. "Don, Officer O'Brien is gonna drive you to my house. Connie is there and I promise I'll be right along."

"No siren," Marty said.

The cop nodded from the front seat of the cruiser and then took off down the street. For now Marty had spent enough time in grief. He knew more would come later.

Doctor Curran approached Marty. "Don't tell me it's another one." Then he looked into the chief's eyes. "Hey," he said. "Are you all right?"

"This is Don Delahunt's house," Detective Taylor interrupted. "His daughter was the murder victim."

"You mean the banker?"

Taylor just nodded.

The medical examiner walked over to the body and knelt down. He gently moved Stephanie's head side to side. He looked up to see Marty. "You don't need me to tell you her death was the same as the others."

Curran stood up and rested his hand on Marty's shoulder. "I'm sorry," he said.

"Look, Chief," Taylor said. "I can handle this, why don't you go home?"

"I had O'Brien bring Don and Marge to my house." Marty's voice was barely audible. "I should be there for Connie. I'll see you in the morning," he said. Then he walked out the door. He lifted his collar and tucked his hands deep into the pockets of his wool coat. The police chief paid little attention to the few people that had gathered in front of the Delahunt house.

The cold air seemed to have slowed him down. Or it could be that his legs just didn't move that fast anymore? Whatever the reason it seemed to take him longer to get home tonight. More than likely it was the fact that he didn't want to face Don and Marge.

The young cop was still there outside the house, his breath visible in the frigid night air. "You could have stayed in the car," Marty said.

"That's okay, Chief. I'm fine."

"Go on. Go home and get yourself some hot coffee."

Marty opened the front door and stepped inside. He remained perfectly still. He wanted to soak up the warmth and security he had always had when he entered the small foyer of his home. Tonight it felt different. The house was warm but the sense of security was gone.

He placed his coat back in the closet and headed down the painted hallway towards the kitchen. The smell of fresh brewed coffee filtered the air. When he reached the end of the hall he stared at the kitchen door. After a deep breath his hand pushed open the door. Connie sat at one end of the table. Her eyes red, in her hand she held a cigarette.

"Are you okay?"

"Would you like some coffee?" she asked.

He nodded and Connie arose from her seat. "I'll get you a cup."

Don hadn't moved since Marty walked through the door. He just stared out the window. His wife sat beside him, her hands wrapped around Stephanie's picture.

"I called Dr. Garr," Connie said. "He's one of the doctors I work with at Norwich. He came right over and gave her something. Oh, and I called Brad's parents."

"I would have done that," Marty said.

"I know," she whispered. "But I wasn't sure how long you would be there. And Marge was just, well, he's out of town anyway. His dad said he would try to reach him immediately. I'm still waiting for his call."

Connie poured her husband a cup of coffee. "And you?" she asked.

Marty looked into his wife's eyes.

"I'm fine," he said. Marty put his arms around his wife and tucked her close to him. Her head lay on his chest. "This is just so sad." Then he gently moved away.

Marty walked over to his friend and placed his hand on Don's.

"I don't know what happened," he said. "We just went to dinner. I mean Stephanie didn't want to come Instead she wanted to stay home and pack." His voice cracked and he choked back tears. "She was just so excited about the wedding."

Marty looked toward his wife. She sat wrapped in her favorite chenille robe. Tears rolled down her cheeks.

"When we came home," Don continued, "the front door was open a crack, which seemed a bit funny, because I remembered Stephie locked it when we left. The house was so quiet. We thought that she had gone to bed. So Marge headed for the kitchen to shut off the light, while I locked up."

When he paused, Marty told him he didn't have to talk about it right now.

"No," Don said. "I have to in order for any of it to make some sense." He wet his lips and lowered his head.

"All I heard was a scream. Then Marge appeared in the doorway. I couldn't make any sense out of what she said. Until I walked in the kitchen and saw my little girl on the floor."

Don placed his hands on the table and looked over at his friends. "We had been teasing her all day," he said. "And just before we left Stephie said, 'You two are gonna miss me when I leave.'" Don's voice evaporated.

Marge whimpered softly and Don immediately turned to her. He gently pried his wife up off the seat and wrapped his arm around her waist. A pathetic smile eased across his wife's face and he stumbled to retain his composure.

Connie quickly ran to her friend's side and placed the woman's arm around her shoulder. Together they walked Marge to the guest bedroom.

Later when Connie walked into her husband's arms, her face mimicked the same confusion he had dealt with so many times. He tenderly rested his wife's head against his chest.

Jesus, he screamed silently from inside.

He suddenly felt the sting of tears in his eyes, and a sharp pain stirred from deep inside his heart. What if that had been his wife lying dead on the floor?

CHAPTER SEVEN

It was after ten the next morning when Marty arrived at the station.

"How are the Delahunts doing?" Jim asked.

"Not good," he said. "And then I had to tell Don that Stephanie's body wouldn't be released until after the autopsy."

"Are they still at your place?"

"No," the chief answered. "Marge's sister, Carol, came early this morning. I guess they'll stay there for while."

"How's Connie been through this?" Taylor said. "I mean being a nurse she must see death all the time. Still when it's a family member or a friend it has to hurt." His voice drifted off and there was just silence left between the two men. They walked to their desks and Marty looked down at the heap of paper. He picked up the top file and stared at the page.

Jim was on the opposite side of the room and stood up. "This might be bad timing," he said. "But is there something about this case that feels familiar to you?" He pulled a cigarette out his pack and placed it in his mouth.

"I don't understand what you mean by familiar," Marty said.

Taylor dropped a file on the chief's desk. "Take a look at this."

"Paula Roache."

"Just look at it," Taylor said. He checked the big clock on the wall. "I have to run to an appointment but I'll be back in a few hours. Look over that file," he said on his way out the door.

Marty opened the folder and began to read the report. He took the pile of photographs tucked under the cover sheet and spread them across his desk. The Roache case had been one of the strangest cases Taylor and him had ever been on. They were partners that night when they walked into the empty house. Marty remembered there was blood everywhere. But they never found a body. They even dug up the cellar and backyard. To this day they had no reports of Paula Roache or her body being found.

Marty continued to check the report and he looked over the photographs and re-read through the original evidence list. He checked each picture, still he had yet to find Jim's connection. He was about to close the file when he noticed two photographs stuck together. He examined it, and what he saw was a folded blue skirt, a white blouse and a pair of panties. They were stacked, not neatly folded but they were placed right next to the pool of blood.

It was a few hours later when Taylor walked back into the office.

"I read through the file."

"It's quite a coincidence, don't you think?" Jim said.

"Yeah," Marty said. "But the ten-year hiatus bothers me."

"Maybe it wasn't a ten-year hiatus. What if he just came back into town?" Taylor said. "Let's think about this. Who else knew about this case besides us? We had minimum press so there was little publicity. And we did most of the investigation."

Taylor with his typical edgy form strolled towards the window. "While I was out this morning I checked on a small lead," he said. Then shoved his body against the cement wall.

"How small?" Marty asked.

"You know the Greek restaurant where the Miller woman worked."

"Yeah, Atheno's."

"I spoke a couple of times with their former dishwasher on the night she was killed. He gave me the name, Vinnie Fiske."

"And."

"He said Fiske used to talk about how he grew up in Ethnic Village. And what it was like back then. Supposedly he got into some trouble and left," Taylor said. "I've checked the town hall, police records. I thought I'd give the bureau a call. But everything comes up empty."

He left the wall and began to pace in front of his desk.

"They found nothing. No Vinnie Fiske or any Fiske registered in this town.

"What about the owners?" Marty asked. "Did you speak with them?"

"Just that night. I thought I'd go down there a little later."

Marty reached for his jacket. "Well, my friend," he asked. "Do you like Greek food?"

"Only if you're buying?"

"You're incredible."

Atheno's restaurant stood on the corner of Tremont and Cedar Street. An inconspicuous place that bore all the trappings of a typical Greek restaurant. Including a large dusty painting of Apollo that stood on the wall between two booths. When the detectives walked in a middle-aged woman with a heavy accent greeted them.

"Can I help you?"

"Hello, Mrs Stanos," Jim said. "I don't know if you remember me. I'm Detective Taylor and this is Police Chief Martin Sacco."

"I remember you," she said. "From the night Dorothy was murdered. You have more questions?"

"We do," Marty said. "We wanted to speak with you and your husband."

"I don't know what else I can tell you but over there you find Nickolas." She pointed to the back of the room where a large man stood in front of a garrish mirror, stacking bottles.

Mrs. Santos walked over to him. "These men want to talk with you about Dorothy," she said.

"I answer all your questions before," he said. He never looked up. "So what do you want now?"

Marty ignored the man's affront and instead politely said, "I'm Chief Sacco. And this is Detective Taylor." He offered his hand.

Nicholas Santos stopped what he was doing and faced the two men. He took a bar rag and wiped his hands. "I remember you from that night."

He shook the chief's hand and then looked toward Taylor. "I spoke with you then. I know nothing new."

Paying little attention to what he said, Detective Taylor asked, "What can you tell us about Vinnie Fiske?"

"Only that he worked here before. Now he is somewhere else. You go find him."

"Look, Mr. Santos," Marty said. "We can do this nice or we can do this difficult. Detective Taylor is gonna start again. If you have the right answers we'll stay for lunch. Otherwise we all need to go to the station."

The old man took a deep breath and rested his hands on the bar.

"Okay," he said. "He told me nothing except that he was a cook in the Navy."

"What about Norwich? Did he ever mention anything about living here or being in trouble?"

"I need a cook," Santos said. "Vinnie was a friendly guy and he knew his way around the kitchen so I hired him."

Mrs. Santos was still at the end of the bar. Until now she didn't say a word. But she turned to her husband and said something in greek.

"I'm sorry," Marty said. "I didn't get that."

"He was a little too friendly," the woman said.

"What do you know?" Santos said to her with a wave.

"Why do you say that?" Taylor asked.

"He always flirt with the waitresses. Some flirt back, but not Dorothy. She don't like him. I think she was a little afraid of him."

"Why?" Marty asked. "was she afraid of him."

She glared over at her husband. "Because she think he followed her home a few times."

"Did she tell you that?" Taylor asked.

"Yes, she told me a few times she saw this man standing next to the broken street light. It was always late after she close up and leave the restaurant. But she never look up at him. Then one night Dorothy walk by and this man says hello. She told me she recognize his voice.

"It make me nervous," she said, then rubbed her arm.

"Did Dorothy ever call the police?"

"No." She smiled. "Besides, what are they gonna do? Stop him from taking a walk?"

Marty turned to the woman's husband. "Do you have Fiske's address?"

"He lives in the boarding house on the corner of Washington and Sycamore. But he's never there."

"How do you know that?"

"Once in a while if the other cook doesn't show up, I call. But the landlord told me he was never there. So I asked Vinnie. He told me he stays in Boston a lot with relatives. And," he hesitated, "I think maybe he gambles."

"You think," Marty said.

"A few times he ask me to give him an advance. He told me he owed the bookies."

"Well," Marty said. "Thank you both for all your help. If you remember anything else please contact either me or Detective Taylor."

"So now you gentlemen have lunch," Nikolas said.

Forty-five minutes later the two detectives walked toward the car.

"I can't eat that food," Jim said.

"Why?"

"It's too rich."

"It was a chicken sandwich for God's sake."

"Yeah but it had cheese and oil and vinegar on it. It's too heavy for me."

"You're probably right," Marty joked. "Because you're used to all that bland food you eat at Lou's Place."

"Forget what I eat, will you. What do you think about Fiske?"

"I think we need to find out who this guy really is."

The town of Norwich, in a sightless effort to ignore the horror that had invaded their community, continued to ready itself for the Yuletide. The merchants who neatly surrounded the common called for a meeting. Despite the somber feelings of the townspeople and the buzzing about the murders, the members of the business community felt that the upcoming holiday season would be a commercial disaster if they didn't play this horrific problem down.

They were well aware that this last murder could devastate the small town industry. Determined to take whatever steps were needed to prevent it, they agreed to help the cause. So the town fathers held an emergency session to determine how to maintain more security for the local people.

"Certainly we will take whatever precautions needed to keep the shoppers safe," Fred Pearson the owner of Pearson's Hardware said to Chief Sacco. "We intend to keep the downtown area well lighted and we want to have volunteers patrol the village area."

Marty didn't like Fred Pearson or his ability to stir up trouble. But he did agree with the assessment for extra security. Still he was not comfortable with the use of an auxiliary group of local men who would patrol the town at night.

"I'll go along with that only if certain guidelines are imposed," he insisted. "Each business can have one volunteer to patrol his area. When the shop closes for the night, the guard goes home."

Pearson looked across the table and stared into Marty's face. "That's pushing your authority, don't you think, Sacco?"

"No, I don't believe so. You see this is a police matter, Fred," he said lifting himself off his seat. "That means the Norwich Police Department is in charge. So if my business here is concluded I have work to do at the station."

Besides the placement of one volunteer per business the retailers did their best not only to maintain a sense of security, but also to woo the customers into a festive mood. The community designed unique displays for their windows. They had a group of carolers stroll the village singing Christmas carols. Other times Christmas music was pumped through the town auditory system.

Even Saint Bartholomew encouraged their parishioners to plan bake sales and the Monsignor sponsored a holly dance with dinner for two at an expensive restaurant for the door prize.

The Ethnic Village had their own worries and dread. After all, two of the three murders had been committed in their neighborhood. The shopkeepers in the lower section of town were even more concerned about the residents' loss of seasonal spirit. In every way both groups of people worked to keep the residents of Norwich secure and festive for the holiday.

It was a great attempt by the business community to alleviate the fears of the public. But even with all the effort of a festive display and plastic decorations there was the realistic truth that the murderer could not only strike again but might even be hidden among them.

The Delahunts had lost their sense of holiday and instead they mourned the death of their daughter. The night before the funeral Marty and his wife attended Stephanie's wake at the Griffins Funeral Home.

Connie saw Marge's blank stare from the doorway, "My heart is broken," she told her husband. "I don't know if I can do this." Her hand tightened around his. Don and Stephanie's Brad stood on either side of the casket. They said their prayers and then Connie approached both men with tears in her eyes. She slowly moved to where Marge sat and seated herself next to her good friend.

Marty too embraced his friend. But they never spoke. Instead the two men just held each other and sobbed. Then the chief walked over to Brad.

The pain on the young man's face was evident.

"I am so sorry," he said. But when he went to embrace the young man, Brad did not respond. Later that evening Marty received an answer to Brad's icy behavior.

"Your sympathies are not good enough, Mr. Sacco," he said. "If the police had caught this man in the beginning Stephie would still be here." Brad's expression was one of agony. "I mean where do I go from here?"

Finally he slumped down in a chair and began to cry. "I'm sorry, sir," he said. "I just don't know what to do."

The next morning a small community of mourners stood in the bitter cold and watched as they lowered the pretty young girl into the ground, while in the background they could hear sobs of a mother's grief.

Marty held his wife so close he could feel the warmth of her breath on his neck. He looked over at the open grave then closed his eyes and listened to the sounds of weeping.

He saw Detective Taylor arrive. Jim removed his hat and walked up the grassy knoll and took his place next to Marty.

A young priest stood on the mound of dirt. "May the angels lead you to paradise," he said. "May her soul and all the souls of the faithful departed, through the mercy of God, rest in peace, Amen."

The priest dressed in a purple robe looked out at the people. "This is a sad time for all of us," he said. "But for Marge and Don Delahunt their life has been forever altered. Please send them your prayers. Thank you all for coming." He closed the missal and slowly made his way around the grave to where Stephanie's parents and Brad stood.

"Father Domenic," Mr. Delahunt said. "Thank you so much."

The priest turned to Marge and placed her hand in his. He leaned over and whispered something in her ear. She nodded her head and Father patted her shoulder before he walked away.

As if on cue, one by one the rest of the mourners sauntered by the grave. Some threw a flower on the lowered coffin. Others stood over the dark hole and moaned a private prayer. Sorrowful neighbors walked up to somber parents. A few people placed a hand on Don's arm or gently kissed Marge, unfettered by the Delahunts' unresponsive glares.

After a few minutes Connie walked over to Carol. The two women entwined their arms around Marge and led her away from the gravesite.

A small reception had been arranged after the funeral. Marty and Jim stayed just long enough to speak with Don and Marge. Marty leaned over to kiss his wife goodbye. "Are you sure you're alright?"

"I'm fine," Connie said. "I'll stay awhile longer. My shift doesn't start till this afternoon. So I'll be home late," she told him.

The two men walked outside to where the car was parked. "I'm glad this day is over," Marty whispered to Jim. "Drop me off at the hospital."

"I ran Fiske's name through the Navy. I found a couple of dozen. So I contacted Jack Ross over at the bureau to see if he could sort them out. None of them listed addresses from Massachusetts, ten had died and one was a colored man."

"Well, keep checking," he said, and shook his head from frustration. "We need every and any lead we can get."

"What are we doing here?" he asked. He parked the car in front of the Norwich Hospital.

"I have an appointment with Kevin Donahue."

"The shrink."

"Yeah. I want to talk to him about the case. See what he thinks. The FBI has been doing a study with a group of psychiatrists. They have actually developed some new theories having to do with suspects that kill more than once. They coined a term for it, sequence killers," he said. "I'm not sure this guy fits into that profile. But maybe Donahue can give me a few answers."

CHAPTER EIGHT

Nina and Millie always walked home by the deserted railroad path. Normally it made little difference if the day was darker than usual, or if the air was colder than normal, but today Millie sensed things seemed different.

She had heard a strange noise from the far end of the field that had frightened her.

"What was that?"

"I don't know," her sister said. "Let's just keep heading for home."

After a few more steps the younger girl stopped and turned to Nina. "Did you see just see someone?"

"No," she said.

The sound of footsteps from behind them froze the two girls. Millie held on to her sister's arm and closed her eyes.

"You idiot," Millie heard Nina say. "You almost scared us to death."

When she opened her eyes Paul was directly in front of them.

"You two are afraid of your own shadow."

"Paul," Millie said with a deep sigh. "I heard an awful sound from over there." She pointed up ahead.

"I've been behind you for about ten minutes and I didn't hear anything." In an attempt to mimic Dracula he curled his lip under his top teeth and raised his hands towards his sister's neck. "Maybe he is here to suck your blood."

Millie giggled. But Nina ignored her brother. She turned and walked ahead of her siblings. They walked a little further and then Millie heard that sound again. She stopped. "There, did you hear it?" she asked. "It sounds like an animal in pain."

This time both Paul and Nina heard the cry. The three of them stood stone still in the middle of the field. Paul moved forward. "Just stay back," he warned.

Out of the corner of her eye Millie saw a figure dash from behind a bush and then quickly disappear. She looked towards Nina. "Did you see him?"

"I saw something," her sister said.

Millie and Nina crept slowly behind. They watched their brother push his way through the tall grass, when Paul suddenly stopped and stared at the ground. The two girls stood still.

"What is it, Paul?" Nina called out. Then they moved forward.

"Don't come any closer," he said.

But it was too late. They were already next to him.

"What's wrong?" Nina said. She stretched to look. "Oh," she said. Then turned away.

Millie saw the color drain from her sister's face. "What is it?" Millie asked on the verge of tears.

Paul shook his head in disgust. "It's just a dead cat."

"What do you mean a dead cat?"

"Nothing. C'mon, let's get out of here."

Nina grabbed her sister's hand and she led her towards the clearing that took them right to Prescott Street. By the time Paul came home they were ready to sit down for dinner.

"Where were you?" Momma asked him.

"I had something to do," he said.

Later that night when the two girls were alone in their bedroom, Millie asked her sister, "Did you see who it was in the field?"

"No," she said. "But whoever it was tortured that poor cat."

A small nightstand and table lamp separated the girls' beds. Nina sat on the edge of the bed.

"Seeing that cat all cut up like that was awful," she said. "Who would do such a horrible thing?" Her hand grasped the chain and she plunged the room into darkness.

Millie rolled over in bed and stared out her window. She couldn't answer that. But she was pretty sure she knew who ran across the field. It was Josef Kerchak she saw disappear along the edge of the tall grass.

For Christmas the Giannetti family had planned a few celebrations. Momma was more than excited. Even though it would take her hours to clean and weeks to prepare for the wonderful holiday.

"Okay girls," she said. "I want you to help me clean the whole kitchen before I make the pasta."

"Why do we have to clean the kitchen before Momma makes it a mess again?" Millie asked Nina one day.

"Because Momma lives by strict rules. If she doesn't follow them, her pasta won't come out right."

"I don't understand," she said.

"It doesn't matter," Nina said. "Just do it."

And Millie soon learned that Nina was right. Her mother did what she believed she needed to do. And she did love to watch her mother cook. So she hovered around the table while Momma kneaded the dough. First her mother placed a sparkling clean white apron around her waist.

Then she put all the ingredients on the table.

"Today I make the raviolis. Later maybe some bread. Before," she told Millie. "I had to do everything that day. Now I thank God for Mr. Orvietti."

Momma was always thanking God for something. This day it was for the second refrigerator Poppa had bought for twenty dollars.

Millie slid her finger against the edge of the bowl and scooped up a little of the riccotta filling that her mother spooned in piles along one edge of the ravioli dough. Then Momma would fold the other section of dough over the filled part, place an inverted glass over each little pile and twist the glass forming the little cheese-filled pies. Millie would then place them one by one on a large platter sprinkled with corn meal.

After they cleaned up from that, Momma would take another batch of dough and begin to make her bread.

"This is the most important part of the meal," she said.

That was true. Millie could never remember a meal that didn't include homemade bread. Most days she could smell the bread in the oven when she turned the corner to her street. And she knew that when she walked into the house there would be a row of bronze-colored bread resting on the kitchen counter.

"Here," Momma said. She handed her a piece of warm bread. "Dip it in the olive oil. It will make your hair nice and shiny."

By the end of the day she could see her mother was exhausted.

"I'm so hot and a little tired today." Momma walked to the sink and dabbed her face with cool water. She sat down in her favorite spot in front of the window because it gave her a view of the street.

"I like to sit here and look out at everybody," she said. "Hey, look, there's Grace Kerchak. She's with her son. I don't know if I like that boy," Momma said. "Sometimes I feel sorry for him. I don't know." She took the dishcloth and wiped her face.

"And you, Millie?" she asked. What do you think about Josef?"

Millie wasn't sure. There were times when she felt sorry for him But there were other times when she hated him. Especially when he made her sister cry. Like the other day when Nina was talking with Alfred Damone on the street corner. Josef walked right up to her and shouted, "Where were you? You promised me you would be there."

Nina was embarrassed. And poor Alfred, he didn't know what to think. His face turned all red and he just walked away.

"Well," her mother asked. "What do you think about Josef?"

"I don't know, Momma," she said.

The old woman lifted herself from the chair. She picked up a loaf of bread and placed it inside a paper bag dusted with cornmeal. Then she rolled all but one in a clean cloth. "This one for dinner. You bring the others down to the freezer?" she asked.

Before she handed the bags to Millie she stopped. She placed her hand on the girl's chin and said, "I have a feeling about this boy," she said with a sigh. "And I want you to promise me that if he bothers you or your sister you tell Paul, you understand."

Millie looked into the flushed red face of her mother. "You promise Momma," she said, her hand still wrapped around the girl's chin.

"I promise."

Then the girl walked down the cellar stairs. She almost did tell Paul about Josef once. It was the time when he was at the bus stop. Nina and her had just reached the corner and out of the blue Josef walked up to her sister and grabbed her by the arm. But Nina pulled away and yelled back, "If you don't stay away from me I'm gonna tell my father."

Millie had asked her sister what that was all about, but she just said, "It was nothing. And don't tell Poppa."

He would just tell Paul and that would be it. It was bad enough he already acted like a centurion around them. Any encouragement and their life would be hell, especially for Nina. It was never mentioned again. As a matter of fact Millie had forgotten about it until just now.

This holiday it was decided the whole family would attend Christmas services. It was Domenic's first time as celebrant for the Midnight service. Poppa was ecstatic over his son's assignment to Saint Bart's and now this. He was beyond joy and insisted that all of them attend Mass. A feat within itself, considering how large the family was and how busy most of them were with their own lives.

Just to organize a Christmas meal was a fantastic commotion.

Millie never understood how Domenic was able to study back then when most of the family was at home. Homework was a tremendous task for her now with just the three of them; truth be told she wasn't nearly as devoted to her schoolwork as he was.

Although she was just a small child she could remember her father's screams of joy when he announced that Domenic would enter the seminary.

"Your brother is gonna attend Saint John's in Brighton," he told the family one night after dinner. "Now I make the attic his room."

"That's not fair. Peter and I have to share a room, why should Dom have the whole upstairs?" Tommy asked.

"Because," he said, "you and your brother are gonna be married soon and leave. But Domenic, he still has to study for a long time and when he comes to visit on the holidays he is gonna need his own place so he can pray in peace."

Poppa was very serious. Even Momma was a little concerned. "What's the matter with you, Salvatore?" she said. "He can pray at the church anytime he wants."

"This is what I want. Do you understand?"

And Poppa didn't listen to anyone's protests. Not even Domenic's.

"Poppa, the other boys are right. I don't need to have the whole attic to myself."

"No," he said. "My mind is made up. I do this my way."

Millie had witnessed her father's unreasonableness many times. Momma even tried to rationalize it one day. "I think he's like his father," she said. "He has a bad temper. Your Poppa told me one time when he was in the field with his father he was so tired, he stopped. Just sat down right there. His father came up from behind him. 'Why you stop?' he asked.

"'I'm tired Poppa,' he said. 'I just want to sit for a minute.'

"His father's face came real close and he looked his son in the eye. 'The only time you stop is if you sick or dead, you understand?' Then he took the butt of the rake and smashed it across your poppa's back. 'There,' he said. 'Now you have a reason to sit down.'"

But Poppa's temper was one thing. His devotion to Domenic was another. Even though he loved his children his first son was the one that took priority over the rest of the family. "I think it's because he always felt that Domenic lost too much when his mother died," Momma explained.

And Millie could see that her mother loved him as one of her own. She had been cognizant of his needs even as a little boy.

"It took him a long time before he felt safe with anyone. But one day he climb on my lap and put his head against my chest. I knew then he would soon call me Momma."

The attic a wasteland of beams and cold walls was a consuming project that enlisted the help of everyone in the Giannetti household. Walls were insulated and covered with paneling, woodwork was painted, the two small windows were washed and a curtain hung. When the family was done Domenic had his room where he could study without the constant irritation of the girl's radio.

But the upstairs bedroom lasted less than two years for Domenic. He spent most of his time at the seminary and was transferred to different parishes across most of the state. By the time he had come back to Norwich he was the attending pastor at Saint Bart's and lived in the rectory. Poppa ended up using the room for storage. And once in a while Millie would climb the stairs just to rummage through some of the old photo albums.

That Christmas the Giannetti family attended midnight Mass and the siblings were excited and proud to hear their brother speak from the pulpit.

"During this most beautiful of seasons," he said, "it is important that each of us give the gift of self."

Millie looked over at her Poppa. He had tears in his eyes and he beamed of pride and joy. She realized that this had to be the proudest moment of his life.

CHAPTER NINE

"A psychopath has no distinguishing traits. He neither looks like, nor talks like a murderer," Doctor Donahue said. He was slouched in the leather chair behind his desk.

"Inevitably, though, there is something in the background that has caused turmoil and research has shown that men who kill women in some form of ritual behavior have suffered rejection."

The doctor removed his glasses and squeezed the top of his nose. "It is hard to pinpoint exact reasons for what we do as individuals. And we are still in the infancy stages of psychiatry."

Marty wasn't impressed by Donahue's generalizations. "What can you tell me about this creep?" he asked.

"I can't give you a specific answer," he said. "Tell me what you have and I'll try to help."

Marty shifted in his seat. "Before the recent murders something happened about ten years ago," he began. "We investigated what looked like a murder on Bay Road. My partner and I arrived at the house to find a bloody mess but no body. Through some old hospital records we were able to determine that the blood type matched the woman who owned the house. Her name was Paula Roache."

"But I always thought that if there is no body, then you can't prove murder," Donahue said.

"That's true in theory. But this case was never solved. We classified it as a missing person. Strangely enough we think we might be able to connect the Roache disappearance to these latest murders."

Donahue's eyes widened. "How?" he asked.

"So far we have three women raped and murdered. Their bloodied bodies grotesquely positioned. Yet the murderer takes the time to fold the clothes of each of his victims and leaves them in a neat pile next to the bodies. We never found Paula Roache's body but we did find a pile of her clothing next to a pool of her blood."

"You are right," the doctor said. "That is a strange connection."

"And that case had minimal exposure to the press. So it's unlikely anyone read about it. Remember there was no body. At the time the clothing we found didn't have a lot of significance. And after a few days the case disappeared from the newspapers."

Marty moved off the chair. "Jim Taylor and I worked the case then and after every lead we came up empty. We couldn't find one piece of evidence that she was dead. It was a sad case to begin with," he said. "The victim's husband had been killed in a terrible accident and her friends were worried about her. Especially after she told them she thought she was being watched. But she never told the police."

"And now you think there is a connection between her disappearance and the man who committed these recent murders."

Marty stood in front of the doctor.

"I don't know," he said. "Maybe I am just grasping at straws. But I will take anything I can get," he said. "What are the chances I'm looking for the same guy? And do you think someone can commit a crime and then stop for ten years?"

"Could it be the same guy, maybe," the doctor said. Then shrugged his shoulders. "Would he stop and then murder again after ten years? What if your murderer ended up in prison in another state," Donahue said. "What if he joined the military and has continued his crimes abroad. There are a number of reasons why he may have or at least seemed to have stopped."

The psychiatrist focused his eyes on the chief.

"What you should try to understand is this kind of a killer doesn't stop. The man who killed these women is an executioner. He's not going to stop, unless someone stops him."

"Jesus," Marty said. "What kind of a person am I looking for?"

"He could be anybody. A clean cut business man or a person who collects trash. That is what makes this kind of a killer so dangerous. Society views him as being crazy, because he is essentially an uncontrollable human being, someone who has tremendous conflict within himself."

"Then you would consider him insane?"

"Not the way the public views the word. It isn't that easy. In the killer's mind these women in some way are responsible for his actions. But even though there is an undeniable rage and a need to lash out, once the act is completed, his senses begin to emerge and his regrets take over, thus the folded cloths. He performs this ritual in his mind as an act of kindness."

Marty lowered his head. "Kindness," he said.

"It is all very complicated."

"If you are expecting sympathy from this man, don't. He does not understand the victim's pain, only his own. But let me address your original question. Yes," he said. "This could be the same man and be cautious because if he is back, he is back with a vengeance."

Donahue held out his hand. "Good luck, sir, I hope you find him very soon."

"I appreciate your time," Marty said.

"If I can be of help again, don't hesitate to call. It's a subject we both share an interest in."

Marty left the office. His heels landed hard against the cement floor and the echo of his footsteps followed him down the long hallway. The only thing he had on his side was determination. *I'm gonna find you, you sick son-of-a-bitch*, he promised. *No matter where you are.*

CHAPTER TEN

It was early morning when Marty slipped on his robe and shuffled off to the kitchen. Something had been on his mind all night, and had kept him from his usual dead-to-the-world slumber. He stood by the breakfast area staring out the window. His eyes followed the dark clouds as they scudded across the sky.

I suppose we shouldn't complain, he thought, *after all, it's two weeks after Christmas and the weather hasn't been that bad.* His eyes scanned the calendar. The date, January 7, was circled in stars. "Today was to be Stephie's wedding day," he said then slouched against the corner of the kitchen wall.

Jeez, I can't even imagine how Don and Marge feel today.

He hadn't seen the Delahunts since after the funeral. Don had taken a leave of absence from the bank and then took Marge up to his sister's place in Maine.

Connie's cigarettes stared at him. He pulled one from the pack and opened the back door. On the deck he took in a long breath of cold fresh air. He held the unlit cigarette between his fingers and massaged the thin stick of tobacco. *Poison,* he thought when he remembered how his lungs used to feel after that first morning cigarette. He couldn't start the day without that thick throaty cough. He had quit the same night he watched his father die from lung cancer. Hadn't smoked since. But every once in a while the urge still gnawed at him.

"Breaking your own rules," Connie said when she suddenly appeared at the back door.

He tossed the cigarette across the yard. "Nope," he said, then turned to his wife. "I just realized it was Stephie's wedding day."

"I know."

She walked over and placed her head against his chest. Marty kissed the top of her head and snuggled his chin against the silkiness of her hair. *If Stephie's death wasn't sad enough,* he thought, *the fact that the murderer's trail was cold made it even worse.* They had next to nothing for evidence. *Nothing!*

After he drove Connie to work he drove to the Delahunt house and parked in the driveway. He sat in the car, his eyes glued to the front door. His body braced against the steering wheel. To see Stephanie's murdered body on the kitchen floor had been one of the hardest things he ever had to do. He was not eager to walk inside that house again.

When he unlocked the front door he felt confronted by the emptiness. For a moment he wandered along the hallway like a stranger who had entered the house for the first time. He shared a loneliness that lingered within the house. Marty brushed up against a small table of framed memories. A photograph of Stephanie and that beautiful smile stole his breath and his eyes filled with tears. Marty felt his shoulders weighted down with sadness and he hesitated at the kitchen door.

He moved around the murder scene. A few bloodspots still remained on the linoleum. To walk the crime scene after the lab boys was very important. A custom he started years ago when he found an overlooked piece of significant evidence.

The police chief felt old when he knelt down to where he had first seen Stephie's body. She had been wearing pajamas that night. That was very unusual for her. Stephanie would never entertain anyone dressed in her night clothes. But there was no sign of forced entry and Don said she had locked the front door after they left. Yet the door was open when her parents came home.

Marty walked into the living room. He and Connie had spent countless hours in this room. Although they could never have children he felt privileged to be able to share different stages of Stephanie's life. Her braces, prom night and he felt sick at heart when he remembered the day she came home all excited about this new guy she had just met.

Marty sat down on the couch. He felt a pain in his heart as he tried to catch his breath. Then he placed his hands over his face and began to cry. This was his time. His time to grieve for that little girl and those new memories he would never have.

The following morning he walked into the station house and met up with Taylor. He took off his jacket and flung it over the hook. "I went to the Delahunts' yesterday. Let's go over the facts," he said.

Jim jabbed a cigarette in his mouth. "All three women were killed by either a trauma to the head. There were no fingerprints anywhere. And we found no forced entry marks."

"But Don told me that Stephanie locked the door behind them."

"Which means she would have had to open the door," Jim said.

"Exactly."

"So what are you saying, she was expecting the killer?"

"No, she was in her pajamas. Stephanie wouldn't have entertained in her night clothes."

Jim took one last drag then stuffed his cigarette in the ashtray. "Okay, so she didn't expect him. But she knew him."

Marty removed his tie and flung it in a desk drawer. "When I was there yesterday I realized you could see right into the living room. What if this guy watched these women?"

"You mean he shadowed them."

"Yeah."

"He picks his prey then studies her habits and follows her," Jim said. "Then when the time is right he kills her."

"Even if that is the case the guy has to have some kind of a pitch for these women to let him in."

"With Dorothy Miller and Stephanie's case I think you're right. In Bette Robinson she always left the door open for her husband. I believe the attacker knew that.

"And these women never made a formal complaint against anyone," Jim said.

"So the killer knew something about all three of these women," Marty said.

"A lot more than we know about him."

"Let's keep in touch with the FBI and see what we can find out about this guy Fiske."

CHAPTER ELEVEN

"Where's your sister?" Momma asked when Millie walked into the kitchen. "Nina had to go to the library. She said she would be home in a little while. What smells so good?" Millie asked.

"I made chicken and potatoes for supper."

On the table sat the entire contents of her mother's sewing basket. "What a mess I make," Momma said. She began to gather all the needles and thread in her hands and place them neatly in the basket.

"I get a call from your aunt today," she admitted. "She's very sick. Maybe it's even that disease everybody gets."

Millie knew what disease. But her mother would never say the word, cancer. "If you don't talk about it, maybe it won't happen," Momma would say.

The girl understood that her mother lived in a secure well-guarded environment, able to exist in that enclosed atmosphere because of her illiteracy. Unable to read English afforded her the seclusion she needed from the outside world. Sure, she heard the gossip and understood there were terrible murders committed in the town. But in her innocence she truly believed that they wouldn't affect anyone in her sphere. It was an unconscious way of keeping oneself insulated.

The winter was long and cold. Norwich was in the full throes of snow and sleet. Normally the cold weather kept most families comfortably warm and secure behind locked doors. This winter the townspeople of Norwich were more vigilant than ever. Including the Giannetti household.

Nina Giannetti was seventeen and popular, but she had never dated. Her father was old-fashioned in so many ways. And his standards for his daughters were outdated, even overly provincial.

In a generation when women married young, Millie's father pushed his values. The younger girls knew that the older sisters weren't allowed to bring home a date until they were out of school. When Rose or Susie met a boy they had to have parental approval before a date. For everyone's sake they agreed it was just easier to follow the rules.

Susie, sarcastic as ever, commented to her young sisters once, "Poppa is so much easier on you two."

But it wasn't true. And if there was any leniency it was insignificant.

And Poppa would raise his fist if either one of them so much as thought about going to the school dance. For Millie it was hard to figure out who was worse, Poppa or Paul. And even though Momma could sometimes persuade Poppa to give in on a lot of issues, dating was one she barely discussed.

At first Nina didn't even tell Millie about her new friend. Then one day out of the clear blue sky she mentioned his name.

"I saw David again today."

"Who's David?" Millie asked.

"A boy," she said. "I met at the library."

Millie stopped kicking the tin can across the tracks. "If I were you, I'd be real careful. You know how Paul likes to squeal."

Their brother basked in his delight to taunt his sisters. Most of the time he would sit behind the wheel of Poppa's car and brag to Nina's friends how he had to babysit his sisters.

"He's not going to find out unless somebody with a big mouth tells him. Anyway I'm going to be eighteen in a few weeks, and old enough to date."

"I won't tell, Nina, I promise," Millie said.

"Tell me all about him."

"He's got blue eyes and blonde hair and he is so handsome."

Millie listened with eager excitement. She had never before seen Nina so excited about a boy. Although they hadn't actually had a formal date, he had walked her home a few times from school and the library. "We always say goodbye at the corner," she said. "Just in case Momma is at the window or Paul is around."

It was two weeks before her eighteenth birthday and she was sick of Poppa's rules. Armed with a rebellious attitude she was about to approach their father.

"Maybe you should ask Momma first," Millie said. "She was able to convince him to let you go to the school dance."

"Only after a holy fit and I had to obey two stupid rules. To be home by 9:15 and Paul had to drop me off and pick me up. Then Poppa asked me questions for an hour."

That was all true. And Millie understood what her sister meant by being interrogated, first Paul would start with the questions.

"So who was that boy I saw you talking to?" would be his standard first question. Nina would usually give him the proverbial "none of your business" to which he always answered, "It's gonna be Poppa's."

One night Poppa kept badgering her about a boy that walked her out of the dance. When she finally came into the bedroom she was crying.

"I want him to die so badly. Can you imagine all these questions about a stupid school dance that ended by 9:00 o'clock?"

The coldness of the season continued and so did Nina's lies.

"I am only going to Delores's for a few hours after school," she would tell Momma and Poppa. And by the time Paul came to pick her up she and David had spent most of the afternoon together. The plan had worked for awhile because Delores's mother worked as a nurse and she changed her shift for a month. But it didn't last and soon the visits to Delores's house stopped.

CHAPTER TWELVE

After a winter of harsh cold the town of Norwich was ready for the transistion into spring. But, however anxious the townspeople were for the change of season the threat of murder was still in the air. While the doors and windows remained closed as protection against the frigid elements, the promise of spring gathered no such refuge. In fact the prey became more accessible. As the nights grew shorter and the days lingered there were new opportunities for the killer who hid in the dark shadows of the innocuous neighborhoods.

Unsuspected and anxious for the arrival of the warm weather Millie's neighborhood seemed to embrace the thoughts of spring. Once the sun became consistent, windows all over Prescott Street were pushed open to let the fresh breezes filter through the houses to remove the stuffy smells of winter.

Millie grew up watching a procession of routine and rituals. Year after year the neighborhood and her family followed the same traditions that had been performed the year before.

Among them were some of her own favorite pastimes. One of those were to watch her mother fill the flower boxes that hung off the porch railings. Every fall Momma would insist the two girls help to fill them with bulbs. A job that seemed tiresome and dull.

But the tedious job of fall turned to be full of rewards because in the spring the sight of colorful blossoms would poke their heads through the flowerboxes.

Momma Giannetti loved the freshness of April and May and she spent many days in the garden with her husband. Each spring Poppa would plant the same list of vegetables: tomatoes, lettuce, potatoes. It didn't matter how much she pleaded. Poppa never deviated. Until one year Momma threatened.

"Salvi, I want the onions this year."

"No," he persisted. "Why do you not understand? They make the garden full of acid."

"Acid or not, I have the onions," she said. "No onion, no bread. Momma was a woman of her word and not surprisingly Poppa planted the onions."

The rest of the neighborhood had their own customs for the return of spring. The porches, once empty over the long winter, were now bustling with women. They would gather each morning to sweep away the dust of cold weather from their porches and returned to the idle practice of long overdue gossip, while their husbands formed groups and played cards in the yard.

The people of Norwich had shared a hard and bitter season. Though some had tasted sadness and tragedy. Most looked forward to spring and were ready to put aside the secluded anger and private fears.

Still others viewed its arrival as more of an intrusion, than a comfort.

George Kerchak had a need to bully his family. His wife, Grace, learned to carry the burden of his rants and raves behind closed doors. But with the warm season that meant it was harder to veil the turbulence and confine the embarrassment.

Sometimes on hot summer nights, Millie and Nina would sit with Momma on the porch outside the kitchen. They could hear the elder Kerchak berate his wife or son. "You stupid bitch," he once screamed. His voice like a dark cloud echoed across the neighborhood.

"Oh my God," Momma whispered. "He is crazy."

Another time the small group heard terrible yells from next door.

"Leave my mother alone," the voice said. "Get away from her."

Momma's face turned pale and she placed her hand over her heart.

"Oh, my God, Poppa," she said. "Someday, something really bad is gonna happen and then that old man is gonna stop."

"Enough," Poppa said. He pointed to Nina and Millie. "You girls off to bed."

Millie walked into the bedroom. She opened the window. Despite the Kerchaks it was a beautiful night full of bright stars and the glow from the moon raced across the yard.

"Nina," Millie whispered to her sister. "Somebody just ran into the yard."

Nina glanced over at her. "Oh, that's just Josef," she said. "He sneaks out to the field at night all the time."

CHAPTER THIRTEEN

With the arrival of the good weather Nina and Millie grabbed their schoolbooks, wrapped themselves in light sweaters and walked to the end of the street. Millie enjoyed the walks with her sister across the field on their way to and from school. In the spring it was filled with wildflowers and lilac bushes that grew along the edges. Millie loved the aroma of tiny violet and deep purple blossoms that filtered the air. One day Nina picked a cluster of lilacs from a branch.

"Here, smell," she said. "If you press the flower between your fingers it will smell just like the toilet water from the drug store."

Millie would soon turn fifteen and this year she began to think about boys and the possiblity of a date. *That was almost impossible*, she admitted. Especially since Paul had approached her one day and asked Millie about Nina's boyfriend.

"Don't you think you should tell Momma about David?"

Nina bent down to pick a handful of violets that had sprouted between the tracks. "Maybe," she said.

"Well you better do it before Paul does," she said. "He knows about David. And you know he's gonna tell Poppa."

"I don't care what he tells Poppa anymore," Nina said. Then stomped away.

April had been rainy and cool but May had begun fairly warm and dry. Then it turned unseasonably hot.

"Tonight we eat on the porch," Momma said. She took a face cloth and moistened her face. "It's too hot for this time of year."

"Set an extra place, Nina," she said. "Domenic, come for dinner."

Millie always enjoyed it when her older brother came over. Tonight she was more than grateful for his appearance because Paul had already begun to torment Nina about David.

"Wait till I tell Poppa about you and that boyfriend."

Nina tried to ignore him but he was impossible and he kept right on with his remarks.

"I know that you lied about why you went to Delores's house."

"Leave me alone, Paul," she shouted.

"Hey, enough!" Momma said. "What's all this about?" she asked Nina.

Paul looked over at his sister. "I think you and Poppa should know that Nina has a boyfriend."

"How do you know if Nina has a boyfriend?"

"Because I've seen them together."

Nina slammed the plate on the table. "He's just a friend, Momma, I know from school."

"Maybe a few other places too," Paul whispered.

It was obvious that Paul had gone as far as he wanted when Poppa walked into the kitchen and asked, "Why you two yell?"

"Nothing," Paul said.

But when Poppa left the room he turned to Nina and sneered. "You two sat awfully close at the library."

Nina ignored his remark but Momma caught on. "Paul, you please shut up."

"Why do you want to get her in trouble?" Millie asked her brother.

Paul quieted down at least for a few minutes then he turned and said, "I know David's sister. The whole family is stuck up. We were in the same class and she would never talk to me. They think they are better than us."

Millie turned sarcastically to her brother. "Did you ever think maybe she wasn't stuck up, maybe she just didn't like you."

"She liked me," Paul said. "Why wouldn't she like me?"

By now Nina had retreated into silence. Millie looked over and saw tears in her sister's eyes. Nina took a step towards her brother.

"I hate you, Paul," she shouted.

"Nina," Momma ordered. "Stop, you go down to the freezer and get me some pasta."

She stood in the middle of the kitchen floor and stared into her brother's face.

"You are a hateful person," she said. Then she made her way past her brother and disappeared down the cellar staircase.

Momma looked at her son.

"What's wrong with you? You like to hurt people and get them in trouble. If you don't leave that girl alone, I promise I'm gonna take the broom to your legs."

Paul turned to Millie. "She's stupid to be with him. People like him only want to use girls from the village. He's just like those college kids."

"What's wrong with college kids?" Domenic said when he walked into the kitchen.

"Nina's been with that kid, David Polanski."

"What do you mean been with?"

"I mean she's going out with him. Sneaking out is more like it."

"That's your sister," Domenic said. "How can you make that remark?"

"I know what I know. I've caught them at the library and I know she met him all the time at Delores's house."

"I don't care, it's none of your business. Isn't it enough that she's almost eighteen years old and still has to answer to Momma and Poppa for every move. Now you want her to answer to you too."

"I just don't want her to get in trouble," Paul said.

Domenic shook his head at his brother. "I know David Polaski. He was an altar boy and he's the head of youth ministry. He's in church every Sunday with his parents. He's a very nice boy. Do me a favor," he said. "Let Momma and Poppa run Nina's life."

Nina stood by the doorway, holding two packages of frozen pasta. She looked over at her brothers. Paul headed out of the kitchen but as he walked by his sister he whispered something. She spun around, tossed the pasta on the table and then ran towards her bedroom.

"What did you say now?" Millie asked.

"Nothing," Paul said. His smugness bothered her and she yelled, "You're a jerk."

"Hey, don't you start with me," Paul warned.

Domenic walked over to his brother. "What the hell is wrong with you?" he asked.

"Okay," Momma said. She stood between her sons. "Do you see the trouble you start?"

Poppa had been in the garden. He placed some lettuce in the kitchen sink and looked over at his wife. "What's this all about?" he asked.

"Nothing, it's over," Momma said. She gave her two sons a look and then said to Domenic, "Tell Poppa what the monsignor asked about the garden."

"Yeah," Poppa, he said. He grabbed his father's arm and led him towards the porch. His voice drifted down the back stairs. Paul turned to leave the kitchen. "Don't you go yet," Momma said. "It's none of your business if your sister has a boyfriend. You let me and Poppa worry about that."

"You don't understand, Momma, Nina's different than the other girls. She's too friendly. She talks to everybody."

"No more talk," she said. "You hear me. No more."

She lay prostrate on the bed when Millie walked in. "Momma wants you to come to dinner." Nina looked over at her sister. Tears streamed down her face. "Why is he such a jerk?"

"I don't know?"

"I don't feel like dinner," she said. "Tell Momma no."

"Nina, you know how Poppa is. Please just sit at the table for a little while."

She sat up on the bed and wiped her eyes. "Okay, just give me a few minutes. I'll be right there."

A few minutes later Nina walked onto the porch. Domenic walked over to her and placed his arm around her shoulder. "Why do you let him get to you this way?"

"I don't know?" she said, then eased her way out of his grip.

Paul was seated next to Poppa on the porch. He didn't even look up when Momma handed him a plate of pasta.

"No more talk," Poppa said. "Let's eat."

Domenic managed to keep some conversation flowing throughout dinner but it was obvious that Nina had nothing more to say to Paul or anyone at the table. She was subdued, withdrawn and ate little.

After dinner and the dishes were washed Millie watched from the kitchen when her mother approached Nina.

"Does Paul tell the truth about you and this boy?" she asked.

"What truth, Momma, mine or Paul's? Do I have a friend name David. Yes." Nina hesitated. "Momma I'm almost eighteen."

"I know," she said. "Tell me about this boy."

"He lives near the library. His name is Polaski. And what Paul said isn't true. He's a nice boy."

Momma stood by the flower boxes. "So did you lie when you tell me you were going to the library or Delores's house."

"No," Nina said. "I did go to the library and I did go to my friend's house. I just didn't say I was going to meet David." Momma pulled a few dead leaves off the plant. "You see you must always tend to these flowers so that they don't suffocate," she said. "And die."

"I didn't do anything wrong with David, Momma."

"I know that." Momma placed her hands on her daughter's face. You're a good girl," she said. "I know you wouldn't do anything bad."

Tears began to fall against Nina's cheeks. "I'm sorry, Momma," she cried. Nina slipped from her mother's grip. Her hand slid across her face and she wiped the tears off her cheek. "Can I go downstairs?" she asked.

"Sure. We don't need to talk anymore." Momma's hand brushed the top of the girl's dark hair. "I speak with Poppa," she said. "Then we see."

Millie stood by the porch rails and watched her sister descend the back stairs. Her sister opened the shed door and walked inside. For that moment while Millie stood in the darkened silence she felt terribly sad for her sister.

"Why don't you come to Mass this Sunday with Poppa," she heard Domenic say. "You could use a few extra prayers."

The two brothers walked onto the porch and Millie turned. "Why do I need to go to church? You're the priest, you pray for me."

"You want coffee?" Momma asked.

Domenic raised his hand. "I do," Domenic said, then preceeded with his conversation. "Poppa took me to Sunday Mass all the time. Each week we would walk up the hill from the neighborhood through the town and into the front doors of St. Bart's," he told his brother. "It was always the same. We would sit in the fourth pew and I would watch everybody that came in through the side doors."

Domenic took the milk bottle from the table and poured some in his coffee.

"Even old man Shaw followed a routine, he would walk down the aisle all the way to the end. He would check each pew for litter. Store whatever he found in his pocket and then he would walk back down to the front of the church and sit in the first pew. After I became an altar boy I realized he sat directly in front of the crucifix. And one Sunday morning I heard him speak to Jesus."

Millie leaned against the porch. She knew that her stepbrother was connected to something far more important than just the Giannetti family. She turned to look at Paul. There he sat, arrogant and puffy with his legs stretched out, his arms entwined across his chest. She didn't understand what compelled him to be so hurtful to Nina. What was it that made him so angry with her all the time?

It was still early and she looked towards the street where some of the neighbors still mingled. Their conversation floated in the air like bits and pieces of dust. Millie looked down towards the shed where Nina was, an old

9x12 cement building which stood at the end of the driveway. She remembered how hard her sister had pleaded with Poppa to let her have just the corner.

"It will be my reading place," she nagged. Until one day he yelled back, "Okay, okay."

But as time went on she eased her way into more space.

"It's only a little space," Poppa told her. "Every time you move something in I move something out," he said. Then he watched her push a large wicker chair through the tiny doorway.

"This is the last thing," she told him.

Although Nina called it her secret place, it wasn't. Everybody from the family to the neighborhood knew about her special corner. It consisted of an old table with a lamp, a small bookcase she found in the trash and of course her wicker chair lined with an old blanket.

Nina enjoyed her privacy. It was no secret that she was moody and a loner. Yet she was friendly. She was passive about many things in life yet she had an incredible passion about life itself. Nina could storm out of the house angry and distraught. But ten minutes later Millie would find her calm and engrossed and sometimes playful.

One time Momma had sent Millie down to the shed to get Nina.

"Momma wants you to come upstairs now. She said that it's too cold for you to be down here tonight."

"Tell her I'm not here. I'm on the moors."

"Where's that?" Millie asked.

"Forget it," she said. She placed her book on the chair and headed out the door. "C'mon, I'll beat you to the steps."

"That's not fair," Millie shouted. "You've got a head start."

"So what?" Nina said. "It's not always about winning."

She bolted up the stairs and waited for Millie. "It's not always about the win," she repeated. "But there are exceptions."

CHAPTER FOURTEEN

The Gianettis' porch door was the alpha and the omega of what Millie considered to be her life. In those simple days she was ruled by consistency mixed with compliance. Her future went as far as the weekend and if she were unhappy about some situation there were all kinds of band-aid remedies available.

"Here," Momma said, "place this pin in the hem until I have time to sew it."

Poppa and Momma dealt with one child at a time and Millie was last. With the other siblings married and out of the house except for Paul, who seemed useless, that left Nina and she was the one always avaliable for any advice Millie needed about school, friends or boys.

After Nina's death Millie had no one. What little dialogue she had with Paul was now lost. And on those few rare occasions that he did share words it was mainly mundane.

"So what's up with you?" he would say with virtually no interest.

As with the rest of the family her parents had never put Nina's death to rest. The holidays were always more of a period of mourning than celebration. Poppa could never start a meal without a toast to Nina; each time he raised his glass Momma would cry.

Just before Millie was about to leave for college, she stood on the porch and looked below at the tiny garage, the cement shed that had impacted her life.

She should have felt excitement at the prospect of a new future. Instead she was anxious and nervous. "You need to be careful," her mother's words warned. "Your brothers aren't gonna be around to help you."

The significance of that expression was something she was about to learn. For Millie without the protection of her family to fall back on and the atmosphere of a large college on the brink of the sixties revolution, she began to realize the definition of the word alone.

By now she was nearing her nineteenth birthday and physically she was comfortably thin, somewhat pretty, and still a virgin. Although she eagerly embraced her academic level, emotionally she was still caught up in the influence of childhood.

Growing up in a large household one observes things. Millie saw at a young age that if and when her brothers or sisters disagreed with authority there were consequences, parental punishments or serious confrontations. So like her siblings Millie learned to repress her feelings. Along with that came the realization that as the baby her opinions weren't important. They were wasted bits of information that didn't amount to anything.

Obvious by her mother's answer to her every comment, "That's nice. But for now the family knows best."

Still her sister's death had blown the family apart. Whatever difference Nina could have made in her sister's life was now gone. Millie's dictum was the same as the rest of the Giannettis. She learned to bury her emotions.

Millie fell into the sixties with its bullshit establishment theories, its drug taking philosophy and sexual freedoms with such intensity that she truly lost track of who she was. Although she had no problem with anyone else doing their thing she never got caught up in taking drugs.

"Drugs can loosen the inner evil in one's soul," she had heard Domenic preach from the pulpit. Words that surfaced even when offered an occasional smoke, and while the abuse of drugs was something she was able to avoid. Abuse was not and she wasted years racking up psychological guilt trips that placed her in malignant relationships.

Beginning with a handsome blonde named Steven Benedict. He had the right answer for every wrong that had ever been done to the human race. As he stood at a small podium in the local coffee shop he held the attention of about twenty students. Millie was one of them. "The small-minded individual who thinks about his own comfort first is what this country is all about," he said. An opinion that was echoed in every corner of a drug-filled campus.

But it was his smile and his green eyes that convinced Millie to believe in his theories and philosophies. She idolized him as if he were God and twenty-four hours after they met she had turned from virgin to a sex-crazed nymph. Two weeks later, inseparable, they moved together into a small apartment.

Steven was her first love and their relationship bordered on her deep need to be wanted, no matter what the outcome. She was committed to him being hers forever. At first she admired his ease with people, his social graces, the way he could walk into a room and snatch anyone's attention.

Because of her admiration she learned to ignore his snide remarks and sarcastic exchanges. But after awhile his attitude about her family began to gnaw at her.

"Your family is strictly puritanical and the essence of traditional behavior. That which our generation must strive to defeat."

"You don't even know my family," she would defend. "Leave them out of this."

At first she thought about him and his comments in the same way she thought about Paul. He was obnoxious. But when their relationship started to falter she began to see a much darker side of Steven. Millie tried to remain silent even when he berated her and attacked her family in front of strangers or friends.

After a dinner at a casual friend's house and a long night of conversation Millie was exhausted and wanted to leave. She was also aware that Steven had drunk more than usual but not to what extent until she approached him.

"Of course," he said, "you must be bored without the usual day-to-day mundane family gossip."

Rather than cause a scene Millie walked away. Still she felt embarrassed and hurt by his careless remark. When they finally arrived home Steven collapsed on the couch and she went into the bathroom to shower.

The tension of the night began to melt away as the water splashed across her body. Then suddenly she felt someone's hands grope her breasts.

"What are you doing?" she asked.

Steven reeked of booze and she couldn't stand the thought of his hands all over her. "I'm exhausted," she told him. "Not now."

He paid no attention to the protest and instead grabbed her by the hair and shoved her against the tile wall. Millie had never seen him in such a violent rage. "What's wrong with you, Steven?" she shouted. "Please stop it!" But he gripped her arm and dragged her wet body onto the floor.

"I don't really care how tired you are, bitch."

He pushed himself on top of her and pressed his lips against her face. She fought him as best she could. But he didn't stop. Instead his hand reached between her thighs and he thrust himself inside. Millie felt sick and confused. When he was finished he looked at her with disgust and rolled over.

She stumbled to the bathroom and recoiled in a corner of the shower. After awhile she reached up and adjusted the water. She wanted it hot, hotter than she could normally stand it. Then she took the soap and rubbed it against her body. "Please make his smell go away," she cried. And the vomit began to rise in her throat.

The following morning she was on the couch wrapped in her robe when Steven woke her. "I'm sorry," he said. "I don't know what I was drinking, but it must have done something to my senses."

"Get away from me."

He tried to put his arms around her. "Millie, you have to believe me, I would never do anything to hurt you. I'm so sorry," he said. His head hung low.

Her strongest desire was to believe him and when he began to cry, she did. She forgave him. He leaned forward and she let him kiss her.

That night was forgotten until a month later. Only this time he didn't just rape her. He beat her so badly she had to be taken to the hospital. Even then Millie still didn't leave.

Whatever excuse Millie rationalized, it took two years before she walked out and even then he didn't want to let go. It took two more years for her to realize that she didn't have to sleep with everyone to forget him.

By now she had become immersed into her studies. And spent much of her time in the library. One day while involved in research she scanned the aisle for a particular book. She couldn't find it. What she did find stuck between two other large volumes was a thin book of poetry by Emily Dickinson. The same book Nina had been reading that warm evening in May just before she died.

CHAPTER FIFTEEN

It was May 8th and unusually warm so early into the season. Millie was seated on the back steps. She placed her elbows on her knees and rested her head. The darkness was just around the corner but for the moment she relished the remnants of a long day. The neighborhood was noisy and people lingered on their porches while their children scattered around the street with jump ropes and baseballs.

Domenic had come to dinner that night and was just about to leave when Momma called to him. "I have a dish of pasta for the monsignor," she said.

"Thanks, Mom," he said. He walked down the steps and turned to face Millie. "Hey sport," he said. "What are you up to?"

"Nothing."

"Where'd Nina go?" he asked.

Millie pointed to the shed. "Guess."

Her brother turned around and looked across to the driveway. He rubbed her head. "Goodnight," he said and continued down the stairs. She watched him walk along the street until he disappeared around the corner.

Millie felt bored and she lazily moved down the steps across the yard. When she opened the shed door it slammed against the back wall.

"Want to go for a walk with me?" she asked her sister.

"Not now," Nina said, her eyes still glued to the book. "You should learn to read," she said and looked up. "Then you would have something to do."

"I know how to read."

"I mean something of value, like this book of poetry by Emily Dickinson."

"It is too nice a night to worry about Emily what's her name," Millie said. She walked out of the shed and slammed the door behind her.

It was really too late to go for a walk anyway. So Millie walked up the steps of the porch, leaned against the railing and looked out at the hazy sky and the stars. One by one her neighbor's lights flicked on in a race against the darkness and she felt surrounded by the quiet of a warm summer night. A slammed door from across the driveway jolted her out of the silence. Her eyes rested on the dark triple-decker that belonged to the Kerchaks. Josef sat on the front stoop. Millie could see his shirt was torn and his hands covered his face. After a few minutes he left and ran across the backyard. *Probably towards the field*, she thought. She wasn't sure how she felt about him. Sometimes she thought he was sad but after seeing him in the field the day Paul found the dead cat, she wasn't sure anymore.

Tired Millie headed for her room. "Goodnight," she said, and waved to her parents on the parlor couch.

"Goodnight, mia amoré," her mother whispered. "Sleep good."

After a cool bath, she pulled down the top blanket and fluffed her pillows, sprinkled some powder on the sheets, then climbed into bed. The fragrance and the silkiness of the talcum felt cool against her body. She rolled over on her stomach and looked at Nina's empty bed. It was 9:30 and her sister still hadn't come upstairs.

Millie wasn't sure it was the loud ticking of the clock that woke her at 2:00 or some other noise. But something had shaken her awake. Nina's bed was still empty, she noticed, then drifted off to sleep again.

But the second time she was awoken the noise was so loud she jumped up. Nina still hadn't come to bed. And Millie was irritated because that meant she had to go and rescue her sister. This wasn't the first time she had been forced out of bed to find her sister asleep in the shed. Poppa would be really upset if he knew that Nina wasn't in bed. One time when she had gone after Nina they had sat on the porch for hours.

"That's the Big Dipper," Nina told her. "That group of tiny lights, that's the Little Dipper."

But Poppa was up early that day and when he saw the two girls on the porch, he ranted and raved at them for two hours. Millie would have rather been beaten than have to listen to her father babble on.

Tonight she moved down the usually creaky stairs as quietly as possible. It was foggy and there was little moonlight to guide her. When she reached the bottom step she noticed the light in the shed was off. That was strange. Normally when Nina fell asleep in the shed the light would still be on.

She raced across the driveway and turned the doorknob to the shed.

"Nina, Nina! Wake up," she whispered. "Do you realize how late it is?"

She took a step inside the cool room and felt this momentary sense of apprehension. Disoriented because of the dark she reached across the wall to guide her. Millie slid along the damp cement and felt something run across her hand and it left her with the chills. She held up one arm in order to search for the overhead light.

"Ohh," she said relieved when she grabbed hold of the pull chain. When the light went on she noticed the empty wicker chair.

"Nina, Poppa is gonna be really mad."

Millie scanned the room for her sister. In the farthest corner of the room she could see the shape of something against the back wall. Millie hesitated before she approached. "Nina," she called. "Are you all right?"

Then she saw her sister. "Oh my God!" she screamed. Nina's pretty face was covered in blood and her nude body was twisted and slumped against the cement. She backed up and ran towards the shed door. Millie tried to scream but there was no sound. In one split second the world had changed. Devastated, and in a state of panic, she rushed for the door. That short walk she made every day now terrified her. Her legs heavy from fear moved in slow motion. And she struggled with each step. At the top of the steps stood a dark figure.

She stood frozen in the middle of the stairway paralyzed by fear.

"Millie, what are you doing?" the voice said.

"Paul," she screamed, then rushed to the top of the porch.

When she reached the landing Poppa was in the doorway. He flung the old door open and said, "What are you two doin'?"

Her body trembled and tears flowed from her eyes. "It's Nina," she cried. "Downstairs."

"What, she fell asleep again in the shed?" Paul said.

"Something's wrong," Millie said. Her voice sounded hysterical.

"What's wrong with you?" Poppa asked. "Paul, get Nina."

"No," Millie cried. There was a thick dryness in her mouth. "Somebody hurt her."

Paul looked toward the shed and rushed past his father down the stairs.

Poppa looked at his young daughter's face. "What did you see?" he asked her. Then he began to follow his son.

Millie tried to run after her father. She saw Paul rush through the door of the shed and she heard it slam against the back wall.

Paul's blood-curdling scream stopped her father. His body suddenly froze. Finally he moved slowly forward. But her brother caught him at the doorway.

"Don't," Paul cried to his father. "You don't want to see Nina like this."

"What do you mean?" the old man said. He broke loose from his son's grip. "Get outta my way!"

Millie could see her father's face through the dim light of the shed, his shadow captured along the cement wall. She stood in the doorway just as her father reached Nina's battered body.

Paul grasped his father's shoulders as the old man fell to his knees. "Who do this?" he asked. "Get me that blanket," he told his son. He placed it across his daughter's body. Her lifeless hand sat on the cement floor and he picked it up. "Who could do this to you?" he asked. He kissed her hand and tenderly placed in on the blanket.

This was all a dream, Millie thought. Just a bad dream and she looked up towards the sky. That's when she noticed her mother. She could see her mother's full body profiled in the faint porch light. "Che cosa," Momma called down.

Paul and Poppa came out of the shed. He stood with his arm around Poppa's waist and helped him up the stairs.

"Salvi," Momma said, confused and frightened. She placed a hand along the railing.

"Salvatore, what's wrong?"

Poppa kept his head down.

"Paul, what's the matter with Poppa?"

The boy's arm reached around the old man's shoulder and he moved him to a chair on the porch.

"What?" she asked again. "Poppa, you sick."

Momma's face was pale and she looked terrified. "Millie, call the doctor for your father," she said. "Paul, will you please tell me what's wrong."

"It's Nina, Momma," he cried.

"Where's Nina?" she said.

"Angela," Poppa sobbed. "Our little girl, she's m-m-morta."

"What do you mean?" Millie stood next to her mother and tried to grab her as she collapsed onto a seat.

"What, did she fall on the cement? Maybe she's just, you know, inconscious," she shouted. "Millie, you please," her mother said. "Please call the doctor."

"Momma," Paul whispered. "Nina didn't fall. She's dead. Somebody killed her."

His words sank in. She looked at her son's tear-stained face and saw the tremble in his lips.

"I need to see my little girl." Momma lifted herself from the chair.

"Not now," Poppa said. "Not this way."

She reached for her son's hand. "You help me, Paul, I want to see my baby."

"You don't want to see her like this, Momma," he said gently.

The old woman stood up and the two men moved quickly behind her. She walked to the porch railing. She stared down at the shed. "Nina's down there alone?" she asked.

"Yes," Poppa cried. Momma leaned toward the flowers in the boxes. She picked off a few dead petals. "They need water," she said. Poppa put his arm around her body and helped her off the porch.

The air shifted from warm and humid to damp and icy. Millie, dazed, walked to her room to find a robe. She was confused and befuddled when she walked back into her bedroom. All she wanted to do was go back to sleep and start the night over again. She gathered slippers and looked at Nina's bed. "You're supposed to be there," she cried.

Millie sat on her own bed and looked over at her sister's. Signs of Nina were everywhere. On her bed lay the curly-haired doll she had had forever, her stuffed animals. A shelf hung on the wall stacked with her favorite books. Nina's purse lay open, its contents scattered across the top of the bureau.

By now her mother's inconsolable sobs echoed through the house. Millie walked into the living room where the normally robust woman was hunched on the middle of the sofa, her face puffy and red while tears streamed down her face. She saw her daughter. "Come," she said and patted the seat next to her. "Your sister's dead," she sobbed. "You gonna miss her too."

Paul looked over at his sister. "I don't know what to do," he whispered. "I'm afraid for them."

"Should we call doctor Shaker?" Millie asked.

"I did," Paul answered. "He's at the hospital. But on his way home he will come by."

Momma looked over at her son. She beckoned for him to come closer.

Then she wrapped her fingers around his chin. "You must make your momma a promise," she said.

"Sure, Momma, what do you want me to do?"

"Don't let them bury my baby without me saying goodbye. Please, Paul." Her face grew stern. Momma tightened the grip on her son's face. "Do you understand? I need to see my little girl. I need to say goodbye."

"I promise," Paul said. He gently removed his mother's hand. "I won't let them bury Nina until you have said goodbye."

Millie watched her father walk into the room. He moved slowly as if he would break any minute. He eased himself onto the couch next to his wife.

Paul took his sister's hand. "C'mon," he said. "Let's leave them alone for a few minutes."

Millie couldn't remember when she called the police but she heard the screeching sounds of sirens. She saw the tires spin dirt in the driveway and stop. Then two young men dressed in blue uniforms leaped out of the car. Paul pointed into the shed.

What came next was chaos. In minutes the yard was filled with policemen, detectives, neighbors buzzing around. Most had been shaken awake earlier by the screams. A neighbor pushed forward from the crowd. "Hey, what's going on?" he asked.

"You don't belong here," a policeman told him.

"I know these people. Are they all right?"

A world of turmoil had been created down below and Millie watched from her spot on the upper deck. Neighbors gathered in clusters and whispered remarks. Some shouted questions, while others stood and pointed at the Giannetti house shaking their heads.

"Was there an accident?" a voice shouted.

She recognized one of Poppa's friends, Mr. Franco. He looked up at the porch. She caught a dim glance of the puzzled look on this face. "Millie, what's happened?" the old man asked. But a policeman immediately grabbed his arm and pulled him away.

The rest of the night was relentless with the echo of police cars and the brightness of headlights that beamed across the driveway.

There was a constant flow of people that appeared and disappeared among the shadows. Family members arrived and the sounds of grief became unbearable for Millie. She did not join them; instead she remained on the porch, disconnected. Her sorrow was too deep, too personal.

CHAPTER SIXTEEN

Marty Sacco didn't want to see another victim's blood splattered all over the floor. He wanted to turn around and run away as fast as he could. Instead he entered the small concrete building.

"It's another one," Detective Taylor said. "Only this one is much younger. Her name is Nina Giannetti."

The chief kneeled next to the victim. He lifted the blanket. "Is this the way she was found?" he asked.

"No," Detective Taylor said. "Her father and brother placed it on her after seeing the body."

"Goddamn," Sacco said, when his eyes wandered toward the familiar pile of clothes. "Did the brother find her?"

"No," an officer said. "Her fourteen-year-old sister found her first. The kid's over there," the cop said. Then he pointed to a young man who stood by the door of the shed.

"Did someone call the coroner?" Marty asked.

"Yeah, he's on his way."

Detective Taylor was by the door next to two men. They were all standing by the back stairs.

"Just that my sister Millie was hysterical," the boy said. "She was so upset I couldn't understand her."

"I'm Marty Sacco," he said, then turned to the older man. "I am really sorry about your daughter."

The old man's eyes were moist with tears. "Thank you, sir."

But the conversation came to a quick halt when they all turned to see where the sudden squeal of brakes came from. A young man jumped out from the driver's side, slammed the door and rushed across the lawn.

"Hey, you, where are you going?" a cop shouted.

"My name is Domenic Giannetti and the victim was my sister."

The cop stepped aside as the young man ran towards his father. The old man melted into his son's arms. "Domenic," he cried. "Somebody kill your sister."

He put his arms around the old man and held on to him tightly as he cried into his son's shoulders. After a few minutes his father released his son and Domenic helped him over to the stairway.

Marty recognized the priest from Stephanie Delahunt's funeral and walked over to him. Domenic looked up at the police chief. "Look," he said, "that's my sister lying in the shed. And I want to give her the last rites."

"Go ahead," Marty said. He motioned to the officer to let the priest through.

It wasn't long before the young priest returned, his face ashen, his voice solemn. He removed the purple ritual scarf from around his neck and placed it in his pocket. "This has been a terrible shock for my family. When will your people be finished?"

"We just have a few more questions," Marty said. "But there is no reason for any of you to hang around down here. My partner and I will come upstairs in a few minutes to take down the statement."

Marty watched as the small group ascended the steps. Half way up the staircase the old man stopped and looked back at the cement shed. He turned to his son. "It doesn't seem right to leave her alone like that. With all those strangers."

"It's all right, Poppa," Domenic said. "She's not alone."

If the Giannetti family still didn't believe what was happening, the coroner's black van arriving would be the defining moment. Two men dressed in white lifted a cot out of the back of the car. Within minutes they were wheeling the young girl's sheet-covered body from the tiny structure.

Every case is different but the procedures are all the same. Marty had spoken only briefly to Millie and Paul. Before he left he wanted to go over what they saw one more time. Generally it was not an easy task. Given the devastation of this crime tonight it seemed even harder.

The two detectives made their way across the porch and into the home of the Giannettis. Marty knocked and waited. The house was typical of the three families that lined the streets in the village.

He peered into the screen door and looked across at the shiny coffeepot that was perched against a back burner.

"Chief Sacco," Paul said and pushed open the door. "Jees, my father and I told you everything we know."

"I'm sorry," Marty said. "I do understand. But we never spoke with your younger sister."

Paul nodded. "Give me a minute."

After a few minutes he came back and invited the two detectives into the parlor. Millie sat next to her mother on the couch. The old man was slumped on a chair. People, family members, he assumed, were circulating around the room.

"We are a big family," Domenic said. "All these people are relatives. We are still trying to reach the rest of the family."

Marty felt true empathy for the Giannettis and he didn't want to be there any longer then necessary. "I just have one or two questions for the girl tonight. If we can have your word that she will come down to the station tomorrow I can have her sign the report then."

"Thank you," Domenic said. The priest looked solemnly at his mother then turned back to Marty.

"How is your mother?" he asked.

"The doctor came by and gave her a sedative so she can get some rest. Other than that I guess she is doing okay."

The priest walked Marty to where Millie was seated. The detective knelt down. "I am very sorry for your loss," he said. He noticed that Mrs. Giannetti held her daughter's hand. He turned to the young girl.

"Hi Millie, I'm Martin Sacco. Would you mind answering a few questions?"

Her voice soft and her face tear-stained, she looked up at the detective. "No," she said.

"Do you remember what time it was when you went to look for your sister?"

"I woke up about 2:30 this morning because I heard a loud noise."

"Do you remember what that noise was?"

"I'm not sure. But I remember thinking it was a door that slammed."

"Is that when you got up?"

"I looked over and Nina's bed was still empty. That's when I got up. I didn't want her to get in trouble with Poppa so I went to the shed."

"Has Nina done this before? I mean fall asleep in the shed."

"A few times," the young girl said. "If my father knew she was asleep downstairs in the shed again, he would get pretty mad."

"Before you went inside the shed did you see anyone?" Marty asked.

"No. It was too dark," Millie said. "Besides I was still groggy and tired." Tears rolled down her cheeks. "I just wanted to wake Nina and go back to bed."

Marty was about to ask her another question when he heard a disturbance in the front hall where Detective Taylor was waiting. It was another relative. Perhaps a brother but he was angry and irrational. Domenic ran over immediately to try and calm the man down.

"Please, Tommy, Momma is in the room."

Marty thanked Miller and motioned for Taylor to come this way.

This may be the most crucial time for correct information. But he also recognized the family's need for solitude. After all they had just lost a family member in a terribly cruel way. He walked toward the kitchen and Father Domenic followed behind. Marty turned and said, "I am very sorry for your family's loss. If the department can be of any help, don't hesitate to call."

Eight hours later, Martin Sacco's weary body strolled down the corridor that led to the morgue, where pathologist Philip Curran was performing the autopsy on the Giannetti girl. The chief was already late and a bit harried when he walked into the windowless room.

In the far corner of the room he could see Curran and Sergeant John Hayes of the Massachusetts State Police.

"Ay Sacco," the ME acknowledged. "You have arrived. We have been waiting for you."

Marty was well aware that he was twenty minutes late. He also knew that Philip could be a real pain in the ass when he was inconvenienced.

"I'm sorry," he said. "It couldn't be helped."

The chief was there to witness and to help assist the state trooper, while he fingerprinted the deceased and removed any personal affects so they could be properly tagged.

Once that was done then Hays could place the labeled items (clothing, jewelry, etc.) into a bag, attach another label with the victim's name and date of the murder. After that the officer of record was to sign the receipt and place it in a tray next to the body. *All very professional and impersonal*, he thought when he looked down at the uncovered body lying on the table.

A Cameo, her face reminded him of one of those brooches.

"Have you come up with anything new?"

"Well," Curran said. "She died from head trauma, just like the others. But this one doesn't seem to have the same sort of brutality attached to it that the others did."

"What the hell does that mean?" Marty asked.

"See these bruises? I think the victim was shaken like this," he said.

He took his hands and demonstrated.

"Are you saying this murder was committed by a different killer?"

"No. There are too many similarities. What I am saying is that the killer didn't seem to be as angry towards this victim." The examiner looked at the face of the dead girl.

"She was a pretty little thing," the state trooper murmured.

"And there is another thing," Doctor Curran said. "This girl wasn't molested in the normal sense of the word. He didn't penetrate her. But we found traces of semen on the body."

"But he did penetrate the other three victims, right?" Sacco asked.

"Yes, but this girl had her period," the Coroner said. "Some of the blood at the scene is from hemorrhaging due to menstruation."

"So he doesn't rape her because he's sensitive," the chief said. "And instead he murders her."

"I just do the autopsies," Curran said. "Motive, that's your job."

Trooper Hayes placed his pile of evidence in a white box. He took a pen and wrote Giannetti Evidence, property of the Framingham State Police. He picked up the box, put it in a bag and headed for the door.

"See you two later."

"This case is really getting to me," Marty admitted.

"I know what you mean. I've seen a lot of pretty girls come through these doors, too many. Maybe it's time for me to think about retiring."

"That sounds good to me," Sacco said. "But not till I catch this son-of-a-bitch." He looked again at the body. "Let me know what else you find, will you?" he said, then walked across the room to the grim hallway that separated the autopsy area from the storage area.

Marty moved past the cold, pale green cement walls. He remembered Taylor's comment about the morgue. It reminded him of his grandmother's house, he had said. "The same sterile sink. Even smells familiar."

He walked past the refrigerated section of the room. He scanned the doors of the gray compartments, most were temporary graves only labeled with numbers instead of names.

He spotted a cubicle further out of its niche than the others. And he attempted to push it back in but somehow it wouldn't budge. A tag dangled from the handle and curiously he looked at it. It was Nina Giannetti's cubicle. With an angry shove he pushed it back and heard the compartment click into place.

CHAPTER SEVENTEEN

Millie had this romantic notion that life stopped when the heart was broken. But when her sister died she found that theory didn't ring true. She learned the body continues to move through the shadows of time. The pain makes little difference.

She also believed that her and Nina shared everything, good secrets and bad ones, trivial or deep. But she now realized that her sister's life was as much a mystery to her as the rest of the world. Each time she remembered those last few weeks before Nina's death, Millie began to realize that maybe Nina wanted to share something but she just couldn't.

"What's wrong?" Millie asked her sister one day. It was obvious she had been crying.

"Nothing," she answered quickly.

Later that same day Millie picked up her sister's book. "Who is Emily Dickson?"

"Emily Dickinson," Nina corrected. "She writes poetry." Poetry was not one of Millie's interest so she placed the book unopened back on the bed.

Two days later she saw Nina run across the yard. She followed her into the shed. "Are you okay?" Millie asked.

Nina was out of breath. She sat in her wicker chair and placed her hands over her face.

"Nina, what's wrong?"

"Do you ever wish you could run away?" she said. "Or maybe just be someone else?"

"I never thought about running away," Millie said.

"Well, I do. I think about it all the time. I just want to go far away from here."

Millie felt sad for her sister. Nina's eyes were moist and her face looked flushed. "Don't ever let anybody steal you away from you," she said.

Although she realized Nina was upset, she was more than puzzled by what she had just said. And she didn't fully comprehend the power of her sister's words. But it was obvious that her sister was in pain.

"Did someone hurt you?" she asked. "Is it Josef again. Please tell me, Nina. What is wrong?"

Nina never answered. Instead she retreated. She closed her eyes and rested her head against the back of the chair.

Millie wasn't sure what her sister's problem was. But she was pretty sure it had something to do with Josef Kerchak. Nina was aware that Josef was always watching her. She had even caught him in front of their bedroom window. Another time Millie noticed a big bruise on her arm and Nina blamed Josef for it.

But no matter how much Millie pleaded with her sister she could not convince Nina to tell her mother or anyone else about him. And she was annoyed by her sister's stubbornness to ignore him, even though he somehow managed to intimidate Nina. So after repeated failed attempts to get her to tell, Millie decided to leave it alone.

After her sister's death Millie told Paul. "I tried to get her to tell someone," she said.

"Why didn't you tell Momma?" he asked.

"Because she didn't want me to."

"Do you think that little bastard had something to do with what happened that night?"

"I don't know," Millie said.

His demeanor quickly changed from anger to melancholy. "I was always so mad at her," he said.

"But why?" Millie asked.

"Because I would hear things about her from other boys."

She stood in the doorway. Paul sat on the edge of his chair, his eyes glued to the floor. He evoked compassion in her. Something she had never felt for any of her brothers. Especially Paul.

"What did you hear?"

"That she was damaged goods."

Millie understood the phrase. "How could you believe anyone who would say that about your sister?" she cried. "I know Nina, she never did anything like that."

"She liked to tease the boys," Paul said.

"So what. All the girls do that."

"I don't want to talk about it anymore," Paul said and headed for the back stairs. "C'mon, I promised Domenic I would take you to the police station."

Millie stopped at the last step and paused. It was as if the breath had been knocked out of her. The shed was surrounded by a yellow tape that read "do not trespass, this is a crime scene." It slithered across the driveway and around the cement structure like a snake.

Paul walked over to her and put his arm around her shoulder.

"Let's go," he said.

"Paul, promise me you won't ever say anything like that about Nina again."

He didn't respond.

They walked inside the brick station house. "My name is Paul Giannetti," he told the desk sergeant. "My sister Millie and I are here to see Chief Sacco or Detective Taylor."

"Wait here," they were told. But less than a minute later the officer came back and told them to follow the hallway to the end.

"See that open door on the right," the policeman said. "Go right in."

Millie straggled behind her brother. She wasn't anxious to talk to anyone. Chief Sacco greeted them at the office door.

"Hello," he said. "You remember Detective Taylor."

"I'm glad you came," he said. He led them both to a seat. "I promise to keep this as brief as possible."

The girl sat down in one of the metal chairs. Marty was impressed with the resemblance between the dead girl and her sister.

"How are your parents this morning?" he asked.

The young girl's expression remained solemn. "The same," she said. "Momma hasn't stopped crying and Poppa just sits on the couch and stares into space."

"And what about you? How are you today?"

"I still can't believe my sister is dead."

"Millie, I want you to try and remember everything from the minute you woke up until you found Nina."

"I told you last night. Something woke me up and I realized Nina wasn't in her bed and went down to the shed to get her. But the light was off," she said.

"Why did that bother you?" Marty asked.

"Because Nina always fell asleep in the shed while she was reading. So the light should have been on."

"So when you saw the light off it made you uncomfortable."

"Yes," Millie said.

"Did you hear anything when you opened the door to the shed?"

"No. I called Nina. And I felt for the light chain."

"After you found the light, what happened?"

"Nina wasn't in her chair. She always sat in the wicker chair. When I didn't see her I thought maybe she went somewhere."

"Where would she go that late at night?"

"Nowhere," she cried. "I just thought that for the minute."

"That's okay," Marty said. "Just tell me where would she have gone."

"I thought maybe she went to meet David."

"Had she ever done that before?"

"No," Millie said. "Never late at night. Just during the day. But she was so mad at Poppa about not being able to date. When I didn't see her in the chair a split second I just didn't know."

"Can you tell me about this David?" Marty asked.

"His name is David and they had been dating for a few months."

"Anyone else?"

"I made a list of a few girlfriends," Millie said. She took a piece of paper out of her pocket and handed it to Marty.

"What about boys? Could she have had a jealous boyfriend?"

The young girl looked over at her brother. He nodded for her to go on.

"There was someone," she said. "Nina told me that Josef Kerchak, he's the boy next door. She told me he would watch her all the time."

"Did you ever see him bother your sister?" Marty asked.

"Once when we were at the bus stop he came up to Nina and said he wanted to draw her. For a school project."

"Did she let him?"

"No."

"Did she ever tell anyone else about Josef?"

"I don't know for sure," Millie said, "but I don't think so."

Detective Taylor turned to Paul. "What about you?" he asked. "Did she ever tell you?"

"No," the boy answered.

Millie gaped at the detectives. "She didn't want any trouble."

"What kind of trouble?" Taylor asked.

"It's just that Josef's father was always yelling and screaming at him. And sometimes you could hear Josef screaming for his father to stop."

Marty turned to the young boy. "Do you know of any other boys that bothered your sister?"

"Yeah," he said. "Billy Weiss and David Polaski."

"You mean Hat Polaski's grandson?" Taylor said.

"Yeah, that's him."

"David wasn't bothering her," Millie said. "They liked each other."

"And what about Billy Weiss?" Marty asked

"He's just a stupid kid from her class. He would stare at her and give her the creeps. He never even spoke to Nina."

"Anyone else?" the police inquired. "A friend or neighbor, even a relative that might have tried to bother Nina or upset her?"

"No. Well, unless you want to count the time my cousin Steven tried to kiss her. Nina told me she had to fight him off. Oh and then there's Uncle Ed," Millie said. She looked over at her brother.

"Who's Uncle Ed?" Taylor asked.

Paul glared at his sister, surprised that she would mention him. "He's my father's brother," he said. "I mean he can be a weasel sometimes. But he wouldn't do anything like that."

"Well it's hard to know what anyone will do under the right circumstances," Marty said. "I promise you we will try to do everything we can."

As the two young people got up to leave, Detective Taylor asked Millie one more question. "Do you remember anything else about that night?"

"I did see Josef outside the night Nina died."

"Outside where?" Marty asked.

"It was late and I was tired, so before I went to bed I went to look for Nina. I found her in the shed. She told me she wanted to finish the last chapter and then she would come upstairs. I left and headed for the porch. That's when I noticed Josef Kerchak."

"What was he doing?" Taylor asked.

"He was on the front stoop. His shirt was torn and he was just staring at the sky."

"Do you remember the time?"

"It was just about dark, maybe 8:30 or 8:45. By the time I reached the top of the porch I heard Mr. Kerchak yell. When I turned around he was there next to Josef. I couldn't make out what he said. But then I saw his father slap him across the face. That's when Josef ran off."

"Did you see where he went?" Detective Taylor asked.

"No, but he probably went to the field behind our house. Where the railroad tracks are."

"How do you know that?"

She shrugged her shoulders. "I don't know."

"What about you, Paul? Did you ever see anything?"

Paul stood in back of his sister. He appeared nervous and fidgety.

"Yeah," he said. "Look, the old man is a nut. All he does is scream or slap the kid around. I've even seen him wack Josef on the back of the head."

"I'll bet you're thankful he's not your father?" Detective Taylor said.

"He's nothing like my old man."

"Did Mr. Kerchak ever bother you or one of your sisters?"

"Not on your life," Paul said. "We weren't afraid of him."

Marty stood up ready to conclude the conversation. "I really appreciate you two coming down to give us this information. I understand how difficult all this has been for you."

Paul noticeably angry glared at the two men. "Do you?" he said. "Why aren't you over at Kerchak's. Why aren't you questioning him."

He said and tugged at his sister's arm. "Let's get out of here."

"Paul," Marty said. "We have to take it one step at a time."

"Yeah," he shouted, "maybe I need to take a few steps of my own."

CHAPTER EIGHTEEN

"I still haven't been able to find anything on that cook at the Athena Restaurant," Jim lamented to Sacco.

"Then he's using an alias."

"I'm telling you, Chief, nothing came up under that name. I even tried looking under the initials VF. But nothing even close to Vincent Fiske."

"Well let's pay the Kerchak kid a visit," the chief said.

When the two detectives arrived at Prescott Street it was easy to see the proximity between the Kerchaks and the Giannetti house. The two families shared a common driveway that measured about twenty feet from either porch. With the warm weather and open windows it would be easy to overhear even moderate conversations. Millie's claim that she was able to tell Josef's T-shirt was torn did not sound unlikely.

The fact that the Kerchaks lived on the third floor was also interesting. Especially the fact that Josef's bedroom was at the back of the house. That meant the boy had a clear view of the shed and anyone entering or leaving.

"You know what's a little strange?" Taylor stated. "Even if this kid didn't want to watch her he could. The Giannetti house is wide open to his view."

"You're right," Marty said. He continued to survey the back of the house and the yard. Then the two men walked towards the front porch. When they approached the stoop they heard a gravelly voice yell to them.

"Hey, who are you?"

"Who are you?" Detective Taylor asked.

An old woman's head popped through a porch window.

"My name is Trioski," she told the men. "And I live here."

"Well, my name is Detective Taylor," he said and flashed his badge. The woman took it out of his hand. "Oh, what do you want here?"

"We are doing an investigation into the Giannetti girl's death." Taylor told her.

"Oh. What about you?" she said to Marty. "You got a badge too?"

"Sure," Sacco said and took his from an inside pocket.

"So, what you want?"

"We just wanted to ask your neighbors a few questions about the Giannetti girl's death," Taylor answered.

"That poor girl. What a horrible thing."

"Did you know Nina?" Marty asked.

"Here you know everybody. She and her sister always around."

"Then you must know the Kerchaks," Marty said.

"Sure," she answered. "I live in this house before they do."

"Then you must know them pretty well."

"I know them enough to stay away," she said.

"I'm busy." Mrs. Trioski shouted before she slammed the window. "I have nothing more to say."

"Thank you," Taylor said.

Marty rang the doorbell to the second floor. "Who's there?"

"We are looking for Josef Kerchak," he said.

A wisp of a woman opened the front door. Her face appeared thin and tired. With a heavy accent she said, "I'm his mother."

"My name is Martin Sacco, and this is Detective Taylor. We are with the Norwich Police Department and we would like to speak to your son Josef."

"Why you talk to Josef?"

"It's just a routine visit," Sacco said. "Your son knew the Giannetti girl and we are talking to anyone who might be able to help us."

She placed her hand to her mouth and said, "What a terrible thing for that girl and her family. "Please come in," she said, then scooted out of the way. "Maybe he knows something."

It was obvious that this woman had led a hard life. There was a large cut on her face and Marty suspected her long-sleeved sweater was to cover up the bruises on her arms. She invited the two men to wait in the living room while she went to find Josef.

"I find him," she promised. She tucked a piece of faded blonde hair behind one ear.

Sacco looked around at the small apartment with its familiar look. It could have been his mother's parlor. She had the same style overstuffed couch with crocheted doilies that lay across the back. He ran his fingers along the front edge of the coffee table and thought about the small gouges on the legs of his mother's worn out furniture. On the small table in front of the draperies was a large ornate lamp. And it all sat on top of a cheap Oriental rug.

His memories dissolved when he heard the sound of footsteps in the foyer.

"Here is Josef," Mrs. Kerchak said, her body obscured by a strong sunlight.

The young man stood a few feet behind his mother. He was tall and lanky and he oozed with a lack of confidence. "Josef," his mother said.

"These are the men who want to talk about Nina."

"H-h-hello," he stuttered, "I'm Josef Kerchak."

The police chief looked at the painfully shy boy and walked across the rug to shake his hand. "Hi, Josef, I'm Chief Sacco and this is Detective Jim Taylor."

"May we sit down, Mrs. Kerchak?" Marty asked.

"Oh, sure," she said. "I am sorry."

Detective Taylor with a discernible eye said, "Josef, how well did you know Nina Giannetti?"

"I don't know." He kept his arms straight and down by his side.

"Well you live in the same neighborhood. You go to the same school. You must have spent a lot of time together?"

"No, Nina didn't like me that much."

"A good looking boy like you?" Marty said. "Why do you think that?"

"I don't know."

Taylor was more to the point with his next question. "Did you see Nina the night she was killed?"

Mrs. Kerchak turned to hear her son's response.

"No, I didn't see anything that night."

"Did you hear anything?"

"No."

"Do you recall what you were doing that evening?"

"I was in my room drawing," he said.

Marty tried to deflect the boy's defensiveness and said, "Oh you're an artist."

"Yes," his mother said. "He is very talented."

"Where do you do your work?"

"In my room. I have a desk by the window because the light is good there."

"Could we see some of your drawings?" Marty asked.

"I guess so," Josef said. "I'll get them."

"No. Why don't you show us your room at the same time."

The boy led the two men down the hallway. When he opened the door Marty was taken back by the neatness and austerity of the room. There was a bed, a bureau and a desk that sat directly under the window.

"This is a pretty neat room for a young man," Marty said.

A metal trunk was at the foot of the bed and Taylor asked, "What do you store in here?"

"Just some of my junk," Josef said. He lifted the lid.

Jim peeked inside. He saw a baseball, a glove and a few other items. "Hey, where did you find this?" Jim held a girlie magazine in his hand.

The boy's mother turned to look. "I found it in the trash," he answered.

"Gee, you have a great spot here," Marty said. He stood by Josef's desk. "And a good view of the Giannettis' yard. You can see the place where Nina liked to go to read real clear. I'll bet you could even watch Nina going back and forth into the shed all the time." He didn't bother to look at the young boy's reaction.

"Is this some of your work?" he asked, eyeing a sketch of a naked young woman.

"Yes," Josef said. His gaze dropped to the floor.

Marty could see that the young man's demeanor was that of someone who was already defeated. His body movements were awkward. Every time he was asked a question his eyes would scan his mother's for approval. The police chief guessed that what he learned from the Giannetti kids was true.

"It was really very nice of you to show us your room," Marty said. He moved towards the doorway.

"I hope Josef helped you a little," Mrs. Kerchak said when she led the two men towards the front door.

"Thank you, Mrs. Kerchak," Marty said. "By the way, we might need Josef to come down to the station."

"Why?"

"It's just routine. You see with so many people we need to eliminate friends and relatives," Marty explained. "I'm sure that as a neighbor his prints are on the shed." He then directed the next remark to Josef. "I mean you must have gone over there once in a while."

"Y-yes."

"Well, there you are." He smiled. "We need to be able to get his fingerprints so we eliminate him."

"Oh sure, I understand," Mrs. Kerchak said.

Both detectives thanked the woman and headed for the car.

"I have to admit that was pretty good," Taylor said with a smirk

"What was?"

Jim pulled a cigarette from his pocket. "All that shit about eliminating fingerprints."

"That, detective, was a ploy," Marty said. "Does that kid look like a threat?"

"Nope."

"Still. I think he knows something."

Jim blew smoke in the opposite direction, then said, "But not enough to be our guy?"

"I don't know," Marty said. "These women died viciously. I mean, Josef Kerchak doesn't look like he has that kind of passion."

"Maybe he just killed the Giannetti girl," Jim said.

"I thought of that," Marty agreed. "But do you think he's clever enough to be a copy cat."

"It's hard for me to believe that he never watched the Giannetti girl from the window," Taylor said. The cigarette dangled in his mouth. "Or that he never had a horny thought. And then there are those girlie magazines in his room. I guess that could make every kid in town a suspect," he snickered.

"You too," Marty said.

"I agree."

"I don't know, maybe he did see something."

Marty leaned back in the seat of the 1952 green Chevrolet. When he was with Taylor he very rarely drove. Sometimes it frustrated him. *But not today,* he thought. He leaned back and closed his eyes.

Years ago he and Taylor had decided that Jim would do all the driving. "That way you can concentrate," his friend told him. "Besides, I don't like the way you drive."

But the chief knew the real reason Taylor insisted on driving. He felt responsible for the death of his best friend. One night when he was with a group of his buddies he let a young friend drive. The boy had just got his license. And when he skidded on a patch of ice he didn't know what to do and the car slammed into a wall killing Jim's friend. "Maybe if I had been at the wheel Pete would still be alive," Jim had said more than once.

When they arrived back at the station the desk sergeant handed the chief a piece of paper. "It's from the priest over at St. Bart's," he said. "He was here earlier."

Please give me a call when you have a minute. It's regarding the burial of my sister. It was signed, *Father Domenic.*

"St Bart's Rectory," a voice answered.

"Father Domenic, please."

"This is him. How can I help you?"

"Father, it's Martin Sacco at the Norwich police station."

"Thanks for getting back to me so soon," the priest said. "I wouldn't have bothered you but I am trying to find out when we can take possession of my sister's body. Actually I called the medical examiner's office myself this morning but so far no one has returned my calls. My parents need to see my sister. I'm sure you understand."

"I do," Marty said. "Let me see what I can find out. And why don't you give me the name of the funeral home."

"Slocumb's," Domenic answered.

"I'll get back to you."

"Chief Sacco," he said. "Do you have any leads yet?"

"Nothing substantial."

"Paul told me you were interested in the Kerchak boy," Domenic said.

"We are interested in any possible connection."

"The Kerchaks are a strange family," the priest volunteered. "Josef is very shy. And his father can be cruel."

"Well, we appreciate any information we get," Marty said. "I'll call the coroner's office right away and get back to you."

"Thanks again," Domenic said.

CHAPTER NINETEEN

Saturday morning Marty walked into the office to find Taylor at his desk. He poured himself a cup of coffee and listened in on the phone conversation.

"Will you see what you have under the name Fubrowski? No, I don't have a first name. Just an initial V. It could stand for Vincent, Victor, I don't know, just run it through."

"What was that all about?" Marty asked when he finally hung up the phone.

"I started running the initials for Fiske. If it is an alias maybe he stayed with the VF initials."

"What have you come up with so far?"

"Nothing," he said and picked up the phone again.

"Mrs. Kerchak, this is Detective Taylor. I was at your house the other day. Yes, ma'am. If you could have Josef come down to the station within the next two hours we would really appreciate it. Thank you," he said and hung up the phone.

"What do you think about this kid?" Marty asked.

"I don't know," Jim said. "I just don't know."

Within the hour accompanied by his father, George Kerchak, Josef was escorted directly into the print room, leaving his father to wait in the corridor.

Chief Sacco stood in the back of the gray room and watched as a policeman asked the Kerchak boy to place his fingers one by one on an inkpad. "Then blot them on the oversized file card," the cop requested pointing to a card lying on the table.

Once that was over he grabbed Josef by the shoulders and stood him against a cement wall. An older man stood behind a camera held in place by a tripod. "Look this way," he yelled to the kid. Josef blinked his eyes against the flash of light. "Okay, now look here," the photographer said. This time Josef shifted his eyes away from the flash.

"I'm done," the photographer told the cop. Marty waved him away and walked over to the boy.

"Hi," he said. "I'm glad you came."

The young boy sat down on the wooden bench next to the door. He placed his hands on his eyes. Marty leaned over. "Those little white lights don't last long," he said. "Listen, when you're ready I'll take you to my office. I'll have your father join us."

"You done it now," the old man yelled to his son when he walked into the room.

George Kerchak was small, wide and tough. He wore a nasty look on his face. "How long you gonna keep him?" Mr. Kerchak screamed at Detective Taylor.

"Sir, please calm down."

"Who are you?"

Marty looked over at Jim and rolled his eyes.

"I'm Martin Sacco," he said. "The police chief."

"Well," he said. "Tell your flunky to stay out of my way."

"Look, Mr. Kerchak, we can do this nice or we can have problems. Why don't you just sit down and have a cup of coffee so that we can talk with Josef for a few minutes."

His face grew tight. "My son didn't do anything," he said. "You just want to railroad him because you can't find the real killer."

"All we want to do is ask him a few questions. If you don't allow us to do that now, here in my office, I will be forced to go to a judge and get a warrant."

The old man stepped back.

"There, now would you like a cup of coffee?" Marty asked.

"No, just get this over with. Josef, come here," he said.

The boy had been standing in the doorway.

"I said get over here," his father beckoned. Josef moved forward and took a seat in front of the chief's desk. He lowered his head and placed his hands in his lap.

"Jim, would you get Mr. Kerchak a cup of coffee?" Then he turned toward the boy. "Josef, how about you?"

"No," he whispered.

"Please sit, Mr. Kerchak," Marty said. He pointed to a seat across the room.

Marty walked behind his desk and sat down. He pretended to look through some papers on his desk while he waited for Jim to hand the coffee to the old man. There wasn't any evidence right now to link the Kerchak boy to the crime. But he wanted to get the kid's reaction to a few questions before he had an attorney. For the moment that was another hurdle he didn't have to jump over. He wanted any information the kid could provide. Later they could determine what was or wasn't relevant.

Jim handed the now more relaxed Kerchak a cup of coffee. Marty pressed a buzzer on his desk and a young woman came into the office. She had a notepad and pen. She took a seat next to Josef.

"This is Miss Davis," Marty said. "She is the stenographer. And she will take down everything Josef says. Now, Josef, would you just tell me again what you were doing on Thursday evening, May 8th 1954?"

"I was in my room," he said. "Like I told you. I sat at my desk and worked on some of my sketches."

"That's right, you like to draw," the chief said. "And you didn't go out at all. It was a pretty hot night," he said.

The boy's eyes roamed across the room and they settled on his father. "Ahh, I did sit on our front stoop for a few minutes."

"Do you remember what time that was?"

"I'm not sure but I know it hadn't gotten dark yet."

"Did you see anyone?"

"No," the boy hesitated then said, "I did see Nina. She went into the shed earlier. I could see her from my window."

"You're a pretty lucky guy," Marty said. "Living next door to two pretty young girls."

Taylor walked over and leaned against the chief's desk. "You must have been the envy of all your friends," he said. "Didn't you have a crush on one of the Giannetti girls?"

"We were friends, sometimes."

"What do you mean by sometimes?" Jim asked.

"I don't know."

"Did Nina have a lot of boyfriends?"

"How would I know?"

"You were jealous of her friends, weren't you?" Taylor said.

"That's enough," Mr. Kerchak said. "You bother my boy no more. Come on, Josef."

The young boy's resigned attitude was so evident in the presence of his father.

"That's fine, Josef," Marty said. "We can finish this some other time. But if you do remember something, anything, please get in touch with either

Detective Taylor or myself."

"You are stupid like your mother," the father said. "How many times I tell you never talk to those girls?" Marty could hear the old man chastise the boy all the way down the hall.

"Jesus, where did that guy come from?" Taylor asked. "Maybe we should be looking into his background."

Marty shrugged his shoulders. "It wouldn't hurt to do a check on him." He'd take anything he could get.

The following day Marty asked Taylor about the fingerprints that were pulled from the crime scene. "What about the blood print we sent over to the State Police lab, any word on that yet?"

"Not yet, but I had Officer Roberts take the kid's prints over to the State lab too," he said. "You never know—we might get lucky."

Late in the afternoon of that same day, Buzzy Wharton, the pathologist from the Framingham State Police lab, called the station.

"Is Chief Sacco there?"

"Hey Buzzy," Marty answered. "What's an old man like you still doing hanging around?"

"I was just about to ask you the same thing. But I'm old enough to know you can always learn something," he said with a snicker. "Which is why I'm calling."

"What do you mean?"

"It has to do with that print you sent over. The one that belongs to a Josef Kerchak."

"What about it?"

"How did your guys know it would match the bloody one pulled off the Giannetti crime scene?"

"Are you telling me you've got a match?"

"Yep. It's the Giannetti girl's blood. And it's Josef Kerchak's print. So I guess you've got a suspect."

"Thanks, Buzzy."

Marty had been pretty sure the Kerchak kid couldn't have committed the other murders.

"But," he told Taylor. "This bloody fingerprint tied him to the Giannetti girl."

Reluctantly, he told Taylor to get a warrant. Then with Detective Taylor and two uniformed policemen they went to the Kerchak house.

"Mr. Kerchak," Marty said. In his hand he held the warrant. "We are here to arrest your son for the murder of Nina Giannetti."

"What you talking about?" the old man howled. "He didn't kill that girl."

The two officers made their way through the house and into Josef's bedroom with Marty and Taylor. While they searched the boy's bedroom Mrs. Kerchak rushed into the room.

"What is going on?" she cried. The boy's father stood in the doorway. His mouth never stopped. Marty listened to him as he used this time as an excuse to reprimand his wife.

"They came to arrest your Goddamn son."

"Why? What did he do? My son is a good boy," she cried. "He didn't do anything wrong. Tell them. Josef, tell them you didn't do this."

"Momma," he said. "I would never hurt Nina."

She looked towards her husband and said something to him in Polish.

"What do you expect me to do," he said, then walked out of the room.

"Detective, my son did not do this. I think you are like the Gestapo," she cried.

Touched by the woman's remark he tried to explain. "Mrs. Kerchak, we are just the police and we are doing what the law tells us to do. We have evidence that places your son at the crime scene." He hesitated and then said, "I would advise you to call an attorney."

The old woman stopped the policeman who held her son's arm. She kissed Josef's cheek. Then she gripped the bannister and watched as he slowly moved down the stairs. "I come to see you tomorrow," she cried. "I promise."

Marty could hear the woman's sobs and her whispered cries all the way to the car. She may have spoke in a foreign language but he understood her pleas. So did her son who sat silent in the back seat of the police car.

When they arrived at the station Marty stopped at the desk and Taylor took him into his office. "We want to speak with him for a few minutes before you book him," he told the two policemen. Marty walked into the office just as Jim removed the boy's handcuffs.

"Would you like something to drink?" he asked.

"No thanks," Josef said then rubbed his wrists.

Marty had a file in his hand. He took out the pictures of Nina and spread them across his desk. He directed the boy over to view the pictures.

"Well," he said, "she died a pretty hard death, don't you think?"

Josef turned pale and looked like he was about to gag.

"You were there that night. You saw her like this, didn't you?"

"No! I don't know anything," he shouted. "I swear to God, Mr. Sacco. I didn't kill Nina."

"If you didn't kill her then explain why your bloody fingerprints were in the shed."

"You see," Jim said, "that places you there and with Nina's blood on your hands, it looks as if you killed her."

Josef looked stunned. He glared at the two men. "I heard a crash," he said. "I knew it came from next door. So I looked out the window. "That's when I saw somebody run out of the shed and head for the railroad tracks."

"Could you see who it was?"

"No, it was so fast. I took my eyes off of him for a second and he was gone."

Marty sat down in his chair and told Josef to do the same. Taylor had just lit up a cigarette and was still perched on the corner of the desk.

"Okay," he said. "Let's start from the beginning."

The kid ran a hand through his hair. He rubbed his chin and then he spoke.

"It was hot and muggy and I couldn't sleep. I kept trying to fall back to sleep but I couldn't. When I heard this loud crash I jumped out of bed and ran to the window. That's when I saw some guy run across the Giannetti yard.

"Do you know what time it was?" Taylor probed.

"No, but I didn't go to bed till after midnight."

"Where were you before you went to bed?" Marty asked.

"I was at my desk."

"Did you see Nina before or after you saw the man run away?"

"No."

"Then what happened?" Jim asked.

"I didn't see anything. Except the light was still on in the shed. I knew Nina was in there. She was always in there reading. She told me once how mad her father gets when she falls asleep in there. He even threatened to lock the doors on her. So when I saw the light on, I figured I should wake her," he said.

"Then you went to the shed to see if she had fallen asleep?" Marty asked. "Was she asleep?"

"Didn't you want to know who had just run from the shed?" Jim asked. "Weren't you a little jealous that somebody had visited Nina?"

The boy's expression changed and his voice cracked. "No! I just wanted to see if she had fallen asleep."

The police chief sat back and watched Jim interrogate the boy.

"Was the light on in the shed then?"

"I don't remember," he said.

"Okay, what did you do next?"

There was a loud knock at the door but Jim tried to ignore it. "Go ahead, kid, what happened next?"

"I-I started to go towards." Again Josef was interrupted and he turned towards the door.

"Who the hell is it?" Marty screamed.

"It's Michael Prendergast from the DA's office."

"Come in," he sighed.

A short portly gentleman stepped into the room. He glanced across at the Kerchak boy, and then with a finger beckoned to the chief.

"I was told you went after a warrant," he said. "What's going on?"

"The bloody fingerprint we found at the scene came up his." Marty looked toward the boy. "When we went to the kid's house we found more evidence."

"Like what?" the District Attorney asked.

"Blood on a pair of pants and a torn shirt."

"Who does the blood belong to?"

"The boys at the lab are looking at the clothes now."

"The fingerprint is good," Prenderghast said. "But the victim's blood on the clothes will tie it up. Can you get a confession?"

"I don't know," Marty said. "The kid insists he didn't do it."

"Do you believe him?"

"I don't know," he said. "He just doesn't strike me as some sex-crazed killer."

"Well keep in touch," the DA said before he headed down the hall.

The chief walked back into the room and said, "You couldn't remember if the light in the shed was on or off."

Detective Taylor picked up the chief's cue and walked around Josef's chair. "You thought maybe she had another boy in there, didn't you?"

"I don't remember what I thought," he said.

"Come on, admit it. You were jealous that she might be in there with another guy," Jim said. "What do you think she was doing with another guy at that time of night?"

"That's not true," he yelled. "Besides, she wasn't like that."

Detective Taylor looked hard at Josef. Sarcastically he said, "Not with you anyway."

Josef looked away.

"Tell me what happened the day you grabbed Nina's arm?" Marty said.

"It wasn't like that" he said.

"That's not what I heard. I was told that you watched her all the time. Is that true?" he asked.

"Is what true? That I saw her all the time? Yeah, I lived next door."

"You know what I mean. Did you watch her?"

The boy remained silent. He turned to the windows.

"Then why did she plead with you to leave her alone?" the chief asked. "Didn't she tell you that if you didn't stop she would tell her brother?"

"I really liked Nina," he sobbed. "I just wanted to protect her."

"To protect her. Protect her from what?" Taylor asked. He handed the boy a few tissues from his desk drawer. "Why do you think she needed protecting?"

Josef's shoulders drooped and he looked exhausted.

"Tell me the truth, son. You were curious that night and you wanted to find out if someone was with Nina. That's the reason you went into the shed, isn't it?"

"No," Josef cried. "I didn't go in the shed."

"You see kid, that's why we get angry," Taylor said and backed away. "It's all about the lies." He anchored himself to the corner of the desk and smiled. "We told you before, we know you were in the shed. We found one of your bloody fingerprints plastered on a cabinet."

"Maybe you'll feel like talking after a good night's sleep," Marty interrupted.

"Yeah, I'm tired," he said after a deep breath. "Can I have my father come and get me now?"

"No need." Jim smiled. "You are going to be our guest tonight."

"What do you mean?"

Jim grabbed the kid by the arm and pulled him towards the hallway. "You see that room over there? Yeah, the one with bars. That's the holding cell or our guest room," he said with a smile. "You can sleep in there tonight."

"But, I didn't do anything," Josef protested. "I swear to God. I didn't kill Nina."

Marty didn't want to book Josef just yet. He still didn't believe the kid killed Nina or anyone else. But he did think he knew a lot more than he was telling. So he decided to keep him at the station for one night. He hoped that would frighten the boy enough to tell the truth.

It was 7:30 the next morning when Jim strolled in with a bag of doughnuts. Marty was already there. "Hey Doherty," he called to the duty cop. "Would you get us some coffee?" The detective tossed the bag on his desk.

"What, did you baby sit the kid last night?" Jim asked. "How did he do?"

"Hand me that bag," Marty said. "Ahh, a jelly donut," he said. He took a large bite and some jelly sat on the edge of his mouth. He licked it off with his tongue.

"Doherty said he cried himself to sleep."

Jim lit up a cigarette. He took a sip of coffee and looked towards the back hall where the kid was confined. "Do you think our Josef had something to do with those teenage sexual assaults?"

"Yeah," Marty answered. "Especially if you factor in that they stopped the same night Dorothy Miller was killed."

"I wanted to give this kid a break. Now, I don't know," Marty said. He stood up and wiped his pants.

"Christ, you're a mess," Taylor said. "You've got sugar all over you."

He handed Marty a napkin. "We know we can tie Josef to the Giannetti murder. And he lives less than two blocks from Dorothy Miller's house. Then there's the Robertson victim. She's another Ethnic Village resident. We have an eyewitness who saw someone running towards the railroad tracks at the end of Prescott Street. No problem so far."

"Then why diversify?" Marty said. "What is his reason to leave the village? What is his motive for Stephanie Delahunt's murder?"

"Good point," Jim said. "Our victims knew the killer. They were comfortable with him. That's why there is no evidence of forced entry."

"Do you really believe that Josef Kerchak is that person?"

Jim looked frustrated. "I don't know."

"Forget him for a minute, what about the Roache case? How do you place Kerchak there?"

"That's another good point," Jim agreed. "Maybe he copied our killer's MO on the Giannetti girl."

"Do you think he's that smart?" Marty asked. "Look, you know as well as I do, that unless it's domestic or passion not many killers work out of their own back yard. Granted," Marty continued, "Nina could have been the victim of Josef Kerchak, but personally, I don't think this kid has it in him. And how did he know about the folded clothes? It wasn't printed in the paper, and he certainly doesn't have any police connections."

After a few quiet minutes Marty smiled at Jim. "Besides, I actually like your other theory better."

Jim was seated with his elbows on his knees. "Which one was that?" he said then rubbed his eyes.

"The one about George Kerchak being a suspect."

"It's possible," Taylor said with a smile. "The FBI are doing a background check on the old man. But did you forget Josef's fingerprint? That places the kid at that crime scene."

"There's no doubt he was in the shed that night. But why?" Marty said.

Sergeant Doherty appeared in the doorway. "Hey Chief," he said. "The kid's lawyer just called, he'll be here in an hour."

"Who is it?" Jim asked.

"You're gonna love this." The sergeant chuckled. "Shapiro."

Leo Shapiro, always cock sure of himself, swaggered into the station house just after 8:30 a.m. With him were the boy's parents.

"Where is my son?" George Kerchak yelled when he stormed into the office.

"He's in a holding cell," Taylor answered. "As soon as you calm down we'll let you see him."

"Your Goddamn right you'll let us see him," Shapiro said. "Have you boys gone crazy? What made you place this kid in a cell over night? I'm gonna have your ass," he said, then slammed his briefcase on Taylor's desk.

"Listen, Leo, we didn't keep this kid over night on a whim. Didn't your clients tell you he was arrested?"

"Arrested! For what?" he said, then turned to face Mr. and Mrs. Kerchak. "Look," he said and led them out of the office. "I want you to wait here until I come and get you."

"But my son," Marty heard the woman say.

"I promise you will see Josef very soon."

Shapiro had a pomposity for irritating people and Jim was no exception. "What's this so called evidence?" he said. "Or did you just lose your senses?"

"How about a bloody fingerprint at the crime scene. Is that enough sense for you?" Taylor snarled.

"Okay girls," Marty shouted. "Let's calm down. It was all in the signed warrant that we gave your client."

"I guess I wasn't impressed," Shapiro said.

Marty shook his head at the egotistical lawyer. He smiled to himself. Shapiro grew up in Norwich. He knew that most people found him crude, arrogant and even offensive. He didn't care. Nothing bothered him. When and if someone decided to give him trouble, Shapiro would just become more determined than ever to win the battle.

"Okay boys," Shapiro relented. "Give me a few minutes. I need to speak with my client."

Marty agreed and led the attorney out the door and down to where the Kerchak boy was. Josef sat on one end of the cot, his knees up against his chest and his arms wrapped tightly around them. His eyes held no emotion. When they unlocked the door, the kid didn't budge.

"Hi Josef," Shapiro said. The thin man walked over to the young boy and sat next to him. "My name is Leo Shapiro, and I'm your lawyer. Can I speak with you?" he asked.

Josef never changed his expression. He nodded yes and then placed his head on his knees.

"Would you leave us alone?"

"Sure," Marty said. He heard the phone ring and saw Jim pick it up.

"Thanks," he said, then hung up.

"The FBI ran those initials," Taylor said. Excited he jumped up from his seat. "They have a description and Navy service record for a Victor Fubrowski from Norwich. I'm gonna take it from there and run a check on him. Victor Fubrowski to Vinnie Fiske, I guess it could work."

"Okay, let me out of here," Shapiro called.

He walked back into Marty's office. "From this point on," he said, "my client talks to no one without me. Do you understand? And before another word he wants to see his parents."

"Okay," Marty agreed. He told Doherty to take the small group and the kid to one of the empty rooms. Taylor was on his way out the door and smiled at the chief. "Nervy little punk, isn't he?" he remarked.

"He doesn't bother me," Sacco said. "He grows on you after a while." Marty took a sip of coffee. "You know what, if I were in that kid's shoes, I'd be thrilled that Shapiro was my attorney."

It was well known that Leo Shapiro would use the law any way he could to defend his clients. There was little interest whether they were guilty or innocent. For him it was all about the winning. Marty had even asked him once if it bothered him to defend vermin. The slick attorney looked him right in the eye and said, "You know what? I sleep real good at night. I'll bet even better than you."

CHAPTER TWENTY

After visiting with his parents for a few minutes, Josef Kerchak emerged depleted with bloodshot eyes. His clothing looked wrinkled and soiled. His hair disheveled, he shuffled behind the duty cop with his lawyer.

"I understand you have something to tell us," Marty said.

Josef eased himself down on to a chair and glanced up at his attorney.

"Go ahead," Shapiro said.

"When I walked into the garage Nina was already dead. There was blood everywhere," he said. His voice cracked and tears ran down his cheeks.

Shapiro gently put his hand on the young man's shoulder. "It's okay, kid, tell them everything."

"Her body was up against the back wall. At first I thought I saw Nina move so I ran over to help her. But when I touched her face, I knew she was dead." His voice fell silent.

"Then what," Marty asked.

"That's when I saw her blood on my hand. I wiped it on my pants and ran," he admitted. "I didn't know what to do. Who to call. I just ran home."

The boy wiped his nose with the back of his hand. "When I got home I realized I had Nina's blood on my pants. I threw them in the back of closet in a bag. I was gonna throw them in the trash but then everything just happened so fast. Mr. Sacco, that's the truth, I swear it."

"What did you mean yesterday when you said you wanted to protect Nina?" Detective Taylor asked. "Who were you protecting her from?"

"She told me that somebody wouldn't leave her alone."

"Nina told you that?"

"Why would she tell you something like that and not her family?" Marty asked.

"I don't know. Maybe she didn't want her father to know."

"Nina told her sister that it was you," Jim said. "That you would sit and watch through the bedroom window. Is that true?"

"Sometimes," he said. "But it wasn't like you think. I loved Nina. I just wanted to see her."

"If you loved her why didn't you call someone when you found her in the shed?" Marty asked.

"Or at least wake your parents?" Jim butted in.

"C'mon, boys, give the kid a break. One at time."

Everyone was silent for a moment. Then Marty repeated his question.

"I don't know why I didn't call the cops. I guess I was too scared."

"Did you think the killer would come back?"

"No," he answered. "I heard someone on the Giannettis' back porch and ran towards my house. That's when I saw Millie standing by the shed."

"Josef, did you turn off the light when you left?" Marty asked.

"I don't remember."

"Tell me what occurred when you saw Millie?"

"It was like a scene from a movie. Everything happened so fast. Millie screamed and ran up the stairs. That's when I saw Paul and old man Giannetti walk into the shed."

Josef rubbed his arm. "All of a sudden the police cars and people were everywhere. After that everything seems like a blur. I closed the door to my bedroom and pretended I was asleep."

Marty felt fidgety. He moved around the room. His hand searched his pocket for that invisible cigarette. The one he could use right now.

"What do you remember about the man you saw run away? Was he tall? Thin. Anything, Josef, at all, Josef, try to remember."

The boy closed his eyes. "All I saw was this black figure move across the yard."

"He's being arraigned at 11:00 o'clock," Shapiro said. "This is enough for now."

Marty agreed. He could see the kid was exhausted. And he didn't think any more questions would give him any new answers.

"I hope the DA's office isn't gonna oppose bail," Shapiro said.

"What are you, stupid?" Detective Taylor remarked. "We got three murders and this kid's fingerprints on the fourth. Do you really think the District Attorney isn't gonna ask for bail."

"I don't care what you've got, my client didn't commit these murders," he argued. "This kid is innocent and you know it."

"Yeah, and you know that for a fact," Taylor said.

Shapiro picked up his briefcase. He grabbed his client's arm. Then he turned to Jim. "I'll see you later, asshole." And he walked out the door with

Josef.

The Monday after Nina Giannetti's murder the town councils for both lower Norwich and the village called an emergency meeting. They sent an invitation to the police chief. Martin Sacco sat in the first row.

Fred Pearson, the owner of Pearson's Hardware and a very vocal member of the town, began the session. "What the hell is going on?" he said. His question was directed towards Marty. "Mr. Sacco, we need you to come up here and tell us what the police department is doing to protect the citizens of Norwich."

Marty moved toward the microphone. "We have hired some auxillary police to patrol the areas. We have…"

"Did you arrest the Kerchak kid?" someone shouted.

"The department is doing a thorough investigation at this time," he answered.

"Well, what about it?" Pearson said. "Did you arrest the kid?"

Reluctantly Marty answered, "Yes."

"Then you have the murderer."

"Technically," he said, "we have a suspect, but all the evidence needs to be corroborated with the State Police lab."

"Then you arrested the wrong man?" another man shouted.

Marty didn't have a chance. He understood that whatever he said was only going to drown him. "We are in touch with the FBI and the State Police. We need to be sure that our evidence is…"

"What is that dribble?" Pearson interrupted. "Give us a straight answer. Off the record you have the Kerchak kid in jail. But you're not sure why? Right!"

Marty stared at the ruddy-faced merchant in front of him. "Off the record or on the record," he said. "We have arrested a suspect in accordance with specific evidence. But that is still under investigation."

Fred Pearson had it in for him ever since he took office. Marty liked to think it was because he beat Fred's brother out of the position. But even if that was part of the reason, it was obvious that the hardware owner was just an arrogant son-of-a-bitch.

The police chief looked over at the crowd. He wanted the townspeople to understand that there was doubt about the Kerchak kid being the killer.

"We have arrested someone," he admitted, "but we need more evidence before we are convinced of his guilt," he said. He handed the microphone back to Pearson, closed his briefcase and headed for the door.

"Wait, Marty."

He turned to see Jack Murphy. He had seen him earlier in the audience. Murphy was a nice guy and they had always gotten along well.

"What is it, Jack?" Marty said.

"This community is frightened. We just want to be sure another murder isn't committed. We don't want to lose anymore loved ones."

Pearson was still at the front of the room. "That's right," he responded into the microphone.

"Don't you think I understand the fear that is in this room," Marty said. "Well just for the record. I do. And I want to find the real killer just as much as you do." He walked through the door and left.

He was grateful he had left the meeting. He didn't want any part of an over zealous group. He knew all it took was a loud mouth and just the right mix of ingredients for a war party. And they already had a rebel rouser with Fred Pearson.

Late the next afternoon the district attorney's office called Marty's office. "I got Shapiro to agree to allow his client to take a lie detector test," Prenderghast boasted. "He balked but I won."

"That's great."

"Yeah, the technician's name is Graham and he should be in touch in a few days. Set it all up, will you, Chief?"

"Okay."

The day of the test a bald gentleman walked into the police station and stopped at the front desk. "Hello, I'm Jeff Graham," he said. I am here to conduct a polygraph test on Josef Koschark."

"That's Kerchak. Let me introduce myself. "I'm Martin Sacco."

"Oh, Kerchak, thank you."

"If you follow Officer Newton, he will show you where you can set up your equipment."

Within the hour Leo Shapiro and the police chief walked in on Graham and his subject. He had wrapped a 3" black band around Josef Kerchak's chest. Then he strapped a blood pressure cuff to the boy's arm.

Doctor Paul Winslow, the state psychiatrist, showed up next. He explained to Josef that he would be the one to ask him the questions.

"I'll be right outside the door," Shapiro told his client. "Just answer the questions as truthfully as you can. Everything will be fine."

First the technician asked the boy a few questions.

"Is your name Josef Kerchak?"

"Yes."

"Do you reside at 10 Prescott Street?"

"Yes."

"Are your parents Grace and George Kerchak?"

He signaled for the doctor to begin his questions.

"Did you kill Nina Giannetti?" he asked immediately.

"No," Josef shouted.

"Did you see who did?"

"No."

Josef glared at the cement floor.

"Did you see someone run from the Giannetti yard on the morning of May 9th, 1954?"

"Yes."

"Did you like Nina Giannetti?"

"Yes."

"Did you kill Nina Giannetti?"

"No."

Two hours later the black band was released from the boy's chest and the cuff on his arm was removed. Marty watched the young man as an officer handcuffed him and led him back to his cell. Josef shambled by. His eyes scanned Marty's face. He wore an expression of confusion, hopelessness and resignation. But as Marty locked onto the boy's pale blue eyes what the police chief didn't see was a killer.

"Well," the psychiatrist said.

"I don't know," he admitted. "I don't think the results are very conclusive."

Marty opened the office door and beckoned the boy's lawyer into the office.

"There isn't enough to go on," Graham explained. "It's just not definitive enough."

"What do you mean by not definitive enough?" Prendeghast said. His voice bellowed in the open doorway.

"Maybe you have the wrong man," Shapiro said. He held his briefcase in both hands.

"Where's the read-out?" the district attorney asked.

"Here," Graham said. "This is the graph." He moved a pencil along the lines. "When asked if he killed her, the needle slows down. That appears to be the truth. But when he is asked if he knows who the killer is, the needle jumps all the way to here. That introduces a dozen theories. I'm sorry," he said. "There is just too much inconsistency to be effective."

"What if we scheduled another session and asked a different group of questions?" the DA asked.

"Not with my client," Shapiro said, and slammed the door on the way out.

CHAPTER TWENTY-ONE

Despite the sun, the dark shadows of mourning had settled into the Giannetti neighborhood. The sensationalism and drama of the murders was on everyone's lips. Nothing so perverse or sexually evil had taken place in the mundane little town before.

The newspapers printed as many details as they morally could. The inept release of facts printed helped to create the public opinion that Josef Kerchak was guilty in not only Nina's death but that he was also responsible for the other murders as well.

The youthful age of the accused killer and the horrible ways in which his victims died caused a wave of fascination. Because Nina was the fourth victim and the youngest she became a martyr. And groups of people gathered around the Prescott Street house. They formed a morbid curiosity that invaded the privacy and the grief of the family for days.

Millie Giannetti's doorbell rang constantly from representatives of different local and inner city newspapers in the hope that they could increase their sales.

Her brother Paul's brusque manner seemed like a Godsend during that time. He guarded the door like a Centurion. There were so many people that stood and gawked at the Giannetti house. A constant presence that neither diminished nor hid from shame when Paul yelled, "Get away from here."

Millie's mother sat at the kitchen table. Her favorite pastime was less a diversion now. She fingered the neckline of her freshly ironed black dress and glared out at the people who lined her driveway.

"Why these people don't go home," she cried.

"I don't know, Momma," Millie said. She walked over and kissed her mother's forehead. "Are you all right?"

"Yes, mia bambina. It's just everything is so black around me." She turned to her daughter. "Why this boy kill your sister?" she asked. Tears flowed down her cheeks.

"I don't know."

"It is so sad," Momma said. "This boy hate my little girl so much he has to kill her. This I don't understand. Why he hate so much?"

It was time to leave for the funeral home. But there was something Millie needed to do first. Every time she entered the bedroom she felt the sting of her sister's death. Nina was no longer there. She wasn't primping in front of the mirror. Or lost in the latest book. She would never be there again. Millie stood in front of the mirror. She picked up her sister's lipstick. Nina had once reprimanded her for using it without her permission.

"If you had asked me," Nina said, "I would have let you."

Millie noticed a few strands of her sister's long black hair. She removed them from the hairbrush and carefully placed them on a handkerchief she kept in the bureau drawer.

There was a soft rap at the door and she heard her brother's voice whisper, "Millie, we have to leave."

The night Nina was killed Paul had taken her book and given it to Millie. She placed it on the bureau. Today she would give it back to her sister.

It was nearly 12:00 o'clock when the little group gathered in the kitchen. A long black limousine pulled up in the driveway.

"The funeral home sent it," Paul told his father.

"Angela," he called from the front room. "We have to go now."

"I'm coming."

Momma walked from the kitchen to the back porch. "Where are your brothers and sisters?" she asked her youngest son.

"They are at the funeral home. Waiting for us."

Momma had felt dizzy lately and the family was worried about her. Once or twice she had even stumbled and almost fallen. So today Paul guided her down the back stairs.

"Give me your hand," he said.

"Go ahead, I follow you."

She took one step at a time until she reached the driveway. Poppa walked her to the car. He placed his hand along the shiny black trunk. When the chauffeur held the door open Poppa helped her in. She clutched the overhead strap and pulled herself onto the back seat.

Millie sat across from her parents. Her mother's chubby fingers wrapped tightly around her black purse. She rested her head against the velvet seat. Her father's usually rosy cheeks were now gaunt and pale. He looked so fragile.

The funeral home was right in front of them. And Millie struggled with unending queasiness in the pit of her stomach. The limousine stopped. *This is real*, she thought.

Until now she had hoped it would just go away, all the police, the people and especially the sadness. But today, in front of Slocumb's Funeral Home, she knew the ordeal would never end. For the very first time she understood what it meant to share her parent's darkest nightmare.

It had been decided earlier that the family would go in together. Everyone would wait for Momma and Poppa. Millie saw her brothers and sisters in small groups by the front door. They were dressed in black, their faces pale. Most were sobbing, some stoic. But they just stood there, like children poised for a leader. Suzy stood next to her husband, his arm around her waist. Peter came alone from New York that morning. His wife stayed home with the babies. And Tommy stood at the curb, his hands clasped behind his back.

The limousine came to a stop and the driver opened the car door.

Paul helped Momma first. She unconsciously pulled at the back of her dress. Tommy ran over and hugged his mother then grasped her arm. The rest of the family waited by the entrance.

Paul reached for his sister's hand and helped her out of the car. Millie began to walk towards the rest of the siblings but stopped to read the sign that was above the entryway: "This is the doorway to Peace." She gripped Nina's book then followed the rest of the family.

When Momma Giannetti reached the top of the stairs she let go of Tommy's hand and grabbed her husband's. Together, they approached the ornate room that held their daughter.

Flowers were everywhere. The bouquets and arrangements were placed all along the walls, in front of and behind the casket as if to frame it. But for Millie the flowers didn't mask the smell of mothballs or the stench of cigarette smoke.

Nina's coffin was at the far end of the room flanked on either side by candles and a heart-shaped wreath. Domenic stood in front. The young priest had been there all day. "Please," Momma cried. "Don't let her be alone all day."

As his parents approached the white coffin, Domenic moved quickly to help his mother kneel in front of the casket. Millie watched her brother make the Sign of the Cross. Then he said a short prayer and everyone whispered, "Amen."

The old woman looked at her daughter. "Mia bella bambino," she cried. She placed her hand on Nina's porcelain face. "Fa Freda," she said. Momma dropped her head against her arm.

Poppa gently stroked the girl's hair. He looked to his son for solace. The young priest put his arm around his father and then the two men helped Momma to the sofa up against the back wall.

Tommy and his wife were next. Then Peter, and so it went in order until they had all knelt next to their sister's body. Paul and Millie were the last ones to approach. With her gentle features and long black hair her sister looked serene and beautiful as she rested in the folds of a pink satin bed. Millie looked to her brother and he lifted Nina's doll like fingers. And she placed the book under her sister's hand.

Millie moved to her place in line. "Millie, that was a thoughtful thing to do," Domenic whispered. "Nina would like that."

She was the youngest and therefore the last. Millie stood alone. Normally Nina would have been next to her. Now she felt isolated.

The family had just a few moments of silence before the sounds of whispers began in the front hall. Relatives, neighbors and friends drifted through. Poppa moved off his seat. He had prepared himself. He stood between his daughter's coffin and her mother to greet the visitors that came to pay their respects.

Nina's wake lasted two days and two nights and by now the Giannetti family was exhausted. But the parent's devastation and outrage was the fuel that energized them to get through this. Each night after the wake Momma would sit in the dining room and lament about Thanksgiving Day.

"I have that boy in my house. Do you remember?" she asked Millie. "How he stared at your sister. Maybe if I didn't invite him here."

It didn't matter how many times each one of the siblings tried to explain. Momma believed that she was one of the reasons her daughter was killed. One night Domenic pleaded with her. But it made little difference.

"It doesn't matter what anyone says. She's convinced that it's her fault," he told his siblings.

If the tiny Ethnic community of lower Norwich was devastated by the murders, they would be traumatized by the accusation that the killer was one of their own. As people knelt to pray for the young girl, their faces carried a look of confusion and despair.

The newspapers had begun to fill their pages with photographs and distorted versions of the Kerchaks. The small Polish family became the center of what was believed to be justified public opinion. Because Josef was in jail he was spared the terrible verbal and physical contact that surrounded his parents night and day. Rocks thrown at their windows crashed on the floors of the upstairs apartment, leaving the couple terrified and shattered.

Mr. Kerchak changed his job as plant supervisor to night watchman in order to avoid the constant disdain that followed him. Grace Kerchak eventually lost her meager job when a group of young boys tossed eggs at the drug store window where she worked.

As the town became defensive and angry the police presence became more visible, even to the point where the police chief assigned two officers outside Slocumb's Funeral Home.

On the morning they were preparing to bury Nina, the family stood patiently as a stream of mourners arrived at the church in order to say their final prayers for the pretty dark-haired girl.

For the fourth time in less than a year Saint Bartholomew's would be the focal point for tragedy. The sense of loss that united the communities was evident by the blend of people who piled into the mahogany pews.

Both sides of Norwich related to the tragic feelings that filled the church. From Dorothy Miller to the Robertson woman to Stephanie Delahunt and now Nina Giannetti, the diminutive town was stunned by the dramatic events that had unfolded before their eyes.

After the mass, Nina's coffin made its way slowly down the aisle and outside to where Monsignor Harrow gave another blessing before the white casket was lifted and placed in the hearse. Traffic came to a halt when the family's limousine led the procession. It wound its way along the main street and past Prescott Street. When the black car pulled into the cemetery they came to a stop and waited for what seemed like an eternity as relatives, friends and neighbors disembarked from their cars. Finally they were able to make their way to the gravesite virtually hidden to them by the hundreds of people who stood side by side. Along with her brothers and sisters Millie followed her parents who were led through the crowd and then seated next to a large gaping hole where Nina's coffin sat on a metal frame.

"We are burying this child with such pain in our hearts," Monsignor Harrow said. He stood isolated on the tiny knoll. "Her soul is on its way to you, Lord." Then he turned to his young priest. "Domenic, would you lead us in the Lord's prayer?"

He moved away from the family and walked up to the coffin. He placed his hand on the casket. "Our Father," he said, his voice hushed. "Hallowed be thy name."

It was the end of the service and most of the people left. Millie lingered behind and watched her parents, the two old people, shadowed the sun, and followed the paths that fell between the head stones.

Paul turned and waved to her. "I'll be right there," she said.

She wanted this time to be alone with her sister. To kneel down and tell Nina how much she loved her and how sad she felt that she was gone. Millie picked up a small handful of dirt that was to cover her sister's body.

"I know you can hear me, Nina," she whispered. Then she tossed the dirt onto the coffin. "I will always remember you."

On the ground she spotted a tiny basket filled with lovely blossoms. Two pink roses stood out amongst the other flowers. There was a card attached with the words, *I'm sorry*. Millie took the roses out of the container and placed them on Nina's casket.

This was a loss that could never be replaced. And she felt overwhelmed by the sadness. Still she believed that now her parents and the rest of the family would find some closure.

Even though she understood that after her sister's burial she was obligated to begin her life again. It soon became apparent that this would not be an easy task especially for her parents. Millie could still sense her mother's pain. It never went away and one day when the girl walked into the kitchen her mother was standing by the table, her eyes glued to the window.

"Momma, what's wrong?" she asked.

"Poppa should fix that garage door," she said. "It slams all the time. And I look up. I think it is Nina. But it's just the wind." Tears filled her eyes and she fell into a chair.

"Oh, Momma," Millie said. "I am so sorry."

"I keep hoping, Cara Mia, that Nina is gonna walk through the door. But, I know she's never coming home. You know how I know that," she said, her face wet with tears. "Because I still feel the pain of seeing her in the coffin."

CHAPTER TWENTY-TWO

Marty Sacco went to the Norfolk County State Jail on an unrelated matter the very same day Josef Kerchak's mother was there to visit with her son. He had been placed in the minimum-security facility pending trial, scheduled for late September.

The police chief felt sorry for the woman as he watched her walk through the front door. *It can't be easy for her*, he thought. *After all, she barely speaks English and now she has to try and understand the legal system.*

Mrs. Kerchak stopped to speak with a priest who was on his way into the compound. Each week a different community sent a priest to the prison to speak with the men. Marty assumed this was Saint Bart's turn when he saw it was Father Domenic.

When he came through the outer door he could hear some of the conversation, and he slowed down his pace.

"I am trying, Father," Mrs. Kerchak said. "But it is so hard to see Josef like this. Still I know he is innocent and I have faith in God that he will be all right."

Father Giannetti studied the woman's face. "I am glad that you have so much faith," he said. His smile was empathic. "Faith can be very powerful."

How bizarre, Marty thought. *Here is the mother of the accused killer of this man's sister and yet because he's a priest, he is required by God to show her patience and compassion.*

The sound of the buzzer opened the security gate and Marty walked through. Father Giannetti was behind him seemingly preoccupied. He watched the priest remove a small black book from his pocket and then disappear around the corner.

Marty was at the facility to gather some information and to visit with an old friend. "Hey, O'Brien, are you in here?" Marty knocked on the office door.

"Chief, how have you been?" a man said, then crawled out of a closet.

"What are you doing in there?"

"I was looking for an old pair of bowling shoes."

O'Brien wiped his hand on his pants and then offered it to Marty. "It's been years," he said. "You look good. You never change."

"I don't know about that. I certainly feel a hell of a lot older."

"Well," O'Brien said, "I miss those old days. How is that son-of-a bitch, Taylor? How the hell is he doing?"

"He hasn't changed. He's still doing the things he always did. Only today he's even more irritable."

They bantered back and forth for a few more minutes and then O'Brien remarked, "Sounds like you got your hands full with these murders."

"That's why I called you," Marty said. "We have this one small lead. His name is Victor Fubrowski. You know Taylor, he'll dig till he finds something. And he did. But the guy's file was empty. I mean there was an arrest record and then nothing. No explanation of the charges, no indication about whether he was arraigned or not. It looks as if the kid just disappeared." Marty said. He leaned back in the chair.

"That's why I called. I remembered you worked Ethnic Village long before I got there. I thought maybe you could help."

O'Brien was perched on the desk. He grabbed a pack of cigarettes from his desk, then offered one to Marty.

"No, thanks," he said, "quit two years ago. Anyway, I know it's a long shot. But I thought maybe you might know something about this Fubrowski."

"Sure, I remember the little sucker. He was a smart kid. Good looking, popular with the girls. But his father was a drunk and his home life was a living hell. The old man did maintenance work for the church, when he wasn't drunk."

He took a quick drag. And the smoke circled around his mouth.

"But he got himself into some serious shit," O'Brien said. "He had a bad temper and liked to beat up on people. He got involved with the daughter of some big time crook in Providence, Joey Mattressi. He beat the daylight out of her when he found out she was pregnant. The old man went crazy and sent his two boys after him. Just like that," he said with a swipe of his hands. "The kid was gone. Speculation was the Mattressi boys got him. Either way he disappeared."

"So you have no idea if he's dead or alive?" Marty asked.

"Once I heard he joined the Navy," O'Brien said. He shrugged his shoulders. "But I never saw him again. As far as the department was concerned, good riddance."

Marty stood up and pushed the chair back against the desk. "Sounds like the Mattressi boys might have done you a favor," he said. "Well, thanks for the information. And if you remember anything else, give me a call, will you?" the police chief asked.

"Sure," he said. He squashed his cigarette out in the ashtray. "Hey, say hello to Taylor for me."

The heads of the town council had contacted Chief Sacco to schedule a confidential meeting. When they arrived at his office he stood up to greet them. "Gentlemen," he said. "Although I am always happy to be of help to the committee, I'm a bit confused about this private meeting."

"We want to know about the Kerchak kid," Fred Pearson said.

"What about him?"

"We want you to speed up his trial and dispose of this case quickly, so that we can go on with our businesses." He turned and slammed the office door.

"I have no control over the judicial system."

"That's not what we mean," Pearson said. "We want you to convince Shapiro to take the prosecutor's deal. Then there would be no trial and this dirty business would go away in time for the holidays."

Marty glared at Pearson. *What a pugnacious asshole this man is.*

"I can't believe you."

"We want to be sure this kid doesn't get off," Murphy said. "Just in case your evidence isn't strong enough."

"It's not like the Kerchak kid isn't guilty," Pearson continued. "I mean we all know the kid is strange. I saw it myself one day when he came into my store with his father. The old man handed the boy a can of nails but the kid reached too late and they fell on the floor. He smacked the boy on the side of the head and berated him for five minutes. You know what I mean. The kid is crazy."

The chief was dumbfounded by Pearson's remarks. He walked over to the door and opened it. "What the hell are you thinking about?" he said. "If you leave within the next two seconds I'll think your being here was just a bad dream. Otherwise I swear I'll find something to book you on."

"For Christ sake, Sacco, why do you continue to stand on legal bullshit with this case?" Pearson yelled.

"It's not bullshit, Fred, it's precedent and the reason I follow the rules is so even scum like you can be protected. Now get the hell out of my office!" He slammed the door. Marty turned his back to the door and leaned against it. "What a bunch of assholes."

CHAPTER TWENTY-THREE

Nina's death changed the simple existence of Millie's life on Prescott Street. Although she was still too young to leave home she never felt comfortable in that house again.

"Why you always running away from here?" Momma asked her one day.

"I just want to keep busy," the girl said.

Her sister's bed stood untouched. The stuffed animals were in the exact same position Nina had left them before her death. Her desk developed layers of dust from neglect. Millie felt guilty for so many things and not touching her sister's possessions was one of them.

The truth is she would do anything to stay away. She visited her older siblings. Millie would baby-sit after school, nights, and on the weekends. She volunteered to wash her sister's windows, floors, anything to keep her away from the house.

Her brothers and sisters didn't care. It was a needed bit of freedom for them. But for Millie it was self-preservation. The longer she stayed away the easier it became for her to forget that night.

And now life was different. The house was not just quiet. It was silent. Fewer and fewer conversations took place. Other than, "Pass me that plate." There was barely a word spoken at mealtimes. And the usual, albeit obnoxious, bantering that one time took place with Paul had completely vanished. He was no longer around and if he did come home he usually ate in his room.

Momma and Poppa had truly isolated themselves from the world. Every day was the same. After dinner Poppa would go to the living room and sit alone on the couch to watch television. Momma would go to her room. Millie would be left alone to contemplate her fate.

Even the Friday night get-together with the aunts and uncles stopped. When and if someone came to visit, Momma would sit in the kitchen and weep over her daughter's death. Millie's home had become little more than a structure, a place to sleep. It no longer felt comfortable. When Nina died the life and the parents Millie knew ceased to exist.

It was the realization that she would no longer have her old life that prompted her to have the courage to leave Norwich and go somewhere far away to college. Her hope was that school would not only remove her from the house but that it would take her away from the past.

But there is a part of the past that she never wanted to forget. Years later she would still remember the walks along the railroad tracks. Her youth may have vanished but the murmurs of a young girl's laughter and silly secrets did not.

Today that field is cluttered by trash scattered along the pilings. But Millie can still feel the spirit of innocence as it blows through the tall weeds.

Before the tragedy she lived a passive, easy existence with little reason to complain. It was not in her make-up to cause an argument or debate a fact. Simply put she didn't want anyone to dislike her. And disagreements caused problems.

As contradictory as it might sound that was what Millie admired about her sister the most. Nina was different than the rest. She had this ability not to care about other people's perceptions of her.

It was her opinion of self that counted. One time Millie went to her sister for advice about a friend, "Celia, lied to her mother," she said. "And she wants me to go along with that. If I don't, she won't be my friend anymore."

"Who cares?" Nina said, then quoted something about being true to one's self.

"What does that mean?" Millie asked.

Nina shook her head. "Never mind," she said. "You do what you think is right for you. Not Celia."

She didn't lie and it was Millie who put a stop to her friendship with Celia. All she ever wanted was to be just like her sister Nina. She began to realize that Norwich was not where she wanted to be. Sometimes she went to extremes and pleaded with her parents to sell the house and move.

"It's our home," Momma said. "You don't move away from your home not with all the memories that still live here, no matter what they are." And so they stayed.

But the rest of the family tried desperately to move on. They needed to put their lives back together. In the hopes that they could forget the trauma of the past.

It was six months after Nina's death that Millie learned about the devastation that had so enveloped her sister. Momma asked her to do a favor.

"Just take you're sister's clothes and put them in the boxes."

Later that afternoon Momma walked into the bedroom. "I came to see if maybe I could help you," she said. Her mother opened the top drawer of Nina's bureau, and pulled out a favorite sweater. It was pink with pearl buttons and it had a soft Angora collar.

"I remember this," Momma said with a smile. "Susie buy this for her last Christmas." She sat for a few minutes and fingered the fur. "I'm sorry," she said. "I can't do this." Momma placed the sweater on the bed and left. That's when Millie realized that was all she had left, her sister's clothes and the memories.

CHAPTER TWENTY-FOUR

Marty walked into the station house and pulled a folder from a metal file that sat behind his desk. He flung his jacket over a chair and yelled to Taylor, "Hey Jim, pour a cup for me, will you?"

He loosened his tie and opened the file cover. There were the usual glossy eight by tens from each case. The pictures were clipped to the folder and he glanced through them quickly.

There was so much blood, he thought, *I have never seen anything like that except for in war.*

Then he put them back in a pile and began to examine each individual photo. When he was finished he took the image and placed it separately on his desk. He was searching for something, anything that would give him a clue.

Paula Roache was the name on the written report. She was a pretty, twenty-six-year-old brunette with brown eyes, married for less than three years when her husband was killed in a car accident. "Jesus," Marty said to Jim when he handed him the coffee. "The poor man went over a bridge that was closed."

"You're reading the accident report for the Roache kid, right?" Taylor asked.

"Yeah, how does that happen?"

"Easy," Jim said. "The state was working on the road and never put up a signal to warn drivers."

"Well, it says here that it was late at night when Timothy Roach's car drove over the non-existent section.

"It was a bad night," Jim said. "Between the rain and the fog. He skidded and his car spun out of control."

"It also says his widow sued the state for wrongful death and by the look of things they were close to a settlement," Marty noted.

"She lost her parents a few years earlier too."

"What about her state of mind?" Jim said. "Think she went over the edge and just left?"

"A bit too dramatic," Marty said. "She led a relatively low-key social life. Was a teacher at the elementary school, volunteered at the church and did charity work for the hospital."

"She's the perfect victim," Jim said. He walked toward the door. "No husband, no family and no body." He quickly swallowed a gulp of coffee and placed the cup on the desk. "I'll catch up with you later," he said and left.

Marty continued his inspection of the photographs. One, then another in between sips of coffee. He pulled a magnifying glass out of his top drawer and moved it across each of the photos. This time he placed the glass over the pile of clothes.

"There they are," he said. "Right next to the kitchen door."

But then he noticed something odd. There was no organization to them. They weren't neatly tucked and folded. Not as they were for the last four victims. This guy had made a point of his victim's clothes being in a neat pile. But Paula Roache's things were just tossed in a pile. *What does that mean? This guy all of a sudden found neatness?* "How does that happen," he said aloud.

Marty buzzed his phone for the desk clerk. "Doherty, come here, will you?"

"Yeah, Chief."

"How long does it take the lab to blow up a picture?"

"A day or two."

"Here," Marty said, then handed him a glossy. "I want you to go through the files of the four women murdered and pull any photographs of the clothing. Then I want them blown up two sizes larger and back on my desk ASAP. Tell that to the lab boys." He grabbed his jacket off the chair and swung it over his back. "I'm on my way over to see Leo Shapiro. If Taylor calls tell him to meet me there."

It was the first time since these murders began a year ago that he felt there was one tiny connection. At this moment the chief would have clung to any possibility.

Shapiro wasn't his favorite man but he was wise, organized and an observant son of a bitch. He had also been the attorney for Paula Roache's lawsuit against the state. Maybe he could recall something about the night of her disappearance.

On his way over to the attorney's office he remembered that night in April and what the two detectives had found when they arrived at the Roache home.

It was early evening when he received a hysterical call at the station. "Please! Something has happened to my friend," a woman said.

"Calm down lady, what's your name?"

"Sally, Sally Fresno. Please hurry."

"Is your friend hurt?"

"I don't know."

"Where are you?"

"I'm in her hallway where the phone is and all I can see is blood."

By now the woman was frantic. "I want you to get out of that house immediately but first tell me the address."

"It's 115 Bay Road. Won't you please come now?"

"We are on our way. Miss Fresno, go outside and wait there."

The two detectives dashed across town and arrived at the house in minutes. A young woman was in front of the house. She looked terrified and paced up and down on the sidewalk.

"Thank God," she said. "Something's happened and I can't find my friend."

"I'm Detective Sacco." He took the woman by the elbow and placed her in the back seat of the police car.

"I was supposed to meet Paula. Then we were to walk down to Saint Bartholomew's to volunteer for the church fair next month. When I arrived the front door was opened. So I just walked in."

"I want you to sit right here." Then he radioed for an officer.

She nodded and slid across the seat. "I called Paula but she didn't answer me. Then I walked into the foyer. That's when I saw the blood. The phone was right there so I called the police."

"I don't care what you hear. Stay here till the officer comes." Marty told her. Then he and Taylor approached the open front door. Jim unholstered his gun. The front hall was dark with only a shadow of light visible from the end of the long hallway.

A small phone table marked the entrance to the living room. Jim hugged the wall with his back and disappeared up the steps. Marty took the first floor.

"It's empty up here," Jim said.

"Here too." Marty placed his gun back in the holster and looked for a light switch. A large black stain was visible on the living room rug. Jim saw a lamp, took out his hanky and switched it on.

"Jesus, that's a lot of blood," Jim said. He bent down and rubbed it between his fingers.

"The kitchen is a holy mess," Marty said. He led Jim through the door.

Taylor looked around at the toppled chairs and broken dishes. "Well, there's no doubt there was a struggle." He knelt down by some clothes and a pool of blood. "Look at this," Jim said. He lifted the edge of a pair of woman's underpants.

Marty spotted the cellar door was partially opened. He signaled to Jim and both men drew their guns. Marty crept down the stairs. His back hugged the cement foundation. He thought he heard a noise from the corner. But it was just the sounds of air blowing in from outside.

"There's nothing down here," he yelled to Taylor. "Just a dirt floor." But there was no sign of a fresh grave. Or even a footprint. Still he knew the lab boys would dig it all up.

They never found anything credible. With all that blood in the house they never found a drop outside. The criminologists dug up the yard and the cellar. Neither Paula Roache nor a body, a murder weapon or a suspect was ever linked to that case.

From time to time Marty did think about it but without a body they didn't have a crime. But if there was a connection it seemed odd that the killer would have stopped with the Roache woman. And even more bizarre was Josef Kerchak, if he did kill these women. Then who was responsible for Paula Roache?

Still what was really troublesome was the fact that somebody was out there. Lurking around the streets of Norwich.

Shapiro's office was on the other side of town in a newly constructed brick and wood building. The land and the original dwelling had at one time been owned by the Archdiocese. It was used as a host center when Saint Bartholomew's and the other area churches invited visiting priests.

But a while back the Catholic Church gave Saint Bartholomew's permission to build a Children's Center and rectory. Still they had to provide some of the funds through various donations. The Monsignor was able to raise money from cake sales, raffles, and car washes. But the rest of the funding came from the sale of the property that Shapiro now owned.

He went up against the whole community at the time. They wanted no part of Shapiro's plans for the proposed building. Leo stood his ground. And the town counsel, namely Fred Pearson, threatened to tie up the property for years. Eventually his request was granted.

Lately, however, the community had become greedier and when Shapiro went in front of the committee to request an addition for the site, things had changed. Now the town was hungry for the tax monies and revenues that any new business could gather. So Shapiro was quickly granted permission to reconstruct. And by the visibility of the engineering tags the excavation would take place soon.

Marty looked through the plate glass window of Shapiro's office and caught the eye of the attorney.

"Hey, what are you doing in the productive area of the damned?" he said with a grin.

"Expanding," Marty asked.

"Yeah. What can I do for you?"

"I need to talk to you about a case."

"Is this about Kerchak?"

"No. You were Paula Roache's attorney?"

"Yes," he said. "That was a litigation suit against the state. We won the case too." He shook his head. "But when she disappeared the Commonwealth tried to locate a family member. They came up empty. So Massachusetts kept the money."

"I was one of the detectives assigned to her case when she disappeared," Marty said. "I just took a shot and thought maybe you might remember something about the case."

"They found my name in her address book. And they called me. I'll tell you what I told the officer back then. She was a nice kid that became a young widow because of a stupid mistake some state workers made after having a few drinks at lunch. Paula had a hard time with her husband's death," he said. "When she came to me with her story I was eager to take her case. I knew it was a winner. I also had an ace in the hole that only five people knew. Something that was going to net her big money and me a great fee."

"What was that?"

"Paula Roache was pregnant at the time of the accident. But when her husband died she had a miscarriage. So the state was responsible for two deaths."

Marty shook his head. "That's too bad."

"I only knew her as a client and what I can tell you is public record. She was a pretty girl, a teacher and she was involved with a few church charities. She was still in love with her husband and other than her students and her girlfriends, there was nobody else in her life."

"After her disappearance you never heard or received anything from her?"

"No. What the hell is this? It's a dead issue. The woman's been gone for over ten years," Shapiro said.

"I don't know. In your opinion, Leo," Marty asked, "was she rational? I mean, would she fake her own disappearance?"

"Not in my mind," he said. "She was determined to go forward with this case. Paula wanted the state to pay for the loss of her family."

He stood up and moved from behind the desk.

"Thanks," Marty said.

Twenty-four hours after he had asked the clerk for the enlarged photographs, they were placed on the chief's desk. He ripped open the large manilla envelope on his way to the strategy room. He took each of the glossy prints and clipped them to the blackboard at the front of the room.

Marty backed away in order to scan the photos. Each one was of the pile of clothes found near the bodies. Every piece of garment was folded and neatly placed. But Paula Roache's blouse was rolled in a ball and tossed.

"Doherty said you wanted to see me," Jim said when he wandered in.

"Yeah, come here and look at these pictures."

He walked over to the blackboard and slowly studied each print. "I don't know," he said. "What have I missed?"

"Look at the way the clothes are folded."

Again the detective made his way along the edge of the blackboard. Jim moved close to the pictures. He ran his fingers along the photograph. "There's a difference in this photograph," he said. "The clothes aren't folded. It looks like the killer might have been in a hurry."

"You're right," Marty said. "But maybe he wasn't in a hurry."

"What do you mean?"

"Look, the psychiatrist said that the suspect places the clothes next to the body to give the victim a little bit of dignity. But maybe he just left the clothes in a heap because he wasn't leaving a body."

"Okay, then why leave them anyway?"

"I don't know. Maybe he left them in a pile because that was the way he did things then. What do you think about this theory? He was taught to fold clothes because he was either in the military or prison."

"You mean he developed a neat fettish," Jim said while he pulled a cigarette out of his pocket.

"I'm saying the killer committed the first crime as a young man. And then he went away or did time. But when he came back he started over again. Only this time he was older and he had been taught a few things. Maybe now he pays more attention to detail."

"So he commits his first murder as a kid." Jim paused, lit his cigarette then continued. "But he stops for awhile and then later carries through with what he started."

"Let's say at a young age after he murders the Roache woman he gets arrested for something else," Marty said. "Maybe he joined the Navy or had to leave the state. Anyway when he comes back he comes back with a vengeance."

"Maybe I'm crazy but both assumptions sound reasonable," Jim said.

"Then that is what we need to look for," Marty said. "I want you to find out within a fifty mile radius who spent the last ten years in prison, or the military. Who was released before August of last year and who has a history of hating or assaulting women. And keep working on this Fubrowski, Fiske guy, will you?"

"You really believe that Kerchak kid is innocent," Jim remarked.

Marty pulled the pictures from the board. "I just don't see him killing these women. If we found his old man's body now that would be a different story."

"You got a point."

Jim had been able to gather most of the information by the next day.

"We're looking at three men from the area that were convicted for either rape or assault during the last ten years," he said. "One is dead and another is back in Walpole State Prison and the other one is some reformed do-gooder who at one time lived about twenty miles from Norwich."

"A reformed do-gooder."

"Yeah. He works with prisoners while in jail and then when they come out, he helps them find jobs. You know the shmeel," he joked. "Anyway, I did a thorough background check and I don't think he's our man."

"Okay," Marty asked. "Why not?"

"Although the guy has an assault record as long as your arm, he doesn't have any complaints from women. To be honest with you, the guys he beat up had records longer than his. And it's his age, right now I think he's over fifty."

"Did you see this guy or talk to him?"

"I talked to him for a few minutes. He was all bent out of shape about one of his trustees. Anyway, I can have one of our guys tail him for a few days. But my gut tells me it's not him."

"You're probably right," Marty muttered. "But humor me. Keep an eye on him."

"Something came in on this Fubrowski lead," Jim said. "He did two stints in the Navy as a cook. What I have to do now is get Fiske's fingerprints off to the FBI so they can do a match. But I don't want to scare him off."

The theory about a return killer had a lot of merit. Somebody like this Fubrowski would have grown up here and would know the town inside and out.

He would know all about the back roads and the overgrown trails that lead from the deserted railroad tracks to the lower end of town. He would know how to get from Ethnic Village to the square and even into the newer neighborhoods without being seen.

The town of Norwich had about 50,000 square miles and twenty thousand of it was yet to be developed. A great area to hide in. Marty reached in his desk and pulled out a map. Norwich looked something like an odd-shaped rectangle, with a few upscale neighborhoods, the business community and the common off to the upper left side. Ethnic Village stood out on the lower section of the map.

Before the turn of the century, the town was centrally located between Boston and Western Massachusetts. It was the perfect spot for a new train station, which over the years expanded and stretched to eventually serve many other communities as well as Norwich. The consequence was the easy accessibility from many different neighborhoods.

Anyone who grew up in that area knew the deserted track like the back of his hand. Marty's fingers traced across the paper. He created a route from all ends of town. *It doesn't matter which end of Norwich you start from. If you cut through the deserted railroad station you'll find your way home.*

CHAPTER TWENTY-FIVE

In the following days, with the ruthless young killer safely behind bars, the town settled into a sense of complacency. The village began to settle back into a normal existence. And the quiet security that had once surrounded the people began again.

But the police as well and the townspeople were no longer naive. They had become aware that the veil of safety had been torn. And their life as they once lived it had now become a little more precarious.

The police chief was not grateful for the temporary peace of mind that had spread across Norwich. He knew if the residents felt safer they would tend to become careless about their security; besides, the detective knew something that the town didn't know. And that was that the young boy sitting in the cell at the Norfolk jail was just a ruse. Josef was no angel, that was for sure. Still murder was a whole other game and Marty just didn't see this kid as one of its players.

"Chief, it's for you," the desk clerk told Marty. He had just walked into the station house. "Take a message," he said, then asked. "Wait. Who is it?"

"That attorney, Shapiro."

"I'll take it in my office," he said. Marty acknowledged Jim before he picked up the phone.

"Leo, what can I do for you?"

"There's something I want you to see. Can you come to my office right away?"

"What's wrong?" he asked.

"Just get over here, and you can see for yourself."

"Hey Jim," Marty yelled, "c'mon, we're going for a ride."

Detective Taylor screeched the wheels of the car against the curb in front of Shapiro's office building. When the two men stepped out of the car, Marty noticed the large excavation shovel frozen in place. They found the attorney, Dennis Black, the town engineer, and Sam Chanowsky, the owner of "The Below Ground Excavating Company" clustered around a big hole.

"What's going on?" Marty asked.

Shapiro's eyes gazed downward in the direction of the hole.

"Holy shit," Detective Taylor said. "That looks like a human skull."

Twenty minutes later Dr. Curran and two of his associates were right in the middle of the pit. "It's human all right," he confirmed. "And this is just an educated guess but I think it's a female." He held the remains in his hands. "And by the looks of the creases in the skull I would say that this person, whoever it was, was killed by a blunt force to the head."

"Can you give me any time frame?" the chief asked.

"My guess is no earlier than five years ago and maybe closer to ten. I can give you a better idea after the autopsy."

The police chief with Taylor directly behind headed for the car. The detective jumped into the front seat and put the key in the ignition.

"Do you remember who owned this land before Shapiro?" Marty asked.

"Didn't the church have something to do with it?"

"Yep, the Archdiocese. After it was sold the bishop gave the money to the old pastor, Monsignor Donovan, to do some renovations on the rectory."

Jim banged his hands on the steering wheel. "I remember that," he said. "They added a few rooms. What? About ten years ago."

"Yeah," Marty said.

"Well, what do you think?"

"The place was empty most of the time. Always dark."

"Kind of like open season," Jim said. "That is for anyone who wanted to hide a body. And Victor Fubrowski's father did maintenance for the church."

The chief was thrilled at the discovery. He knew that if the remains turned out to be the gravesite of Paula Roache, his theory would have a life. He also realized it would be the strongest evidence they had to eliminate the Kerchak boy. This could be the link they needed.

Marty decided to call Shapiro. He wanted to set up a meeting with the kid.

"Why?"

"Listen, Leo," Marty argued. "I just want to talk to him. Besides, you'll be there if you feel he needs any protection.

"Okay," he said. "Meet me there around three."

The afternoon turned out to be cold and soggy. The chief put his collar up and ran from the car into the atrium that surrounded the jail. Once the guard buzzed him in. He walked along the drafty outer chamber and waited to be buzzed again into a small anteroom. There he saw Shapiro in the hallway.

They were led into a room with nothing but a few chairs and metal table that was bolted to the floor.

"What am I doing here?"

"I need a few questions answered," Marty said.

Josef entered the room. The door clicked shut behind him. He was thinner than Marty remembered. His head was shaved and he looked haggard.

"Hello, Mr. Shapiro," the boy said.

"Hi kid. Do you remember Chief Sacco?"

The young boy gazed at Marty with cold, disinterested eyes. A tired smile slid across his lips. "Hello, sir," he said.

"I know you told us everything about the night of Nina's death. But I thought maybe you might have had time to remember something new, anything," Marty said.

The young boy turned to his attorney. "Mr. Shapiro," he said. "Can I ask you something?" Shapiro moved closer to his client. He bent down and bowed his head. Josef whispered something in the lawyer's ear. The attorney nodded and after a few minutes told the boy to "Go ahead."

"What is it?" Marty asked.

"I knew Nina was in trouble," he said.

"You saw her murderer."

"No, I mean I knew that she was being forced," the boy said. "She was being forced to have sex," Josef blurted out.

"Start from the beginning," Marty said.

Josef looked ashamed. He lowered his head for a minute then he said, "Everything you said was true. I did follow her. I watched her all the time. It's all true," he said. "I couldn't help it. I really liked her and I wanted to be with her. But Nina wouldn't go out with me. I was jealous. I admit it. I acted like a jerk."

He gazed down at the floor. "It was the week before she died when I approached her. She was alone. I could tell she was crying. I walked over to her. She was on the wall near the old railroad tracks. I decided I was gonna tell her I was sorry about the way I had acted. When I got closer she became frightened and backed away."

"Why was she afraid of you?" Marty asked.

"It wasn't me she was afraid of." Josef began to cry.

"Are you okay?" Shapiro asked the boy.

"Could I have a glass of water?"

Marty reached past his briefcase and picked up the plastic pitcher and poured some water into a paper cup. "Here." He waited for the boy to drink a few mouthfuls then he said, "Please go on."

"I asked her what was wrong. I told her I wanted to help. That's when she told me. She said she was afraid. Because someone wouldn't leave her alone, she said he forced her to do all kinds of awful things and now she was gonna tell on him."

"Wait a minute, Josef. Why would a girl that admitted she doesn't like you tell you something so horrible she couldn't even tell her own family."

"That's just it," Josef said. "She was too ashamed."

Nina acted desperate that day. Like she didn't know what to do. I don't understand why she told me. Maybe she knew I did really want to help."

"And the day you grabbed her by the arm did you want to help her that day too?"

"It wasn't like that," Josef said. "You have it all wrong. The next day when I saw her on the corner I went over to her just to talk. She saw me and ran away. I caught up with her and took hold of her arm. I told her that if she told me who the person was I would tell him to leave her alone. Nina began to scream at me. She acted as if I was crazy. 'Get away from me,' she said."

"What did you say to her?"

"That I just wanted to help her, to be her friend. Then Nina said, 'Everything I told you yesterday was a joke. It was all a joke on you,' and she laughed. That's when I grabbed her arm."

"Did you believe it was all a joke?"

"No. I don't think so. I mean she was so upset. Crying and everything, I really believed her."

"There is one more thing," Shapiro said.

"Yeah. What is that?"

"How important is my client's information?"

"I don't know yet, why?"

"We want something."

"I figured."

"Go ahead, kid," the lawyer said.

"It was me," the boy admitted, "I was the one that chased the girls and put bags over their heads. But I swear that was all. I never meant to hurt anyone."

It was obvious the kid was telling the truth. And what he said so far seemed to fit. "Tell me, Josef. What made you stop?"

"It was about 7:30 and I was hanging around Depot Street for a girl to walk by, when I noticed this man toss his cigarette. After awhile when I looked up he was still there, under the street light. I couldn't see who he was but he creeped me out. Anyway, I figured he was a cop, so I started to leave. Then I saw him reach up and unscrew the light. The corner went black."

"And you didn't see anyone else?" Marty asked.

The boy shook his head.

"No, but I saw the same man later. I was on the front porch, hidden by the big bushes. It was so dark and he moved so fast. He couldn't have seen me."

"You're sure it was the same man?"

"It was him. I know it was him," Josef said.

"Did you see where he went?"

"The railroad tracks."

"Is there anything else?" Marty asked. He grabbed the handle on his briefcase.

"That's all I know. I swear, Chief Sacco."

"Thank you, Josef. I'll be in touch," he told Shapiro.

Marty walked into the courtyard of the prison. The rain may have ended but it was still cold and damp. He rushed into the car and headed for the station house.

"All the paperwork is back," Doherty told the chief when he walked past the reception desk.

"What paperwork?"

"The coroner's. You do recall the body they dug up at the lawyer's office a few weeks ago?"

"Is it on my desk?"

"I gave it to Detective Taylor."

"Is that Curran's report?" Marty asked.

"Yeah, it's Paula Roache all right," he said waving the file. "Its all in the ME's report." He handed it to the chief. Marty took it studied it and then tossed it on his desk.

He walked over to the window and stared out at the park. "I love this place," he said. It didn't matter how dreary the town looked. Or how big a pain in the ass some of the town members could be. He truly loved it there. He watched a young couple stroll along the park. He saw two old ladies stop to converse. He saw the sun move behind the clouds.

"I saw the Kerchak boy today. He told me some new things. Oh and by the way, Jim," he said, "your hunch was right. The kid was the one that bagged the young girls."

"You weren't surprised, were you, Chief?"

"Josef also told me about this guy who stood under the street light and watched him. He thought the man was a cop. Later he saw the same man head towards the railroad tracks."

"What made the kid think the guy was a cop?"

"Because the kid thought he was being watched. He also said the guy unscrewed the streetlight. That's when Josef went home."

Taylor gulped a sip of coffee. "So he never saw his face."

"You think this guy killed Miller and our boy saw him run away towards the tracks."

"Could be," Jim said. "We still aren't much further ahead."

"Yes, we are," Marty said. His attention diverted towards the window. Darkness had crept over the town. "I haven't told you the rest of our conversation. Josef told me that Nina hinted about being sexually molested."

"Hinted?" Taylor asked. "What did he mean, she hinted?"

"She told him that somebody had forced her to do things."

"And you think that's the connection to her murder?"

"I don't know, maybe."

"That could be a stretch. I mean you know that most molestation is domestic," Jim said. "It usually ends up being some dirty family secret nobody wants known. Which is the reason we hardly ever convict anyone of it."

"You're right," Marty agreed. "Then why was it a secret? Nina told Josef she didn't want to tell her family. She was ashamed and didn't want them to know."

CHAPTER TWENTY-SIX

Millie was only fifteen when she found Nina's journals, but she was old enough to know that they opened a door that should have remained closed. The realization that her sister was sexually abused focused itself on the mainstream of her existence. As if Nina's death hadn't caused enough inner turmoil, the fact that she had endured constant molestation left Millie with emotional guilt and heartache. If what her sister had written was true, then her home as she remembered it was little more than a lie.

Her mind didn't want to think that it could have been any one of her brothers or worse yet, Poppa. *No!* Her heart would cry out with rejection.

She reread each and every page dozens of times caught up in the turmoil that Nina must have endured. Millie heard the heavy breathing of the molester. She felt the hot sweaty breath on her face, his hands groping over her body.

Uncle Ed, she thought as she remembered the way he used to gawk at them each time one changed a bra size. *But molestation*! And why, why wouldn't Nina tell Momma? That was the question that haunted her. What would have possessed her sister to keep this terrible secret quiet for so long?

In fact Millie would later learn through her own need for answers that it was quite normal to hide sexual molestation. It was while trying to deal with her own abusive relationship that she realized what it must have been like for her sister. The constant struggle to please. The moral confusion, and the secret shame that she carried with her. Millie hid herself in many ways, first promiscuity and then academically. In Nina's case she ran away to a world full of literary fantasies that kept her confined and secure.

Still the real question that continued to nag at Millie was if the sexual molestation could have had something to do with her sister's death.

Yet she wasn't comfortable enough to share those personal thoughts and words with the detectives. To bring in the police felt so intrusive. But she needed to speak with someone she could trust. And who would feel much the same way she did about having Nina's best interest at heart.

"Hello. This is Father Giannetti."

"Domenic, its Millie."

"Millie, is everything all right?" he said, surprised.

"Yes. Could I come in to see you today?"

"Sure, I'll be here all day."

"I have to do some errands for Momma. But I should be able to be there sometime in the afternoon."

"Okay, I'll see you then."

She arrived at the rectory and Mrs. Carr, the housekeeper, escorted her to Domenic's office. "Father Dom," she said when she tapped on his door. "Your sister is here."

"Hi Millie," he said, while still seated at his desk. There was a pile of papers in front of him. "Come in." He shoved the files to one side and moved away from his desk. "I'm sorry, I have just been so busy with all these reports for the parish."

Millie had never been to her brother's office. And she had only seen him in his collar at Mass. Most of the time he dressed like the rest of her brothers. "I didn't think you had your own office," she said.

"Does it intimidate you?" he asked.

"A little."

"We can go somewhere else to talk if you would like."

"Oh no," she said. "This is fine."

"What can I do for you," he said. "Did something happen to upset you today?"

"It's Nina."

Domenic looked solemn. "Are you still concerned about Momma?"

"No. Well, yes. But that's not why I'm here," she said. "You see a few days ago Momma asked me to clean out Nina's closet and drawers. She is gonna donate them to the church. That's when I found these."

Millie reached into the paper bag and pulled out the books. "I wish I hadn't read them. But I did. Now I don't know what to do about it."

Domenic with a confused look on his face took the books from his sister.

"I've placed markers in a few spots for you to look at," she said.

It was obvious to Millie that her brother was shocked, hurt and embarrassed by the page he read. Domenic closed the book and remained silent.

"Are they all like this?"

She nodded. "Do we have to tell the police?" Millie asked.

"I just don't want Momma and Poppa to find out. I think they have been through enough."

"I agree."

"I don't know how helpful these could be to the police. After all, how could there be any connection?"

"All I think about is how terrible it must have been for her."

Domenic leaned against the front of his desk. "It would be better if you thought about Nina at peace. Because she is," he said. "It is not going to do you any good to remember her in such pain. But I do understand how you feel," he said. He sat down in the seat next to his sister. "There is nothing we can do accept pray for ourselves."

"I know," she said. Tears fell from her eyes. "I think about her all the time," Millie said.

"I know. I do too."

She wiped her face. "I have to go. Momma will be upset if I'm late."

"Are you sure you're okay?"

"Thanks Domenic," Millie said. "I do feel better."

"I am sorry you had to find these," he said. He placed the journals back in the bag and put them in a drawer. "I know Nina wouldn't have wanted that."

There was a light tap at the door. Mrs. Carr called to Domenic. "Father, you have a phone call,"

"I'll only be another minute," he said.

"Whatever you are feel is okay," he told his sister. "I know you are confused and hurt. But try to understand that Nina is happy now. No matter what has happened it is over."

"I know you're right," Millie said. She kissed her brother on the cheek, and waved on her way out the door.

Millie walked out of the rectory and turned just in time to see the huge oak door slam shut. The girl stepped quickly along the stone walk. Her shadow moved against the cement. She turned and looked upward where the steeple loomed. Millie eye's focused across the street to the entrance of the cemetery. Nina was buried there among the plants and blossomed flowers.

"I'm sorry," she whispered.

Millie's parents still grief stricken, settled into a routine of daily visits to Nina's grave, speechless mealtimes and a mother's nightly sorrow behind closed doors. Paul was rarely home. Instead he worked days and took night classes in order become an electrical engineer. The result was a repetition of silence and boredom for Millie.

Domenic made the attempt to come once a week for dinner and it was obvious that it pleased her parents. Momma and Poppa made an effort to be more sociable on those nights. Momma would take care to prepare either pasta or a roast chicken and after dinner both parents would spend a few minutes at some lighthearted banter.

"You do the Mass this week?" Poppa asked.

"Yes. Momma, why don't you come to church with Poppa this Sunday and hear my homily?"

"Why you want the building should fall down," she joked. It was the first time she had laughed in weeks.

But that was all there was. After that they would both go back to their own method of grief. Despite his parents' obvious decline, Domenic made the visits. For Millie it was a break from an otherwise lonely dinner. Most of the time they would sit and chat about nothing. Still she enjoyed and was grateful for all the conversation.

"What you have been up to lately?"

"Nothing, just bored," she said.

"No boyfriends?"

"How can I have any boyfriends. I'm not allowed to date."

"Where is Paul?" he asked. "I never see him anymore."

"He has school tonight."

"It must be pretty lonely here for you."

"It's okay during the week while I'm in school," Millie said. "I'm so busy and my friends help a little. It's the weekends that are the worst. Momma doesn't want me out of her sight."

"Maybe if I talk to them, it might help. I remember what it felt like stuck in my room all the time."

"That's different, you wanted to study."

"It doesn't matter. There were times when I felt bored and confined."

"It was so noisy back then. Everybody was always here. You all lived at home then."

"That's true," he said with a smile. "It was certainly chaotic."

Millie's elbows rested on the table. Her head was placed in her hands.

"Why did you decide to become a priest?" she asked.

"It had a lot to do with Poppa," Domenic said. "Every Sunday I would watch him at church. He was so committed to Mass and God. I wanted to understand who it was that deserved that kind of admiration, so I studied the competition." Domenic poured a bit of brandy in his glass and swirled it around. "As I began to strengthen my faith, I too felt a deep devotion and that is what pushed me to devote myself to God. But as with anything," he said, "there are periods of restlessness and even a sense of being disconnected from the outside world."

"Are you glad you became a priest?"

"I am," he said. He checked his watch. "But, I need to go, otherwise Monsignor Harrow will begin to worry. You see, I too must check in all the time."

Before he left Millie asked him about the diaries.

"I've decided not to give Nina's journal to the police."

"I'm glad I don't think Nina would want us to do that," she said.

Millie waved goodnight to her brother and watched him head down the back stairs from the kitchen doorway. When he reached the bottom step he paused to look over at the tiny shed. Then continued on. It was something Millie had done so often.

Nothing was the same anymore, not even the upstairs porch. Her mother didn't care about the tulips and crocuses that used to hang over the railings. Now she planted flowers in the cemetery. Once in a while she would go with them to kneel at Nina's grave and say a prayer or two. But Millie wouldn't stay. Most times she would leave her parents there and walk home.

One day after spending two hours at Nina's grave she decided to walk home. Just as she reached the top of the porch she heard someone call to her. She turned quickly and saw two men below.

"Can I help you?" she asked.

"Millie, do you remember me?" the police chief asked.

"Yes. But my mother and father aren't home right now."

"We actually wanted to speak to you. But we can wait until your parents are here if you would feel more comfortable."

Paul was in the doorway of the kitchen and he saw his sister and heard the conversation. He ran to the railing.

"What do you want?"

"We would like to talk to your sister and to you."

"Does that mean you haven't found my sister's killer?"

Marty chose to ignore his remark. "I don't know if you remember us, Paul. I'm Chief Sacco and this is Detective Taylor."

"I know who you are."

"I don't like this long distance conversation. Can we come up and speak with you?"

The two men walked up the stairs and entered the porch. "We won't keep you long," Detective Taylor said. "We just need for you to clear up a few rumors we heard while doing some investigating. We would like to separate the facts from the gossip."

"What kind of gossip?" Paul asked.

Millie was by the porch door. She stood with her arms folded across her chest.

"We've received some information recently and I need to verify if it is true."

"About Nina?" Millie asked. "What kind of information?"

"Did your sister." He looked over at the young girl. "There is no easy way to say this," he said. "Did Nina ever mention anything about being sexually molested?"

Millie walked to the table and sat down. She placed her hands over her face and began to cry. She nodded her head.

"What are you saying?" her brother asked.

He turned and looked at the two detectives. "Who told you that?"

"So you don't know anything about this?" Detective Taylor asked.

"Millie, what are they talking about?"

She turned to her brother. The color had drained out of his face. He looked confused and hurt. *Domenic told me he wouldn't give the journals to the police.*

"It's true," Millie said. "I read her diaries."

"What do you mean it's true? What diaries?"

"I don't understand?" Paul cried. "What are you talking about?"

"I came across Nina's diaries while I sorted her clothes to give to the church. That's when I read them."

"Read what?"

"Nina had a diary and she wrote about how someone was touching her all the time."

Paul looked at his sister. "Did she say who it was?"

"No." But Millie's eyes grasped her brother's and she remembered his remark about damaged goods. She turned away and looked toward the floor. Tears welled in her eyes.

"Your sister left a diary," Marty said.

"Yes, isn't that how you found out? My brother Domenic gave them to you. Isn't that why you're here?"

"No," the chief answered.

"I told you we were here because we heard something from someone and we wanted to verify if it was true. I think," Marty said, "you just did that."

"Does Domenic still have the books?" Jim asked.

"Yes," she said. "When I found them I didn't know what to do so I called my brother."

"So you gave them to Father Giannetti?"

"Yes, that's right. I didn't know what else to do."

Paul had been silent for most of this time. He sat with his arms folded against his chest, his expression cold and brooding. "Who told you this?" he suddenly blurted out.

"You know I can't tell you that."

The boy moved off the chair. He walked to the other end of the porch.

"Thank you," Marty said, then the two men walked down the steps. But as they began to descend, Marty heard Paul.

"You and Domenic find something like this and don't tell anyone else in the family."

"Only because of Momma and Poppa," Millie said. "You know how they have been lately. If her dying wasn't enough this would finish them off easy."

Millie knew her brother was right. She walked over to the railing and stared down at the empty shed. This was something so private to her sister that she never shared it with anyone. Not even with people she trusted. Now her sister's memory would become nothing more than gossip for the whole town.

CHAPTER TWENTY-SEVEN

"It's 12:15," Taylor announced. "What do you say we go for some lunch?"

"What did you have in mind?" Marty asked.

"Athena's, and I'm buying."

"Now I am worried," the chief joked. "You're too cheap just to buy lunch."

Taylor stood by the door, his arms folded on his chest. "Christ, I can't fool you," Jim snapped. A nasty smiled crossed his lips. "That's why you're the chief and I'm only the detective."

"All right," Marty said. "I'm game?"

"Remember I told you I needed to get Fiske's fingerprint? Well, I'm gonna try and intimidate Nick Spanos into getting us something with his prints on it."

Mrs. Spano greeted them at the door of the tiny café.

"Gentlemen, you back for more questions?"

"No, we're here for lunch," Taylor said. "I wanted to try some more of your good food. By the way, who's cooking today?"

She seated the two men by a window, handed them each a menu and said, "Vinnie."

After a few minutes she came back for their order. "What would you two like to try?"

"I'll have the chicken soup and a lamb sandwich," Marty said.

"Make that two." Then Taylor asked if Nick was around.

A few minutes later Nick Spanos, plump, sweaty and wearing a scowl, walked to the table. "Tell me you called me over just to compliment the meal," he said.

"We just need a small favor," Taylor said. "Something a business man like you would want to help with."

"I don't do no donations."

"No money," Taylor said. "We just want to get help with this petition." The detective pulled a large envelope out of his coat pocket. He placed it in front of Santos.

"What's this all about?" Nick asked.

"It's a petition to extend the benefits for the police department."

"This gonna cost me money."

"No, it's gonna cost the state," Jim said.

Marty figured Jim had doctored a legitimate petition. It was a simple thing to do and nobody ever really read them anyway. And he was pretty sure neither would Nick Santos.

"So you come down to the village just to get me to sign it."

Marty looked past Jim and into the face of the overstuffed man. "I heard you had a pretty good lunch," he said. "I wanted to try it."

"Okay," he said with a sigh. "Let me read this petition."

He read the first line, then skipped to the back page. "So I sign here," he said.

"Yeah. Do you think you could get some of your help to sign it too?" Jim asked. "We need a lot of names."

By the time the two detectives had finished lunch Santos came back.

"I get you five more names," he said. "A few waitresses and my wife."

"How about the guys in the kitchen?" Jim asked.

"What, are you crazy? They can't even read. When I asked Vinnie to read it he handed it right back to me with greasy fingers."

"Oh, that's okay," Jim said. "Thanks anyway."

After they left the restaurant Marty said, "Hey, sport, thanks for lunch."

"Well I figured you could get it next time," Taylor said with a chuckle. "Besides I got what I came after."

"That was pure genius," he said.

"It worked out even better than I expected," Jim said. "Well, where to?"

"Saint Bartholmew," Chief Sacco said. "We have an appointment with Father Giannetti."

When they arrived at the church they were greeted by the Irish housekeeper. "Chief Sacco," she said. "How are you?"

"I'm fine, Mrs. Carr. What about yourself?"

"Good," she said. Her eyes glanced upwards. "Thank God. Are you here to see Father Dom?"

"Yes."

"You can wait right here," she said and directed them to the bench outside his office.

Mrs. Carr knocked on the door. It creaked opened and the old woman whispered something.

"Show them in."

Father Giannetti smiled when he greeted the detectives. "Gentlemen, what can I do for you?"

"We wanted to talk with you about Nina's diaries," Marty said.

He motioned for the two men to sit down.

"Father, we spoke with your sister Millie earlier and she told us about the journals that Nina kept."

"Yes, I have them," he admitted.

"Why haven't you given them to us?"

"I just don't see the connection to her murder," he said. "Whatever happened in my sister's life with relation to these incidents surely has nothing to do with her death. Especially since you have three other women who died in the same manner as Nina."

"Father, you know that any evidence that relates to the victim that is intentionally kept from the police is considered an obstruction of justice."

The young priest stood by the window. He began to pace in front of his desk.

"If the press gets a hold of those diaries," he said. "My family will suffer Nina's death again. Only this time I fear it would be worse for my parents. I wasn't trying to obstruct justice, I simply wanted to protect my parents."

"I do understand that," Marty said. "Look, give us the journals and we will just go about our business. I give you my word that the department itself will not leak any information to the press."

"I'll tell my family this evening," Domenic said. "If you'll excuse me. I'll get the diaries for you now."

Jim was restless and he moved off the chair. He strolled to the back of the small office and picked up a book from the priest's desk. "This guy likes poetry," he said with a smirk.

The police chief looked across at the neatly arranged desk of Father Giannetti with envy. "So do I," Marty said.

"Well, I believe the priest is right about what could happen if this story were to get out. The press would do a number on the family," he said. Jim pulled a cigarette out of his pocket.

Marty picked up an ashtray and handed it to Taylor. "I agree. It could get awfully messy."

"And we have almost no control. You know these guys even listen in on the phone conversations."

"Then I guess everyone is gonna have to be a bit more vigilant," Marty said.

Father Giannetti opened the office door and stepped back into the office. He handed a bag to Marty. "They are all in there."

"I assume you've read them."

"No," he said. "I flipped through a few pages. I hadn't been able to convince myself to read them yet," Domenic said. "But I only flipped through a few pages. If you just give me tonight to tell my parents before any other information is released I would be grateful."

"That's fine," Marty said. He tucked the journals under his arm. "It will take us a day or two to read the material anyway." He offered the priest his hand in friendship and thanked him again.

When the two detectives left the office, Jim turned to Marty and remarked about the sound of their shoes against the shiny wood floors.

"It's because the room is hollow," Marty said. "It just echoes."

"Yeah, well churches and rectories give me the creeps. They purposely keep the rooms dark and dull to intimidate little kids."

Marty looked to his friend. "Well," he said. "Then that explains the dilemma."

The housekeeper stood by the front door and waited for the two men.

"Good afternoon gentlemen," Mrs. Carr said.

"The weather seems to have changed," Marty noticed. She was in a struggle against the wind to hold the door open. "Let me help you," he said.

"Thank you," she said, then scooted inside. "It started out like a nice day. But now with this wind and those dark clouds I think we are in for some heavy rain."

Jim was already in the car when Marty opened the passenger's side door. He checked his watch then said, "I have an appointment with Donahue."

Jim was remarkably quiet for the drive until they reached the hospital entrance.

"Why don't you come in with me?" Marty said.

"You want me to meet with the shrink because why?" Jim asked.

"You know I don't like these scientific witch doctors."

"I want you to hear what he has to say. It might give you some insight into the investigation."

"Yeah. But not today," he said. "I have an appointment."

He dropped Marty off on the corner of Newcomb and Washington Streets. The chief looked up at the old building. There was nothing of architectural interest about the brick hospital. It was a drab building. Almost like a box with windows. Once inside he walked the long corridor that connected the hospital to the mental wards.

"Thank you for seeing me right away."

"Actually, it's a relief," he said. "My day has been full of routine upsets and I welcome a brief change. Well, what can I do for you?"

"I know that I do not have to remind you that anything we say is in confidence," Marty said.

"Of course," the doctor agreed.

The police chief pulled the journals out of the original bag in which he received them and placed them on the doctor's desk. "These belonged to the last murder victim," he said. "A young girl named Nina Giannetti. I wanted you to look them over and then give me your opinion."

"Have you read them?" the doctor asked.

"Yes," Marty said.

"Then tell me what you think."

Marty hesitated before he answered. He wanted to be sure he placed enough value on the young girl's thoughts. "I believe she was lonely, frightened and desperate." He moved closer to the desk. "Maybe I'm just doing a spin in the dark with this. But I'm hoping that these diaries can lead me to her murderer."

Donahue reached across for the books.

"I placed a few tags in specific sections I found of special interest," Marty said.

"Before I can give you any opinion, I would need to read them all."

"I understand that," Marty said. "I'll leave them with you."

"There is something," he said, after flipping through a few pages. "Did her mother give you these?"

"No. She knows nothing about them."

"That makes sense to me. These letters are for her mother. But because the girl feels that she shares the burden of responsibility she never actually gave them to her mother."

"Why would she feel guilty?" Marty asked. "It's obvious she was sexually molested. So why does she feel responsible?"

"That's the very point. Molestation is like a robbery. It takes the child's fragile self-esteem and replaces it with a guilty self-image. Thus the child feels responsible."

"And that is why she could not tell her mother?" Marty asked.

"Maybe the girl believed she would be a disappointment to her mother.

Or maybe she felt her mother knew and didn't try to stop it. If the victim sees herself as part of the blame she is not going to tell anyone. As long as it remains a secret she can hide from it. But," he said, "there is something to be said for her diaries, isn't there?"

He closed the book and said, "Give me about a week. Then I will be in touch."

"I appreciate anything you can do that would be of help," Marty said.

"Well," Jim asked when he arrived back at the office. "Did the shrink have anything to add?"

"You should have been there. You could learn something," Marty said.

He looked towards Jim. The detective stood at the window. He leaned against the cement wall. He was poised in his favorite position. His head rested against the wall and his arms crossed against his chest. His cigarette rested on the windowsill and the smoke misted upwards in long thin strips.

Taylor was a thinker. He kept his thoughts and hunches to himself. He never showed his hand until he was about to strike.

"This is a very dirty business we are about to engage in," Marty said.

Jim picked up his cigarette and took a drag. "We've been in this dirty business for years."

"Not like this," Marty said. "If that girl was molested by someone other than a family member, we will have to interview every male in Ethnic Village."

Jim glanced toward the chief. "I agree that the son-of-a-bitch who was diddling with that little girl should be caught and put behind bars. But, there is no proof he's the same guy who committed the other murders. Christ," he said, then pulled another drag off his smoke. "I'm not even convinced that Kerchak is innocent. Case in point," he said. "The kid's been in jail for six months, and nobody else is dead."

"I agree with you in some of your theories. But don't insult my intelligence. You don't believe this kid is guilty any more than I do. Otherwise why would you be so interested in this guy Fiske."

Maybe, Marty thought, as he sat back in his seat, *he hasn't killed anyone else because he's playing with us. Or he is just so confidant even relaxed, over the fact that we have the wrong man. Maybe for the moment he's just killed out.*

"No, you're right," Jim said. "There is a connection. I'm just not sure it includes the Giannetti girl."

"You think her death is a copy."

"I'm not sure," he said. "There is something about it that is different. I can't even figure out my own hunch yet." He was ready to toss his cigarette, but Marty rushed the ashtray to the end of the desk. Jim still threw the cigarette on the floor and stomped on it.

"Why did you do that?" Marty said. "You know, you can be a real asshole at times."

"Yeah," he said. "That's what my ex-wife tells me."

He leaned down and picked up the butt and flung it in the ashtray. "There, is that better?" he asked.

"Anyway," Jim said. "Let's say the father or one of the brothers was the one that molested Nina. Then this would have happened before, to the other girls. Wouldn't you think?"

"I don't know. I mean that is usually what happens. Then the secret becomes the family's. But this girl never told anyone. If it had happened before, she wouldn't have anything to hide," Marty said. "Then why wouldn't she tell her mother?"

"What if it was the father?" Jim said, then he began to pace the room.

"I just don't see the molester's connection to her murder."

Marty placed his head back on the chair. Jim reached for another butt. Then he flung the empty pack into the trashcan. "I hate these things," he said.

"Then quit."

"If I do," Jim said, "I'd end up with a flask in my pocket."

Detective Taylor's phone rang and he rushed to the desk. "Yeah."

Marty heard him say Steve into the receiver and assumed it might be Steve Sullivan from the bureau.

"Okay, thanks," Jim said. He hung up the phone. "That was Sullivan over at the bureau. They got a fingerprint match from that phony petition I sent them. Vinnie Fiske is Vincent Fubrowski," Jim said. "He joined the Navy in 1944."

CHAPTER TWENTY-EIGHT

She was surprised to hear his somber voice on the other end of the phone. "Hello, Millie, is Paul around?" Domenic asked.

"Sure, hold on. It's for you," she yelled to Paul, then handed him the phone. "I can't, I've got school tonight. Okay, okay," he said. "I'll be here."

Momma was standing in the kitchen when her son walked in. "What's the matter?" she asked.

"Domenic is coming over. I'll be here for supper too," he said, then he walked into the back hall and closed the door to his bedroom.

The darkness began to roll in earlier every night with the end of summer. Still, it wasn't unusual for Momma to keep the back door open. But tonight she was cold and rubbed her arms for heat. "Fa fredda," she said just before she closed the door.

"I guess summer is over," Domenic said when he heard his mother's comment.

"Summer has been over for me for a long time."

"How's Poppa doing?"

She shrugged her shoulders and mumbled. "Ehh."

"And you?"

"I don't know anymore. I used to think I was strong," she said. "Now I'm not so sure. Maybe someday soon I'll be lucky and take a long nap."

Millie knew what her mother meant. All she ever talked about was dying. "When I see the death of my own children," she said, "then I live too long." She smiled sadly at her stepbrother. Domenic left the porch and walked into the living room where his father sat alone on the couch.

"Come on," Momma said. In her hand she held a large platter of pasta and roast chicken. "Sit down and mangia."

Normally the Giannetti boys would eat a mound of pasta. But tonight their appetites seemed to pale. Paul played with his food while Domenic picked at a few forkfuls of spaghetti.

"My pasta no good tonight," Momma said.

"Of course not," Poppa said. "It's delicious."

Paul put down his fork. "It's not your food, Momma, I'm just not that hungry."

Once dinner was over and the table was cleared, Millie put on a pot of coffee. Poppa limped to the cabinet and retrieved his nightly ritual of brandy. He picked up the bottle, poked his fingers inside a couple of glasses and carried them back to the table. Then he poured three drinks.

Momma handed Millie a plate of Italian cookies and she scanned each confection carefully in order to choose just the right one. Then she placed the dish on the table and sat down next to her mother.

"So Domenic," Momma said. "What is wrong?"

"Why do you think something is wrong?" he asked.

"Because I know my boys. Paul doesn't go to school. You call at the last minute to come for dinner and then you don't eat. You think I'm stupid," she said. "Now tell me what is wrong."

Domenic put his elbows on the table and lowered his head to his hands.

"What's the matter with you?" Poppa yelled to Momma. "Leave the boy alone."

"No, she's right, Poppa," he said. "I have something to tell you both."

Momma looked over at her son. Her face drained of what little color she had. "I don't want to hear any more bad news," she said.

Domenic began quickly. "Nina kept a diary," he said. "A day-to-day journal of everything that happened to her."

"So what," Momma said. "Nina was always reading."

"Let the boy speak," Poppa said.

"This is different," Domenic said. "In this book Nina wrote about terrible things that happened to her." He turned to his father. His voice softened and he said, "Nina wrote that she was being molested."

"What do you mean?" Momma asked. "She was raped."

Millie watched her stepbrother as he tried to explain. His lips trembled and his eyes filled with tears. "She wrote that it happened all the time. Even when she was a little girl."

The old woman wrapped her face in her hands. "But Nina never told me. Why she didn't tell me this?" The old woman turned to Millie. "And you, did she tell you?"

"No," Millie said.

Her mother's expression changed. "Millie, what about you? These things happen to you too?"

She shook her head. "Nobody ever touched me."

Poppa's body went rigid. He picked up his drink and swallowed it. He closed his eyes and then sat still for the longest time. Then Millie saw tears run down his cheeks.

"Do you know who did this?" he asked.

"Nina never wrote who it was," Domenic said.

"Why she never told me?" Momma kept wringing her hands. "Who would do this?"

"Josef Kerchak," Paul said. "I want to kill him with my bare hands."

"You don't know if it was him," Domenic said.

"Yeah, well the cops said they heard that about Nina. And Josef is the one who is in jail. I'll bet he's the one who told the cops. And how would he know if Nina never even told Momma."

"Tell me, son," Poppa said. "Why do you tell us this now? She is dead. Why does your mother need to hear this?"

"Do you think I wanted to tell you?" Domenic said. "I had to. The police know and I didn't want either of you to hear this from someone else."

Poppa's gaunt image stared at the three children from across the table.

"When this all gonna end?" he cried. "The newspaper's gonna print this about Nina. Make it look like she did something wrong." He lifted himself off the chair and grasped the table. He poured himself another drink, picked up his glass and walked into the parlor.

"What does it matter anymore?" Momma braced her hands against the table. She lifted her body from the seat, then looked towards her children, her face full of deep lines, her eyes clouded. "No matter who did this. Even if you know. It's not gonna bring my little girl back. Jesu Christ, help me," Momma said, then she turned and left the room.

If only I hadn't found those books, Millie thought. *If only I had kept them to myself. Poppa was right, why did anyone need to find out about this?*

"I'm worried about Momma and Poppa," Paul said. "Why did we have to do this?"

"It's all my fault," Millie said. She wanted to run away. Not face any of what has happened. But she couldn't so instead she began to pick up the dishes on the table.

"No," Domenic said. "This is not anyone's fault. I think Nina wanted her diaries to be found." He looked at the table and placed one dish on top of another. "C'mon, Paul, let's help clean up."

Later when Millie was alone in her room, she thought about what Domenic had said. Maybe he was right. Maybe Nina did want the books to be found. But how could she? Nina didn't know she was gonna die.

Since Nina's death Millie had seen a tremendous change in her parents. She watched the years melt off their lives. Still she was not prepared for what came next.

Once Momma and Poppa were told about the diaries, the whole family was called together. It was to be a day of emotional pain. Some of her brothers and sisters seemed cruel by their lack of empathy. The careless comments that floated across the family dining room table left her stunned.

"I don't believe any of it," Susie said. "Nina was always in a fantasy world. She probably copied the letters from some book."

"How can you say such a thing," Rose said.

"C'mon," Tommy said. "What does it matter now?"

For days, one by one, the Giannetti children, relatives and friends, were called into the police station. The police interviewed uncles, cousins, godparents, and friends. They even interviewed Chief Polanski's grandson. Marty had known the boy forever and when he came into the station he immediately knocked on the chief's door. "Hi, Mr. Sacco."

David was a handsome boy. He came from a good background and Marty was positive he had nothing to do with any of the murders.

"Come in," he said. After he shook the boy's hand and exchanged a few pleasantries, he said, "I'm sure you know why you're here."

"It has something to do with Nina's death."

"I know that you two were friends before she died."

"Yes sir."

"How long had you and Nina been seeing each other?"

"About three months," he said.

"Did her parents know?"

"No," he said. "Nina wasn't allowed to date or even talk to boys. Every time we tried to see each other her brother Paul would give her a hard time. Finally she…"

"What?" Marty asked.

"She began to sneak out so we could see each other once in awhile."

"Did that bother Nina?"

"Nina was a really nice girl," he said. "She didn't like doing anything behind her parents' backs. But she would get really get mad, because her father wouldn't let her do anything or go anywhere without her brother Paul. And he was nasty too. She told me he teased her all the time."

"Where did you go on your dates? I mean if Paul was always around what did you do?"

"Sometimes we just walked or went to the movies. But most of the time we did our homework together at the library."

"Did Nina ever confide anything to you about being threatened or anything else?"

"Just that her brother always told on her. She did tell me that if her father found out about us she would probably be in big trouble."

"Where were you the night Nina was killed, David?" Marty asked.

"It was very warm," he said. "My brothers and I slept in the basement with a few of our friends."

"I want to thank you for coming by," the police chief said. "It was nice to see you again. And if you think of anything, no matter how unimportant you think it is, please, call me."

David was half way out the door, but he stepped back in. "There is something," he said. "I don't know if it means anything. But one night when Nina and I were in a hurry to get back to Delores's before Paul got there, there was this man on the corner. When Nina saw him she became frightened. I asked her what was wrong. She just said, 'He's always around.' When I asked her what she meant she just said, 'Never mind.'"

"Did you ever question her again about this man?"

"Yes, but she told me he was just somebody from town that she saw all the time. And he made her skin crawl."

"And did you see him again?"

"No," David said.

Marty had called the Giannetti home to find out when the two women would be able to come to the station. He felt he wanted to speak with Millie again about that night.

"We can come to your office after school on Wednesday," Mrs. Giannetti told him. He had prepared himself to be extra gentle with the old woman and to keep them there for as short a time as possible.

As the two women approached the police chief's office, Millie began to feel a slight intimidation. Standing in the farthest corner she spotted Detective Taylor. He smiled at her as she walked through the door.

"Come in, Mrs. Giannetti." Then he turned toward Millie and said, "We really appreciate this visit."

Detective Taylor lifted his hand and signaled to somebody in the next room. Within seconds the police chief walked in.

"I have to leave," Jim said. "I'll be back in a while."

"Good day, ladies," Marty said, then left.

"It's nice to see you again, Mrs. Giannetti. And thank you for taking the time to come down to the station."

The old woman sat in the chair. She never changed expression. There was no smile. Just a dead look into the police chief's face. He tried to avoid her stare and looked toward the young girl.

"Millie, how are you today?"

"Why are we here?" the old woman asked.

"Please Momma," the girl said. "I understand why we are here."

"Good," Marty said. He walked to back of his desk. "Although, I am sorry to have inconvenienced you. You understand it is important that we see everyone."

His eyes wandered to Mrs. Giannetti. "I don't mean to minimize your daughter's death," Marty said. "But there were four women killed."

Millie understood why her mother was resistant to being there. She knew something the police chief couldn't possibly know. That Momma's interest into their investigation was limited. In her sense of reality it mattered little about the other killings. All she knew was that whoever they caught would not be able to bring her little girl back. So therefore what did it mean? In Momma's defense, she couldn't understand the level of it could happen again.

"Do you ever remember having a discussion with your sister about her diaries? Even in a hypothetical context?" Marty asked Millie.

"She never told me anything."

"How about anger. Did she ever get mad at anyone? Maybe one of your brothers."

"Are you serious?"

"I don't mean brother/sister anger," he said. "I mean the kind that can cause you fear or intimidation."

"Nina was always angry with Paul," she said. "But that's because Paul was a jerk." The young girl lowered her eyes. "But she never told me anything about what's in her diaries."

"Mrs. Giannetti," he asked. "If I were to ask you who you would think could do this to your daughter what would you say?"

She stayed silent for little more than a minute. The she turned to the police chief and said, "I don't know who could do something so bad to a little girl. But I know it could never be anyone in the family. You need to look on your streets for this animal," she said.

It was obvious to Marty that she was uncomfortable with their discussion about this subject. "I don't want to talk to you anymore about my daughter. She's dead. You leave her alone." She stood and motioned for Millie to move. "Enough," she said. "We leave now."

The young girl looked at the police chief. "I'm sorry," she said.

"That's all right," he said. Marty placed his hand on the girl's shoulder and led them to the door. "Thank you again, Mrs. Giannetti," he said. Marty stood in the doorway and watched them walk down the corridor and out the front door of the station house.

He sat back at his desk and picked up Nina's file. It had been almost a week since he had given the diaries to Dr. Donahue. If he didn't hear from him soon he would have to put a call into the psychiatrist's office.

When the buzzer on his phone rang he picked up the receiver.

A familiar voice bellowed from the other side.

Marty was momentarily sidetracked by the appearance of Jim. He stood in the doorway, a cigarette planted between his lips.

"Leo, what can I do for you? I can be, what's up?"

He looked over at Jim. "Okay I'll see you around then," and hung up the phone.

"What was that all about?" Detective Taylor said with a smirk.

"Never mind. Where have you been?"

"I was over at records," he said. "Did you know that the town of Norwich lost three kids to the big war? Pretty high odds if you consider the population."

Marty was always amazed by the lanky cop's wide range of interests. Jim was a born nitpicker, someone who was never satisfied, always looking for more. His attitude didn't work well for his life. But it was great for the police department.

"What were you doing at the record department?"

"I wanted to check out something," he said. He pulled a tiny package of peanuts out of his pocket. "What's on for this afternoon?"

"Father Giannetti was supposed to come in today. But he can't so we are gonna meet him at the rectory. And we are gonna meet up with Shapiro around three."

"Shapiro, what does he want?"

"I don't know."

"What about the priest? Why do we need to go to his office? Isn't it customary for people to come to the station anymore."

"Listen to you," Marty said. "You sound like an old lady. He asked us to meet with him at the church because Monsignor Harrow is ill, and it's the housekeeper's day off. He just didn't want to leave the old man alone."

"What is it about the church that bothers you so much?"

"I told you they do things to purposely intimidate people. Every time I go near one I feel like I did when I was a kid. And the nuns, they were the worst. Mother Francis was always on us about confession. I used to hate Saturday mornings," he said. Because we had to go into the little boxes and tell the priest what we did all week. I hated to go into one of those things."

"I did too," Marty admitted. "But I got over it."

"Mrs. Carr," the police chief said. "I'm surprised to see you. Father told me you had the day off."

"Originally. But I needed a different day," she explained. "So I decided to work today instead.

The two men followed her to the priest's office. They stood in the hallway until he answered the woman's knock.

"Your appointment is here," she said.

"Thank you," came a voice from inside.

Father Domenic opened the door and greeted the two men. "Please come in," he said.

Detective Taylor walked in first and Marty followed. "How is the monsignor doing today?" he asked.

"Thank God, much better. I'm sorry about the confusion. I could have come to your office."

"That's not a problem, Father," he joked. "Jim, here, likes to drive me around."

Marty looked over at Taylor who stood against the office door with a serious stare.

"Anyway, I only have a few questions."

"Of course."

"Did any one of your siblings talk about being molested as a child?"

There was a look of confusion on the young priest's face. "No," he said. "Never. None of my sisters have ever approached me."

Detective Taylor moved from the door and stood near the desk. "What about your brother Paul?" he asked.

"I'm not sure I understand the question. Are you asking me if he talked about being molested?"

"That or," Marty said, "could he be the molester?"

"Of course not," Father said. "My brother is quick tempered and a bully. But he's not capable of doing anything like that."

"Like what?" Jim asked.

"Molestation or murder."

"You know better than me, Father, that everyone is capable."

Father Domenic moved away from his seat. He pushed the chair back and stood up. "Yes, Detective," he said. A look of anger swept across his face.

"I agree, but not everyone acts on those emotions. We have a large extended family and if you are asking is it possible, I would have to say of course. But if you are asking is it probable, my answer is no."

His expression softened and he said, "What I don't understand is why you are so caught up with who molested Nina. Shouldn't we be more concerned with her murderer?"

"We think there could be a connection," Marty said.

"You think the same man that molested my sister killed her and the other women."

"Father, did Nina ever mention being followed or threatened?"

"No. I'm sorry," he said. Father Domenic looked down towards the floor. "I didn't mean to cause any problems with the investigation. I didn't think of Nina's diaries as evidence," he admitted. "I was concerned for my parents. I saw them as more grief for them."

"That is understandable," the police chief said.

"I don't have any information that could be of help. Nina never mentioned to me about being followed. For that matter she never hinted about any trouble."

Marty was ready to leave. He looked over at Jim and gave him the eye.

"Well, we do appreciate your honesty and your time," he said.

"It's 2:15," Marty said. "Let's just drive over to Shapiro's office and see if he's there."

"Sure," Jim said. He turned the car around and headed outside of the village.

"What did you think?" he asked.

"About what?"

"Last night. Did you watch television?"

Marty ignored the queston. Jim's voice rambled on like whispers in the background. He paid no attention. His mind was centered on Josef, Nina Giannetti's journals and the reason for Shapiro's call.

"So what did you think?" Jim said. Only this time his voice rumbled.

"I-I don't know?" Marty said.

"Well," Jim answered. "I'm not sure who deserved it. But I thought Marlon Brando was pretty good in that waterfront movie."

"What," Marty said and turned toward the driver.

"I asked you what you thought about last night's Academy Awards."

"Jesus, Jim, you drive me crazy. I didn't watch it."

Taylor pulled into the driveway of Shapiro's office. "This guy does pretty good for always backing the loser."

Marty shook his head. "Can you just listen," he said. "No wisecracks, okay."

Leo was on his way out the office when he spotted the chief.

"Hey, you didn't have to come to me," the attorney said. "I have no problem walking into a police station."

"We were in the neighborhood. I thought I might catch you."

"Come on in," he said. He unlocked the door and the three men stepped into the office.

"I was looking through some of my old files," Shapiro said. "I wanted to store them away. When I came across a few notes from Paula Roache. That's when I remembered the kid."

"What kid?" Marty asked. "Josef Kerchak?"

"No. When I was Paula's attorney she mentioned a few times about being watched. I told her to call the cops. But she said it was probably her imagination and she didn't want to accuse anyone if she wasn't sure."

"Did she know who it was?" Jim asked.

"No, she thought it might have been one of her students. I made her promise that if it continued she would tell the police. The afternoon before Paula disappeared she left me a note. She must have dropped by my office on her way home from school. But I wasn't in. So I never saw it."

Shapiro hesitated. He lowered his eyes and shook his head. "My secretary innocently placed the note in the folder and then she must have forgot about it. After Paula disappeared the file was placed inactive and put away."

Leo picked up his briefcase that sat next to his desk. He opened it. "I just happened to go through the file this morning and I found this. Here," he said.

Marty opened the envelope and took out the folded piece of notepaper.

Dear Mr. Shapiro

I have decided to take your advice and contact the police. Last night when I returned home late from a long day at school I saw him again. Only this time he didn't hide behind the large oak. Instead I could see his face when he leaned against the tree. He never took his eyes off my bedroom window. I felt frightened and vulnerable.

A few times I peeked out to see if he had left. But he was still there.

I decided to phone the police and went into the front hall. But that's when he left. I didn't sleep all night I was so terrified. It was as if he were in my house.

When I first saw him I recognized the face. But it wasn't until the morning that I realized who he was. He's been to my house a number of times. You see he is one of the delivery boys for the local grocer.

Although I am obligated to work at a charity for a few hours early this evening, I thought I would ask you to come with me to the police station. I should be home around 7:30. I will wait for you to call. I really appreciate all your help and hope that is an agreeable hour for you.

Paula Roache

Marty turned the note over to Jim, who read it and then slipped it into his pocket.

The attorney closed his briefcase and held it with both hands. "I wish I had been there," he said.

"This could be a real tangible piece of evidence," Marty said. "Something that could possibly link Paula Roache to the new murders."

"Good," Leo said. "If that's true then my client cannot be guilty. Do we agree on that point?"

"I agree," Marty said.

"Would you let me know if you come up with anything?" Leo said. Then he added. "I know, off the record."

Marty nodded with a fraction of reluctance.

Once outside Marty looked towards the car. Jim was already seated behind the steering wheel. When the chief approached Taylor pulled a cigarette out of his pocket. He had that look on his face, that cock-sure arrogant expression.

"What," Marty said.

"Dorothy Miller told Mrs. Santos almost the same story about some guy who watched her. Then he would disappear," Jim said. "But Paula Roache recognized him because he had delivered her groceries. If he's the guy then he would have been in his late teens or early twenties back then. That would make him somewhere in his thirties today."

"And Dorothy Miller put a face on her peeping tom," Marty said. "Yeah," Jim agreed. "Vinnie Fiske's face."

"Do you remember who owned the grocery store ten years ago?"

"I'm sure it was Sam Knight," Jim said. "A peculiar little man who was paranoid about insurance so he wouldn't let anybody who wasn't twenty drive the grocery truck."

"Jesus, Jim, I love you."

CHAPTER THIRTY

Nineteen fifty-four was almost over and despite the fact that Norwich was having its problems the world kept on spinning. We were awed by the works of Ernest Hemingway, James Michner and a real life legend—Pablo Picasso still painted at the age of seventy-four. We saw war correspondents nightly who fed us news about Korea. We thrilled to Mr. Baseball and his marriage to the female heartthrob of the century, Marilyn Monroe. There wasn't one teenage girl who didn't think Marlon Brando was the sexiest man alive. Elvis Presley joined the list of draftees and Jimmy Dean had one more year to live.

In Millie's house it was her father who was enthralled by the newest wonder of life. Poppa said it's like "a radio for the eyes," but Momma called it a chatterbox.

Whatever it was thought of back then, television was to become a national observation area for everything. That included the local news.

If the murders of these women weren't enough of a tragedy, Nina Giannetti being the youngest victim gave the press even more reason to exploit the murders. Because of the local news arena the Giannetti family was besieged constantly by out-of-town reporters. Which included *The Boston Globe*, *The Daily Herald* and a weekly newspaper that covered ten surrounding towns. It was called *The Transcript*. It reached its peak by the coverage it gave to the murders, especially Nina's.

They played up the death of the young girl and her large Italian family. Each week they would toss out a headline. "Giannettis Being Questioned in Sister's Death."

Photographers hounded them. They were everywhere. They scurried through the yard and shot photographs of the shed, the family on the porch, on the back stairs, even of the parents at the grave.

In the funeral home they snapped pictures of the dead girl as she lay in the casket. During the funeral they set their cameras to snap as the mourners entered the limousine. Then they would splash a collage of photographs across the front page for days.

Nothing was off limits. One day when the doorbell rang Millie opened the door to find a young man on the front stoop. Her teenage passion was fully aroused when he, well dressed and handsome, smiled at her.

"Hi. Are you Millie Giannetti?" he asked.

Her face red, she managed to stutter a hello. "Yes, that's me."

"My name is Michael Hogan. And I came specifically to see you."

"Why?"

"You were Nina's sister?"

"Yes."

"The one who found the body?"

Millie realized he was just another gossipmonger. "Please leave," she said, then started to close the door.

But the reporter shoved his foot between the opening. "Tell me your thoughts about your sister's death," he shouted.

Paul must have heard the commotion because he ran into the room. He saw the man's foot stuck in the door and slammed his heel on top of it. "Who the hell are you?"

"Hey," the man shouted. "My name is Michael Hogan and I am with *True Crime Magazine*. Asshole, get off my foot. Look," he said. "I'm willing to offer you a good sum of money for your story."

"Get out of here," Paul shouted. "Otherwise I'm gonna step on more than your foot. Do you understand?"

He opened the door and released the reporter's foot. But Hogan still persisted. "How about a hundred bucks just to talk to the girl?" he yelled through the door.

The reporter finally left the porch and Millie watched from the living room window. He walked down the stairs and gaped into the shed. He even lifted up the cover of one of the trashcans. After a few minutes he parked himself in his car and stayed there for hours, just staring at the house. He left before it got dark. But the next day he was parked in the same spot.

Millie felt saddened and puzzled by the people who preyed on her family's grief. And she found out it didn't matter whether she spoke to the reporters or not. Most made up stories anyway. And that man Hogan from *True Crime Magazine*, well in less than a month, he had printed the story of Nina's death and he wrote excerpts from her diary about the molestation.

The police department denied him access to the journals. Yet he claimed his information was documented. Millie believed it was based solely on town gossip. What made it so incredible was his appearance on the local radio station. When he was interviewed he spoke as if the victim's family had given him permission to print the article. At one point he even made the statement: "We at *True Crime* have tried to be as sensitive to the Giannetti family as possible."

Nina was killed in May, and months later Millie was in the throes of a new life. The school year just started. Her intention was to continue as before. That was easier said then done.

Everything was a reminder of how life was before her sister's death. Nothing was simple. The excitement of new classes, a trip to the library or a glance at a new boy didn't have the same meaning. Nina had always been part of that. Now simple daily routines became struggles.

The two girls had spent their best times engaged in conversation to and from school. Millie still had to make that walk but it was just a lonely effort. And the loneliness wasn't something that could be absorbed by the few friendships she had.

At the better part of fifteen Millie knew she would not be able to date for years. She even thought a relationship with a boy could help her deal with Nina's death. Maybe even learn to accept it. Certainly she would still grieve. But to converse with another person, someone she could trust to understand her sorrow, would make a tremendous difference.

Instead she was forced to let her solitude fester with little exposure to a world outside the Prescott Street home.

By now Poppa had become paranoid about anyone who came near her. For everyone else dating was a national pastime. But each time she pleaded her case it fell on deaf ears.

"It's just a school dance, Poppa," she would plead. "Teachers and chaperones will be there to watch us. I promise to come home right after the dance."

Poppa would look her in the eye and tighten the muscles in his face. "No, you understand. No."

Momma would sometimes feel empathetic and plead on her daughter's behalf. But he would not budge. "No. This girl gonna stay home until she marry."

"Look Poppa," Paul said. "I'll take her to the dance. I'll even stay with her and then bring her home."

At this point Millie was grateful for Paul's interference and agreed to go with him. One night her father relented. "I let you go this once," he said. "But only with Paul."

Millie went but that was the last school dance she attended. The intimidation level of her older brother constantly by her side was an incredible stigma. To attend the school dance with an older brother once was enough humiliation for a lifetime.

With Paul she may not have liked it but she knew what to expect. He had always been blatant about his over protectiveness. So she paid little attention to his presence when she saw him outside the school or library.

But when one of her friends recognized Domenic, Millie believed Poppa had gone too far.

"Isn't that your brother?"

"I can't believe my father," she said.

"That's your brother?" a new classmate asked. "My brothers don't look like that."

"He's a priest," Millie's friend Sylvia said with a giggle.

"Well he doesn't look like a priest."

"Yeah, but he is," Millie said. Annoyed, she rushed across the street to where Domenic stood.

"I don't believe this," she screamed. "Did Poppa ask you to spy on me too?"

"Hey, calm down," Domenic said. "I was with a parishioner who lives three doors down from the school," he said, then pointed to a white house with brown shutters. "I took a chance that you hadn't left yet and decided to wait for you. That's all."

Millie slowed down her pace. She turned to her brother. "I'm sorry," she said. "But Poppa's got me paranoid. He won't let me do anything."

"I understand. Still, Millie, with everything that's happened you do realize he's just worried about you."

"That doesn't make it any easier. I know he wants me to be safe," she said. "But I'm tired of being teased about my brother always being around. Last week one of the new girls even came up to me and said. 'Well at least you'll have a date for the prom.' I was so embarrassed," Millie said.

It didn't matter how much she tried to understand or rationalize her father's concern. In her mind he would destroy any life she could have. And she resented that and at times her momma and poppa. Sometimes she even resented Nina.

By mid-October Millie was surprised that her mother hadn't started to prepare for the holidays.

"They not the same any more," Momma told her. "When I think how much has changed in one year."

She stopped what she was doing and pulled out the chair by the kitchen table. She hadn't sat there much lately. "I don't care about the neighbors no more. Not since that boy kill my daughter."

Once Millie said to her mother, "Maybe Josef didn't kill Nina."

"What do you mean? Why the police arrest him? You think they have nothing to do but put people in jail. Of course it's him," she said.

"I just mean."

"Never mind, no more talk."

For most of the Giannettis, Josef Kerchak was Nina's murderer. It mattered little whether he killed the other victims. But for Millie the most confusion was centered around her family's lack of empathy when it came to Nina's molestation.

"It happens," Momma said. "It's not right. But what are you gonna do?"

Millie's earlier years had been those of complete support for her parents' wise and trusted opinions. Her mother's response was difficult for the young girl to accept and she was troubled by the indifference that seemed to take over. It was true the family had always been able to repress anything that bothered them. The usual answer was to place the problem under a rug somewhere in the back of the mind.

But somehow this was different. It felt wrong to sweep away what her sister was forced to deal with for so many years. Yet as bad as she felt about their apathy, she didn't for one minute believe that anyone in her family was responsible for the abuse Nina suffered. After all neither her or the other siblings had ever been molested.

Then why Nina? She must have asked herself that a million times.

And she just didn't believe it was one of her cousins or Uncle Ed, for that matter. Sure he could be a leech, but something that deceitful.

Millie even tried to see Josef as the offender. He did have some weird habits. Yet it was easier for her to believe it was Mr. Kerchak that did it. After all he was a threat, even to his own family.

What Millie didn't realize was that her convictions about Josef's innocence would soon be fact. And on the night of November 3rd, 1954, it became obvious that Josef Kerchak was not the murderer.

CHAPTER THIRTY-ONE

He moved quickly along the street in and out of the shadows. He was extra tired tonight. But he was fast and a good thing too, because of that damn cop.

His body picked up speed and his breath rose in front of him. The more he ran the more rejuvenated he became. He had reached the field now and raced across the railroad tracks. He used them as a guide in the dark. When they twisted toward the right, so did he. That's when he knew he was almost home.

"Chief, it's Swenson. You better get over here quick."
"What's going on?"
"I'm at the bakery," he said. "I think we have another murder."
"Jesus H. Christ," Marty screamed. "Get Jim on the phone," he said to an officer.
"We'll be right there."
It wasn't even 7:30 in the morning. Marty had decided to go in early to clear up some things on his desk. He drove by Jim's house and picked him up.
"What's up?"
"Swenson, the night duty cop called about a murder."

Walter Swenson made the rounds for the business area of Norwich. It was generally a nightly routine where he would check doors and peeked through windows. With the recent trouble he had become extra cautious.

In the five years Marty had assigned him to that duty, he had never encountered anything more than a few mischievous kids.

He stood in the cold air and spoke with the police chief.

"It was my last check," he said. "I always went to Janette Owens's, at the end of my shift around six. Most times she came in early for the morning rush. Most of the time when I knocked on the back door she would unlock it and let me in. Janette always had coffee and one of those big muffins for me. But this morning it was different," he said. He stopped for a minute to catch his breath.

Marty knew for months that Swenson had a crush on the pretty owner of Crumbles Bakery. And his early morning visits for that cup of hot Java were just an excuse to be with her.

"Earlier just before I knocked on her door, I saw someone in the back near the parking lot. So I yelled to him. Then he whizzed by me. I thought it was a kid about to steal something. I followed him for a few blocks but he was gone. When I came back I noticed Janette's back door was partially opened," he said. "I yelled to her. But there was no answer. I yelled again. But nothing, so I pushed the door open and walked in. I didn't see her. But something in the oven was burning so I grabbed a potholder and pulled out a batch of cookies. They were burned to a crisp."

Cold air rushed out of his mouth when he spoke and Marty didn't see the look of detachment in Swenson's face. Instead he saw concern and bewilderment, the same look that he usually saw on the faces of victims' families.

"None of this seemed right to me," the cop said. "So I walked to the front of the store. Janette wasn't there. I decided that she must be in the bathroom and walked to the back of the building. I knocked on that door," he said. "I kind of hesitated before I opened the door but…there she was."

Marty walked into the little toilet area. Clean except for the splattered blood. He glanced down at the familiar scene. The woman sat sprawled against the back wall. Her large eyes glared back with an empty stare. Marty guessed that the once pretty blonde's head had been smashed over and over against the cement wall her body rested against.

He knelt down. This time he didn't check for a pulse. It was a stupid habit. Besides the coroner's men were already there.

Janette Owens was a pretty woman. Maybe in her late forties, she had been widowed early in life. The bakery was her business and it had helped her raise her daughter. But she worked hard.

He glanced around the room to find the killer's card, the gruesome clincher. There it was. Just as expected, a neatly folded pile of clothes next to a pool of blood. The clean white apron that Janette always wore was folded perfectly, immaculate except for a tiny spot of blood.

Marty walked outside. Jim was by the ME's van with a cigarette, not too far from where Walter Swenson sat on the ground by a stack of wood, his head bent onto his knees.

"That poor bastard," Jim said. "He's gonna see that woman like that every day of his life."

"Have you talked to Curran yet?" Marty asked.

"No, I saw his men go in but not him. He'll be right along," Jim said. He threw his butt to the ground. "I guess you were right," he said.

"About what?"

"That Kerchak kid."

As promised Dr. Philip Curran had the autopsy report on the chief's desk in less than a week. It not only proved exactly what he thought it would, it pissed him off.

"Now what?" he said.

"Chief, a few of the town members are here to see you."

"Not now," he told the desk clerk.

But it was too late. The group was in the doorway.

"Pearson, what do you want?"

"We want this son-of-a-bitch caught. That's what we thought happened when you arrested the Kerchak kid."

Marty bolted from behind his desk. "Get out of my office," he said. "I don't need your arrogant self-righteous attitude right now."

Detective Taylor heard the commotion and ran into the chief's office. Taylor walked over to Pearson and stood in his face. "What the hell are you doing here, Pearson," Jim said.

"We want to be kept informed."

"You know what, let me inform you about this. If you don't get the hell out of here I'm gonna write you up for berating an officer."

Jim placed his hand on Pearson's shoulder and pushed him toward the door. "Now you and your buddies get out of the chief's office."

"Hey, you better not manhandle me."

"What are you gonna do, have me arrested?" Jim slammed the door and turned the key in the lock.

Marty had already sat back down behind his desk. "You realize it's almost a year to the day for Dorothy Miller," he said. "And ten years for Paula Roache."

Both men fell silent.

The small town of Norwich had just had its sixth murder. And except for a few small leads they were stumped.

"Maybe we should bring Fiske in."

"On what evidence?" Marty said. "If we bring him in then have to let him go, he's just gonna run again."

"Wait till Shapiro gets a hold of this," Jim said.

"But he's right Goddamn it. His client has been up there for something he didn't do. He's been fair with us," Marty said. "Even if we can't release Kerchak yet, at least the kid will know he's not going to stand trial for the other murders."

The phone on the desk buzzed and Marty yelled. "I don't want to talk to anyone, I don't give a shit who it is."

But Jim had already picked up the receiver. "Yeah, hold on," he said.

"Does that mean the shrink too?"

Marty grabbed the receiver. "Give me that," he said.

"Yeah, this is Sacco."

"I'll be there." After he slammed down the receiver. His eyes latched right on to Jim. "Don't make any plans," he said. "I want you there too."

Later that afternoon an anxious police chief and a skeptical detective walked into the sparse office of Dr. Kevin Donahue.

"Hello," he said.

"Let me introduce Detective Taylor," Marty said.

The two men shook hands and the doctor offered them each a seat.

"I'm sorry it took me so long to get back to you, especially in light of this new murder. But there were things in the journals that left me puzzled. So I had to reread them a few times.

He picked up one of the diaries and opened it to a bookmarked page.

"This child was besieged with guilt," he said. "It's as if in some way she felt responsible. In my opinion this girl thought that she had seduced her molester and for that she should be punished."

"Punished? How?" Marty asked.

"By God. By her family, that's one of the reasons she wasn't able to discuss this with anyone. In her eyes she was the one who should be blamed. You see the most telling aspect of this," he said. "Is that the child was even too terrified to speak face to face with her mother. And there could be a number of reasons why. Possibly shame, embarrassment, but my own theory is it wouldn't have mattered. I believe that it would have caused such turmoil in the family or that it would have been carefully disposed of." The doctor looked over at the two men. "Perhaps even both."

"And here," he said. While he turned the page. "She makes references to the fact that he is always around. "He watches me all the time. I know he is there even when I cannot see him."

"In your opinion, is it possible that this girl was murdered by the same person who molested her?" Marty asked. "I'm not sure, you see I believe this girl was molested by a family member. Could that person be the murderer? If she threatened him, maybe," he said.

"What I am almost certain of is that if this child didn't get help she would have eventually committed suicide. It was a very sad reading," Doctor Donahue said.

He placed the diaries back in a bag and laid them on the desk in front of the chief. "Very sad indeed."

"I have a question," Jim said.

"Sure?"

"If a member of the family is prone to molest," he asked. "Would he have a history? I mean it's not something you just wake up one day and do, is it?"

"That's a good question," Donahue said. "But the answer can be vague. You see the molester might find something in his victim that no other person has been able to offer him before. Let's say he needs to fulfill a sexual weakness. He is not in charge of his desires. He is like a machine that needs to be oiled in order to get through the day, unfortunate analysis but true."

"Okay, then she tells him I've had enough. Leave me alone. What then?"

"He will break down, do whatever it takes."

"Maybe even kill her?" Marty said.

"Or someone else," Jim answered.

"He could. Violence can be motivated by passion or self-preservation or even self-defense." Dr. Donahue continued. "You must remember—that kind of violence is predisposed. In other words he was capable all along."

Once back in the car the chief looked down at the pretty flowered cover journals and then turned to a page Donahue had bookmarked. *He is watching me all the time.*

Jim was in the driver's seat and he pulled the steering wheel to the right. "Do we go back to the Giannetti house?" he asked.

"No."

"Right now our evidence is based on one man's opinion. And for the sake of an argument let's say the psychiatrist is right. A family member is Nina's molester. And we accuse someone. Who is going to press charges? And who are we going to accuse, the father, or one of the brothers."

"Then what are we gonna do? Just sit and wait for it to happen again?" Jim's frustration was well understood.

"You know one mistake will blow our whole case. I don't want to take a chance on that. If the man who molested the Giannetti girl is not the murderer, then it isn't gonna matter if we catch him right away. And if he is the murderer I don't want to scare him away."

"I want you to keep on this guy Fiske or Victor, whatever the hell his name is. And put a loose tail on him. I don't want him to know we're following him."

Officer Doherty handed a manilla folder to Jim. "I did that background check you asked for."

"Great, I owe you."

"Victor Fubrowski was born in Norwich, in 1922. He was raised in Ethnic Village on Temple Street, by his parents, Serya and Olga. Went to Norwich High School. From what this report shows he was a pretty good student. And he ran track, what a coincidence," Jim remarked.

The detective walked around to the back of his desk. "He was busier as he got older," he said. "Petty theft, breaking and entering. Later he did a few years in reform school for assault and battery. Then he disappeared. That must have been when he joined the Navy."

"Which all coincides with what O'Brien told me," Marty said.

"Well, that's a neat little pile," Jim said.

CHAPTER THIRTY-TWO

Janette Owens's death threw the town into overdrive. The citizens were seething with well-proportioned anger. The women were more frightened than ever, and the business community was incensed.

"Swenson was patrolling that very area," cried a voice. "It boggles the mind that the murderer would be so blatant."

The community leaders planned meetings in garages and cellars. Their intended purpose was to arouse the residents enough to cause pressure on the police chief and his men.

It was no surprise to Marty that the most vocal member of the group was the general hardware owner, Fred Pearson. He was an agitator and he always found something to sputter about. Most of the time his roars went unheard. But in light of the recent issues his remarks were focused on the most vulnerable of problems and the townspeople listened with expanded interest. It was a well-known fact that the arrogant shop owner didn't think much of Ethnic Village or its people. He had tried to talk the town members into the purchase of parcels of land, in order to eliminate the lower section of Norwich. He wanted to turn it into a shopping area.

"It's the way of the future," he was quoted in the town paper a few weeks back.

Pearson overlooked a small crowd of people he had gathered in his store. "Let's face it," he insisted. "Most of the trouble starts in the lower section of town and we need to arm ourselves to defend our homes, and businesses."

But the local residents who lived in Ethnic Village also began to congregate after a concerned business friend from the other side of town contacted his friend, Micheal Persocco.

The trusted friend told Mr. Persocco about the assembly and how Mr. Pearson was sure that whoever had committed the murders was from the lower section. "The European community would never give up one of their own," Pearson had warned a group of listeners.

It was at that point that Mr. Persocco convinced the small community of local vendors to have their own encounter. People from every ethnic group and representatives from the different neighborhoods were there to address the concerns that had been raised.

Poppa found out about it and insisted that Millie and Paul go with him and Momma.

The younger Giannettis stood against the wall of the somber room as groups of Polish, Irish and Italian spoke to the audience. They listened to the words of the small council that made up the committee from Ethnic Village. "If this continues it could damage our way of life," a gentleman said, "we depend on the upper area of the Norwich Community for more than half of our business and we don't want to lose that revenue," Mr. Persocco said. "But this isn't just about the money."

Millie's point of view was from behind a beam that held up the corner. She was restless and couldn't be still. It was a sea of faces. People she had known her whole life. The Mercarios were there, and the Tracers. While she looked around at the familiar, she was struck by two people seated in the back row. It was the Kerchaks. They were well hidden and secluded under the shadows of light, quiet and obscure. They sat silent and stone faced caught up in the clamor of angry voices that surrounded them.

It had been a while since Nina had seen them. Mrs.Kerchak sat with a bandana around her head, her face swollen and red. Her eyes pools of emptiness. Mr. Kerchak stared straight ahead. He too had aged. Somehow he didn't appear to be as oppressive as he once seemed. Instead his cheeks were hollow and his shoulders slouched. Millie felt a kinship with the old people. She felt that they had aged in the same dramatic way as her parents.

Momma was seated less than twenty feet away from them. She was still convinced that Josef was Nina's killer. Even now when it was obvious to everyone else that the police were after a different suspect. Millie was concerned about her mother's reaction if she should see the Kerchaks. So Millie decided to move closer to her mother and she would try to deflect her mother's attention. She was sure that the meeting was near a close when she heard one of the members ask for volunteers.

"We do not want women young or old going anywhere at night. The council will arrange for escorts if there are no men in the house," he said.

"We want to form a group that will be in constant touch with the police department."

A representative from the department stood up and spoke for less than a minute about the presence of police in the neighborhood. "It will strengthen ties with the department."

After an hour a board member finally closed. "We will continue again next Tuesday," he said. "Now if there is anyone interested please write your names on this paper."

While Millie went to escort her parents out of the building Paul walked up to place his name on the list.

As the assembly disbanded tiny groups of people stopped and gathered to talk on the way out of the hall. Millie took hold of Momma's arm and tried to guide her out a side door but Poppa stopped to talk with a neighbor. It was too late. Mrs. Giannetti stopped dead in her tracks. She looked at Mrs. Kerchak still seated in the chair, her head low. Momma peered down at the woman who sat like a specter among the crowd. Mrs. Kerchak slowly lifted her eyes and gazed upon the face of her adversary. Tears flowed from her eyes.

Millie watched breathless. Her mother didn't move. She remained stone faced and silent for what seemed like an eternity. Then Momma in a tender manner placed her hand on the shoulder of Grace Kerchak. After a few more seconds she reached for Millie. She took her mother outside where they caught up with Poppa and Paul.

Millie was taken back by her mother's act of empathy. Later that evening she approached her about it.

"Because," her mother said, "we have a lot in common. We have both lost something very precious."

Although her mother's academic capabilities were limited, and Momma had only the basic understanding of the law, she could at times be highly versed in the moral concepts of life. Could she have raised her children with a better view of what to expect? Yes. Did she always do the right thing? Probably not, but Millie understood that what she did share with them was her knowledge of love and her ability to forgive.

Two qualities that helped her parents to survive the rest of their life.

CHAPTER THIRTY-THREE

Martin Sacco knew that this last murder could trigger a town riot. He had heard rumors about the private enclaves and the neighborhood watches. But up to this point they had been carried out peacefully and they helped the residents to feel safe.

Every area faces crime but murder in a small community is generally a lifetime deal. However, Norwich had seen five in a little over a year and because of this the police chief wanted to give the townspeople as much room as they needed.

He also reasoned that with the Kerchak boy in jail it kept him safe from Pearson and the other radicals that didn't care whether he was guilty or not; he felt that Josef could be good fodder for a commotion.

In reality Pearson and his followers were trouble. And Marty's idea of a safe harbor for Josef reversed itself. Pearson was able to use the Kerchak boy's innocence against the police chief. He called a town council emergency meeting and requested the chief's presence.

"What the hell are you boys up to?" Pearson shouted at Marty.

"What does that mean?" Marty asked.

"The Kerchak kid, that's what," Pearson said. He stormed out of his chair and walked up towards the front of the room. His finger pointed at the chief.

"You told us this was pretty well wrapped up and now this. What are you guys—a bunch of incompetent fools?"

"Look," Marty said. "This is an ongoing investigation. And that means that I do not owe you or anyone else an explanation. Frankly, Mr. Pearson, our evidence is none of your business. And I question your motives," he said. "I believe you have more at stake than just the good of this town."

"I resent that," Pearson said.

"Resent it or not, it's the way I see it." Marty was about to sit down but he paused and then said, "Jesus, Fred, you've been at me for months. You should know better."

Marty peered into the crowd. "I do understand your concerns and fears."

"Do you?" a voice called.

Marty looked toward the back of the room and saw Edna Kelly. She pushed through the members and made her way to the front of the assembled group. The older woman stood less than twenty feet away from him. Her dark steely eyes fastened to his.

"Do you," she repeated. "Do you know what it is to walk into a dark house at night and realize that you may suddenly not be alone. Can you," she asked, "even imagine what it feels like to be a woman and be raped? Do you know what it must have been like for those women to know they were about to die?" Edna Kelly stood straight in front of Marty. Her back faced the rest of the group.

"No, sir, I do not believe you do," she said. "Yes I do think you understand my concern. But there is no way, Martin Sacco, that you can relate to my fear."

The police chief was speechless. Miss Kelly turned and walked away. Someone in a moment of mercy adjourned the meeting. Marty picked up his jacket and left the room.

The petite woman had definitely hit him with a one-two punch. She was an active member of The Norwich Business Community. She had owned Edna's Bridal Shop for more than fifteen years and she had been a good friend of Marge Delahunt's. Her viewpoint was more than just fear.

When he walked into his own house he remembered what Edna had said. Exhausted and weary, he looked around at the darkness. He eased his body onto the couch. Marty wanted to grasp what Edna meant when she said, "You can never understand my fear."

But he was a cop, for Christ sake, trained to see things in a more pragmatic way. That didn't mean he couldn't feel pain or see sadness in people's eyes, he just looked at it from a different level.

He tried to imagine what it must have been like for Stephanie Delahunt and Nina Giannetti. He could hear the slow breaths of his wife in the bedroom a few feet away. He suddenly gasped for air.

"You're right, Edna," he said. He had begun to understand her fear. Because he envisioned his own wife alone in the house while a killer waited in the dark, ready to strike.

The weeks that followed Janette Owens's death were full of noise and emotion fueled by the overreaction of the Norwich Business Community. But it soon became evident even to them that if they kept up the negative clamor they stood to lose a lot of money.

On the other hand Ethnic Village was grateful for any distraction that would take the focus off of them.

It was no secret that the two very distinct different neighborhoods tolerated each other. And because of the murders the fear that surrounded the two areas had less tolerance and more visible daily bias.

The one place that continued to be a refuge for both sides was Saint Bartholomew's. Each Sunday as people put differences aside, the church would overflow with parishoners.

Millie watched and listened when her stepbrother appeared on the dias to give the Sunday homily. His speech, though punctuated with Bible verses, was an echo of the sentiments that had overtaken the town. "Through such times of violent turmoil we must grow stronger as a community. I will pray for all of you," he said.

Domenic's voice full of emotion and compassion filled her with pride.

When Millie left the church that Sunday morning she was a little surprised to see the chief of police in the doorway of Saint Bart's.

"Does he always come to Mass, Poppa?"

"I don't think I see him here before. But it's always good when a person comes to church."

Sunday dinner was no longer a big family affair even when Domenic came. But today Momma had promised to make a nice big dinner.

"I make everything you kids like," she said. "Pasta, chicken and sausages. And a big salad for me."

Millie was almost finished setting the dining room table when she heard her mother say, "Domenic, you see us at church?"

It was the first time in months that her mother sounded light-hearted.

"Yes," he said.

The extra workload had begun to show on her brother lately. Monsignor Harrow's illness had put more than the usual pressure on Domenic. Except for a few visit from other priests he was doing most of the masses and the sick calls.

Instead of his jovial good nature, Millie saw a somber and exhausted Domenic when he arrived for Sunday dinner.

"You give a nice homily," Poppa said.

"Thanks," he said, then took a smaller than usual plate of pasta.

"You feel okay?" Momma asked.

"I'm fine," he said. Domenic forced a smile. "I'm just a little overworked."

"Now they give you more responsibility," she said. "And no help. Why don't you call the Archdiocese. Maybe they will send somebody."

"I'll be fine, Momma. All I need is some of your good food."

The family dinner was quiet and for Millie a disappointment. She had anticipated a fun day of conversation and relaxation with her brother. Without Domenic's normal spontaneity everyone just dissolved into their own quiet stillness.

"So Monsignor's been ill, huh," Paul asked.

"Yes and he make Domenic do all the work," Momma said.

Millie ate her meal in between the peppered conversation. She was frustrated and lonely for the better times. She missed all the siblings and the big family dinners.

"Hey, I have to study for a big test tomorrow night," Paul said. He waved goodbye to his brother and walked into his room.

"I have to go too," Domenic said.

"Okay," Momma said. She stood on her toes and kissed her son's cheek. "You don't look good, Domenic, promise me you take care of yourself. I'll say a prayer for you tonight so you feel better."

"Thanks, Momma."

Millie watched Domenic leave. He opened the back door then suddenly spun around. "Goodnight Millie," he said. "Will you say a prayer for me too?"

"Why? You're the priest."

"But you're the angel," he said.

Millie heard the sound of her stepbrother's feet as they scraped against the wood stairs. The meal ended and the day was over. It had disappeared without any diversion. It was just another empty Sunday.

The next day when she came home from school she was surprised but happy to see her mother's face in the kitchen window.

"Hi Momma," she said. Her hope was that Momma had waited for her with baked bread and olive oil. But when she came into the house there was no smell of fresh bread. Instead what she saw was Momma by the window with tears in her eyes.

"I think maybe I sit by the window today. But I don't like to do this anymore," she said. "I'm cold." Momma rubbed her arms for warmth.

She walked over to the front door closet and put her coat on. "I don't know what's wrong," she said. "All day I feel cold in my bones."

There were no windows open, and no visible drafts. Still she complained for the rest of the day.

"I don't know why," she said. "But there is such a chill in this house."

CHAPTER THIRTY-FOUR

A day after his run-in with Edna Kelly the chief decided to bring Fubrowski in for questioning.

"Fiske is in the interrogation room," Taylor told the chief. "He was a busy little bastard while he was in the Navy."

"What do you mean?"

"I just got this from the bureau," Jim said. "Here, read for yourself."

The two men hurried into the 9x12 windowless room and sat down at the gray metal table.

"So," Jim said. "You liked the female sailors."

Fiske kept his eyes down, his two arms outstretched in front of him. "So I like broads," he said, then shifted in his chair. "What's the big deal?"

"I think it was more than like," Jim said. "Let me see. Oh, yeah. 'Fubrowski would stand against the tree and watch us through the window of the female barracks. He wouldn't move for hours and then suddenly he was gone. It was a constant and it scared the wits out of most of the women.'"

He tossed the file on the table.

"So you found out my real name," Fiske said. "Besides they were never able to support those charges."

"You're right," Marty said. "And lucky too."

Fubrowski sat relaxed in the metal chair. He reached in his pocket for a cigarette. "What am I doing here?"

"We were lonely, Victor," Jim said. "We wanted you to spend the day with us."

"I didn't do anything." He removed the butt from his lips. "I just came back to help my old lady."

"What about Dorothy Miller?" the chief asked. "Did you want to help her too?"

"I had nothing to do with that broad's death. I haven't killed anybody. Anyway I wasn't even near here when she died."

"Oh so you have an alibi," Taylor said.

"I was in Boston, with a group of friends."

"What friends?" Marty asked. "Why would I even believe you had any?"

"I can give you their names. I met them in the city about 7:30 that night. I was with Billy Chanowski, Mike Flannigan and a guy they called Big Moose."

"They sound like a real reliable group," Marty said.

A few hours later he told Jim to let him go. "We've got nothing," Marty said. "I've got a call into Boston. Just to see if they come up with anything on those friends of his. But I don't want to come down too hard, not just yet. Make sure there's a tail on him. And notify the State Police. Just in case he decides he wants to leave town."

"You know," Jim said. "Fubrowski and Giannetti grew up together, went to the same high school, competed in track. One of the brothers at Saint John's Seminary told me that Domenic was so good in track that he actually put himself through college."

"Yeah," Marty said.

"Look, I know this is a long shot. Well, I spoke with Brother Joseph. He used to teach a few of Domenic's classes. He offered me a few bits of information. Giannetti was a favorite of Monsignor Harrow's. Father Harrow back then. He even sponsored him for the track team. Then he helped him gain entry into St. John's. But before that he helped him get a part-time job."

Marty eyed the smoke from Jim's cigarette. It floated across the desk then wound its way up to the dingy ceiling. He turned back to the window and watched as the tower from Saint Bartholmew's cast a shadow across the cemetery.

"You know Connie and I haven't seen Don or Marge for almost a year."

"Where are they?"

"Connie got a card a few months back. Said they were somewhere in Maine."

"How is Connie?" he asked.

"Good."

His eyes fixed on a stately woman. From where he stood she reminded him of Stephanie Delahunt. With her long blonde hair and her fur collar turned up against the wind. She held a white box by a string that looked like one of those pastry boxes from Crumbles. *How ironic*, he thought.

He wondered about the other families, like Ed Robinson and Janette Owens's daughter still so devastated by her mother's death. In a small community such sadness cannot be ignored.

He loved this town, the common, the business area with its old-fashioned streetlights. He had seen the changes over the years, a few new enterprises owned by young people on the way up. He heard the complaints made by the school system, too many students, not enough teachers and even less money. And he understood why people had become suspicious of strangers. Why they no longer stopped to chat with their neighbors. The whole town had suffered because of these crimes. Even the obnoxious Fred Pearson had decided not to run for the town committee next year.

Jim spun around in his seat. "What do you say? Should we interview Giannetti?"

"Yeah."

CHAPTER THIRTY-FIVE

"Father Domenic has already left," Mrs.Carr said. "He had to go out of town for a few days."

"Did he say where he was going?" Marty asked.

"Not to me but the Monsignor may know."

"Could we speak with Monsignor Harrow then?"

"He's been so ill lately. Just give me a moment to see if he's able."

Monsignor Harrow looked ill. He had lost a lot of weight and he looked fragile. "Chief Sacco, it is nice to see you again," he said, his voice barely above a whisper.

"We came to talk to Father Giannetti," Marty said, "but your housekeeper said he was out of town. We wondered if you knew just where he went?"

"As I understand it…wait," he said, lifting papers and files. "I have the note here somewhere. Here, it is." Monsignor handed a piece of paper to Marty. It read that he was to leave for a day or two to help a priest at another parish.

"Do you know where?" Jim asked.

"No and that's a bit confusing," Harrow said. "Normally a request like that would be made through me. But it must have come last week while I was sick. Father Domenic was so busy he must have forgot to write where he would be. If it's necessary I can always call the Bishop.

"Is everything all right?" the priest asked. "His family has been through so much lately."

"Nothing like that," Marty said. "We just needed his opinion with an issue."

"Anything I can help with?"

"No," Marty said. "But let me help you." He took hold of the elderly priest's arm and helped him to a seat.

"Thank you," he said, when he regained his composure.

"If you hear from Father Giannetti would you ask him to give me a call?" Marty said.

"I'll do one better," Monsignor said. "I'll put a call into the Bishop for you and find out where he was sent."

Outside by the car Jim commented about Monsignor to Marty.

"He's pretty sick, don't you think?"

"Yeah," Marty said.

"So then why would the Archdiocese send Father Giannetti to another parish?"

"That's a good point. Well, Monsignor said he would call the Bishop. "Let's wait and see what he has to say."

"Look," Marty said. "It's almost lunch time and I'm hungry."

"I could go for one of those Greek chicken sandwiches. But only if you're buying."

"Would we want it any other way," Marty said.

Mrs. Santos didn't greet the two men; instead a young girl met them at the front door.

"Where is Mrs. Stanos?" Jim asked.

"She and Mr. Stanos are in the kitchen."

"Where is their regular cook?" Marty asked.

"I don't know? Vinnie hasn't been around for two days."

The detectives left their seats and bolted through the kitchen door. Nick was at the counter with a knife. A pile of meat sat in front of him. He took the knife and slammed into meat.

"Where's Fiske?" Jim asked.

"Two days ago he called in sick. I haven't seen him since."

Marty rushed to the car and radioed to the dispatch. "Find out who's on Fiske's tail."

"It's Gorman, sir. I can try to reach him by radio."

In less than a minute the dispatcher was back on the line. "Tom checked in an hour ago. He told the duty cop that Fiske was still wrapped up tight in his room at the boarding house." Gorman said, "He's done nothing but sit in his car for a couple of days."

"Call Gormam, tell him Taylor and I are on our way. And send two uniforms just in case."

The cheap boarding house stood on the main street that ran through the center of lower Norwich, a gray building badly in need of paint. The officers shoved the trash away that cluttered the stairway to the entrance. Gorman led them up one flight and pointed to a door with the number five painted on it.

Jim knocked hard.

There was no answer. He knocked again and this time he yelled through the door. "Fiske, open up. It's Detective Taylor."

All he heard was a moan. "Fiske, are you in there? Open up, it's the police."

Marty whispered to the two cops to be ready to shove in the door. When it opened an emaciated Vinnie Fiske stood in the doorway.

"What the fuck do you want," he said. "Can't you see I'm sick?"

Fiske practically fell over. The two officers grabbed him and placed him on the bed. Marty walked into the dingy room. Dirty clothes were everywhere. The room smelled of vomit and urine so thick Marty gagged. He looked over at Fiske, his body pale and sweaty. On the night table next to the bed was a tray full of dirty dishes.

"How long have you been like this?" Marty asked.

"I don't know. Maybe a couple of days."

"Have you seen a doctor?" Jim said.

"No," he said. He tried to sit up. "Leave me alone, will you?"

"Yeah," Marty replied.

"Stay put," Marty told Gorman. "Let me know if he leaves that room."

"Have you heard anything from Shapiro yet about the Kerchak kid?" Jim asked.

"No," Marty said.

Earlier Jim had gone to see the judge about the Kerchak boy. Josef had been in jail for months. And Marty wanted him released. He felt the kid's family life had already left him with a damaged psyche. And he wanted to do whatever he could to help Shapiro get the charges dropped and the kid released and sent home. But he hadn't heard anything from the attorney in a few days.

"Then everything must be fine," Jim said. "Otherwise Shapiro's big mouth would be flapping all over this town."

It was five o'clock and Marty was exhausted. He was just about to walk out the door when his phone buzzed.

"Hello, Chief Sacco. It's Monsignor Harrow."

"Yes, Monsignor."

"I'm sorry it has taken me so long to get back to you. I did call the Bishop right after you left. But he just returned my call."

"That's not a problem," Marty said. He slipped back on the chair behind the desk. "Did he tell you where he sent Father Giannetti?"

"Well, I guess I misunderstood," he said. "Bishop Keene told me that Father Dom wasn't assigned anywhere. It is a bit odd but he must have just gone on a personal journey for a day or two. The best I can do is give him your message when he calls."

"Thank you, Monsignor, I would appreciate that." Marty placed the receiver back on the base.

"Where is he?" Taylor asked.

"On a personal journey," Marty said. "That's what the Monsignor called it."

"That bastard has been right under our noses all this time."

"Hold on," Marty said. "We have even less evidence against him than we do with Fiske."

"Something about that guy always bothered me," Jim said. "From our first conversation."

"I even checked him out with FBI."

"Yeah. What did they have?"

"Nothing."

"Of course they would have nothing. He's a priest. I'm going home," he said and picked up his jacket. He turned to Jim. "Either way, all we have is a priest who might be away for a few days and a hunch. None of it is gonna get us a conviction."

But Jim wasn't satisfied. He took a cigarette out of his pocket.

"What about the Giannettis?" he said. "Maybe they know where he is." Marty held his coat to his chest and sloped against the wall. "I don't know."

"Maybe he told his brother Paul."

"I don't think so."

"What if he just hinted something to the mother. Something she didn't even pick up."

Marty knew Jim was right. He could have slipped a remark to someone in the family.

"First thing in the morning we'll go out to the house and talk with the mother and father."

"Hey Chief," Doherty called out. "Something just arrived for you by special delivery."

"I am never gonna get home," Marty cried. "My wife doesn't even recognize me anymore."

"Go home," Jim said. "Whatever it is it can wait till the morning."

He took the envelope from Doherty and placed it on the chief's desk. Marty walked out the front door.

The next morning when he sat at his desk he remembered the package. He picked it up. On the front it read to Chief Martin Sacco. There was no return address and no postage marks. He tore the top corner. Inside was a letter. He removed it and unfolded it. Then he did what he always did he scanned the last page for a signature.
"Jesus H. Christ," he yelled. "Doherty come here."
"What's the matter?" Jim said.
"What is it, Chief?" Doherty said.
"Who delivered this package yesterday?"
"I don't know, it was left on my desk when I came back from lunch."
"What?" Jim asked. "What is it?"
"It's from Domenic Giannetti."
He perched himself against the desk and began to silently read the letter. *Chief Sacco: I don't expect you to understand what I have done. That is not my intention for writing. It is just my way of trying to cleanse my soul.*
"Read it out loud, will you?" Jim asked.
"Yeah, yeah," Marty said.

> *I have lived in two separate worlds for as long as I can remember. One full of anger and hate and the other seething with terrifying confusion and religious despair. Even as a young child I knew that I would have to live in the presence of a divinity in order to release my soul of the evil that existed within it.*
>
> *I have always been haunted by the shadow of my mother, a bonding so strong that I felt isolated by her death. In many ways I blamed my father for her death and the insecurity that I was left with when he, too, abandoned me by scattering his affections into another life, one that kept me alone and even more isolated.*
>
> *When Nina came along I believed she was my soul mate. She was quiet and, unaffected by the rest of the world, a loner like me. Nina was so young. So easy to love, something of my own that I could use to help me do what I wanted in order to be free. I needed her pure soul to cleanse my own. She was my sanctuary. The only true innocence I have ever known. I believed her to be*

the purest moments in my life. And because of her I had to rid myself of the evil temptations that were constantly moving around me.

I knew those women wanted more from me than I could give. Each one of them was sent as an enticement to pull me further away from the life I had chosen. Each one worked their destruction in different ways trying to gather me in little bits and pieces. Mrs. Miller wanted me to help her regain the sanctity of the church after her divorce. Mrs. Robertson was unhappy in her marriage and couldn't tell her husband. And young Stephanie Delahunt, she was perhaps the worse of all. Always calling to ask about the wedding. "What should we use for an entrance song?" Or some other mundane question. When I arrived at her house that night, she acted so sweet, so welcoming. But I knew different. I told her that her game was wasted on me. I knew what was in her heart and I was going to drive away the evil.

Marty stopped for a minute. He felt outraged. His words left the police chief with a sense of disgust and sickness that was somewhere in the deep crevices of his own soul. He pulled a handkerchief out of his pocket and wiped the sweat off his face. He cleared his throat and then continued.

One night while I went for a walk I saw the shed light still on. When I walked in she was asleep. I sat there quietly to watch her. She was so beautiful, so clean. I leaned over and kissed her face and she awoke immediately. But she was angry and told me to leave her alone. All I wanted to do was talk. But she didn't want me near her.

"No," she yelled, "I don't want you to touch me anymore." She cried, "This is all wrong."

I told her it wasn't wrong. I told her not to worry because it didn't matter God loved her.

I tried to explain how it was through her that I was whole. That she cleansed my mind and heart. But she wouldn't listen. She kept crying louder and louder.

"We're bonded," I said. But she screamed, "I hate you, I hate you. You disgust me." Her eyes were so cold and full of revenge.

It was then I realized Nina had been corrupted.

"I'm going to tell Poppa," she threatened. I knew that she had to be stopped like the others. "Please, Nina," I begged. "Be quiet."

She went on and on about Poppa and the church. So I had to stop her. You do understand that, Chief Sacco. I couldn't have her tell Poppa. So I had to do what I did. Finally she fell against the wall, limp. When she died I knew it was over for me.

"What a sick son-of-bitch," Jim cried.

I realized with Nina's death that any good I had found was now lost to me. That neither she nor my collar had ever shielded me from the burning desires. Nor had they been able to insulate me against the rage. Still the priesthood had helped me to vanquish a guilty conscience, for each time I had destroyed the consuming demons I found a refuge within the shadows of Saint Bartholomew's steeple.

After my stepsister's death I was haunted by each of the women. They invaded my mind and put limitations on my soul. And in the end I knew it was only a matter of time before they would be able to destroy the very essence of what I am. Nothing could save me any more. Not now when the only pure thing I ever knew lay like the others in a bloody heap against the cold floor.

Marty folded the letter and placed it on his desk. He didn't have any words. He just stared out the window at the tower of Saint Bart's.

Jim was always the more pragmatic. He pulled a cigarette out of his shirt pocket. "How are we gonna deal with this? This one is gonna be tricky," he said. "The newspapers are gonna blow this right out of the water."

CHAPTER THIRTY-SIX

It was a clear November day when Millie looked at the sky and thought about the coming holidays. She knew the season would be different with Nina gone but she was forever hopeful. At nearly seventeen she had an imagination and the brightness of a future still burned within her dreams.

That afternoon she arrived home from school and was thrilled to find Momma in the kitchen. "Here," she said.

Millie took the freshly baked piece of bread and dipped it in the olive oil on the table. "Momma this is so good. You haven't made bread in a long time."

"I know, Poppa asked me this morning," she said. "Millie, do me a favor. When you go to your room will you please take the laundry basket?"

She dunked another piece of bread. Millie headed for the back hall. She felt good dipping the bread in the olive oil; it made her think of earlier times. It was comfortable for her. She picked up the laundry basket and saw the police chief and the detective approach the back porch.

"Hello, Millie," Chief Sacco said. "Is your brother Paul here?"

"No, he's at work. What do you want with him?"

Momma heard the voices because she called, "Who is it?" When she saw the two men there she walked onto the porch.

"What do you want?" she asked.

"We just needed to speak with your son. Can you tell me where we can reach him?"

Millie wrote his work number on a piece of paper and handed it to him. She watched them walk down the steps and then get into the car and pull away. She could sense there was something wrong. She could tell by the look on the police chief's face. *What now?* she thought. *What did Paul do?*

Her brother never really showed any empathic emotions. He was into that man thing. Be strong and never let your guard down. But today when he arrived home his face was wet from tears. Whatever the cops wanted was gonna make for an another banner day in the Giannetti household.

"Domenic did it," he screamed from the back door. "I can't believe this."

"What did Domenic do?" Momma asked. Poppa strolled in behind her.

Paul looked disheveled. And he spoke in breathless phrases. "He wrote a letter to the police," he said. "He told them he was the one."

"What?" Poppa said. "The one what?"

"He said it was him that molested Nina. That he's the one who killed all those girls."

Poppa lifted his hand. "Stop it," he said. And smashed it against Paul's face. "I don't want to hear no more."

Millie's brother fell on his knees. "It's true, Poppa," he said. "Domenic is the murderer. He killed all those women."

The room became charged with chaos. Momma plopped herself on to the couch. "Are you crazy?" she said. "Who tell you this?" Her face grew tight and she glared toward her son. Tears fell from her cheeks.

"Why? Why would Domenic do such a thing?"

"Because he is crazy," Paul said.

"No," Poppa screamed. "You are the one. And you try to blame your brother."

Paul burrowed himself into a corner. He sat with his legs up against his chest and his head rested on his knees. "How do you know this?" Millie asked.

"The police have a letter from Domenic. I read it."

Paul shook his head. "You think I wanted to believe it," he said. "I told them it was a lie. Somebody just made it up. But I knew it was Domenic. I recognized his handwriting."

Up until now Poppa had paced the parlor floor. Now he sat in the large chair by the couch. "You think I'm gonna believe this about my son," he said. "No. Never, I don't care who tell me this. Unless Domenic tell me to my face I'm no gonna believe any of it."

He closed his eyes and leaned back in his seat. "Why? Why they blame my son for something like this? He's a good boy, always work hard and study."

"Jesu Christ," Momma said. She lifted her hand in the air, her face full of bitterness, "You haven't given us enough to struggle with. Now you give us this."

Millie was dumbfounded. She began to cry. "Did you call Domenic?" she asked Paul.

"Yes." He nodded. "I tried to reach him but he's not at the rectory. And Monsignor doesn't know where he is. That's why the police came to see me. They thought I might know where he is. He ran away because he's guilty. He murdered all those women including our sister. My brother is a rapist and a murderer!" the boy yelled. "The priest is a sick fuck, a poor sick fuck!" he shrieked, and ran out of the room.

Millie ran towards the kitchen door and down the back steps into the fresh night air. The cool clean air fell against her skin. *Domenic killed those women?* Her mind traced her brother's words. *Including our sister.*

It was clear to her now. Nina would never have told on Domenic. He was the one who had made their parents most proud. Poppa held him up as an example. He was the one who had climbed the mountain and found success. "Poor Nina." In order for Domenic to leave her alone she would have to destroy Poppa.

Millie cried all the way to the old deserted railroad station and walked along the edge of the tracks. She balanced herself on the wood ties and wandered along the field and the high brush slapped against her leg the way it used to. Each piece of broken glass she saw reminded her of her sister. And how Nina must have felt. She paid little attention to where she was. Until she finally looked up and realized she was at the entrance of the cemetery where her sister was buried.

The specter of Saint Bartholomew's was visible by the old-fashioned streetlight. The shadow of the tower flowed across the stone landscape like a black veil.

Millie walked across the graves until she came upon her sister.

"Nina," she cried. When she knelt down next to the plaque to pray her knees rested upon the cold wet grass that surrounded the grave. She outlined the letters of her sister's name with her finger. She saw the basket of flowers and took out the small envelope that lay on top. She placed it in her pocket.

"Please God give Nina peace," she cried. Her voice echoed against the emptiness. "Help my brother Paul who has suddenly become the bearer of all this sadness."

And she begged God to spare her parents of anymore grief. Millie did pray for her stepbrother, but mostly she prayed for herself, hoping that she would be able to forgive Domenic. Because she knew that if she couldn't it would eventually destroy her.

The girl returned to Prescott Street and walked up the back steps. She wandered into the kitchen and glanced toward her Mother's chair. A small night-light cast a grim shadow on the empty seat. It seemed all so dreadfully clear, she thought as she opened the door to her bedroom. She sat on the bed and took the envelope out of her pocket. What she read became the foundation of despair towards her brother.

> *If I could have saved you from myself I would have. It was never my intention to hurt you. In the eyes of God and everyone, including myself, I realize now there is no excuse for what I did to those women. Any explanation would only sound like the deranged defense it is. I will surely burn in Hell for all these acts and deservedly so.*
>
> *But I had to reach you beyond the grave, Nina, because I will not meet up with you in some form of heavenly slumber. And I couldn't leave this world without letting you know that I realize now what I did to you was wrong. But in my own demented way you were mine. When I touched you I believed it was because I had something of my own to love.*
>
> *Domenic*

Her stepbrother's words placed her into a reality she couldn't escape. He was the molester, the murderer and the killer of dreams.

She walked to the bureau and opened the top drawer. There it was, the tiny white envelope she had found on the day of Nina's funeral. She placed them both on the bed. They were the identical. Even the handwritten words across the front were the same. *I'm sorry.*

CHAPTER THIRTY-SEVEN

Yep, this is a hard one, the chief admitted quietly. *I don't even want to think about poor Monsignor Harrow or the Archdiocese for that matter. I can't even imagine what this town will be like when the papers cover the trial.*

When he took the job as police chief he thought of it as his port of entry into quiet retirement, Marty reflected wearily. Now this case had definitely placed him closer to retirement.

"I'll be at home!" he said. Marty walked out the door and down the steps of the station house. Maybe it was time to get out of police work and do the things Connie had always talked about.

"Do I know you?" Connie said. A big smile crossed her lips when she greeted her husband.

"Very funny."

"How about you and me do dinner and a few drinks?"

Connie and him hadn't spent this much time together in months, he thought as he watched his wife walk across the restaurant floor. He enjoyed his wife and the steak dinners. After a few drinks they went home, watched some television and then they settled into bed together.

It was the first time in weeks Marty had been to bed and actually slept; until the next morning when the phone woke him at 6:30 a.m.

"Hello," he grumbled into the receiver.

"Chief, we've got something," Jim said.

"Christ, not another body?

Yeah, I'll be there in ten minutes. Be ready?"

Marty hung up the phone and rubbed his face with his hands. "Who now?" By the time Jim came he was outside on the sidewalk.

"Who is it this time?"

"The body was found at Saint Bart's."

Not that sweet old lady, Mrs. Carr, he thought. Five minutes later the wheels of the police car screeched at the curb in front of the church.

"Who called you on this?" Marty asked.

"Doherty was at the duty desk when the hit came in. He called me."

The massive oak door of the church opened. "Hi Chief," the uniformed officer said. "Wait till you see this." He led Sacco and Taylor towards the tower.

The three men rushed up the musty staircase in the old section. It was cold and the wind howled through the eaves.

"It feels like a graveyard in here," Jim said.

Two more cops stood in the doorway. "Who found the body?" Jim asked.

"The night watchman," he said. "He's over there."

Jim walked over to speak with the night watchman but Marty moved towards the bell tower. He opened the door of the anteroom and then pushed open the door to the tower. Wood rafters ran across the ceiling joists.

The police chief walked to the middle of the room and looked up twenty feet to the top. Hanging from one of the rafters he saw a body. It dangled from a rope. Wind filtered through an open section which caused the body to sway back and forth.

"Get him down," he shouted.

Jim wandered in and looked up. "It was old Kennedy who found him," he said. "When he went to the tower for the usual 6:00 ring. He noticed one of the bells was stuck. So he pulled hard on the rope but it wouldn't budge. That's when he walked in here and found him."

Marty watched the men on the ladders as they tried to manipulate the priest's body from the rafter. They placed him on the stainless steel dolly. Domenic Giannetti was dressed in a white robe that barely covered his feet.

"It was his only way out," Jim said.

Marty wasn't surprised that the young priest took his own life. It must have seemed like his only choice. He walked over to where his body had been placed. A small brown bag hung from a sash around his waist. Marty slid the pouch off the belt and opened it. The he emptied the contents in his hand.

"Thirty pieces of silver," Jim said. "Do you remember the story of Judas?"

Marty nodded yes.

Everybody knew what happened to Judas. "He was paid thirty pieces of silver to betray Christ. But he was so full of guilt he hung himself."

"Well, this is Domenic's thirty pieces of silver," Jim said. "It's his payment to the devil in order to enter the gates of hell."

Marty put the coins back in the bag and placed it in his pocket.

"I need some air," he said. He walked away from the tower and ran down the narrow steps of the steeple. The cemetery gate was open and he walked in. Here among the dead was that final peace. Yet for the living that kind of peace is incomprehensible to understand, a complex irony. Much like Domenic. He seemingly worked so hard for something that was nothing more than a contradiction.

Jim drove the car up to the cemetery gate. Marty sat on a stone wall and watched him light up a cigarette. *Now there's a contradiction in life.* He smiled and walked towards the car.

He slid across the passenger's seat and said, "I guess we should tell the Giannettis."

"How will we phrase it?" Jim said. "Your son committed rape, murder and finally, suicide. He was a priest who dishonored his vows and the Ten Commandments."

"Someone even the devil doesn't want," Marty said.

CHAPTER THIRTY-EIGHT

The Giannetti family knew when they heard the doorbell ring at 7:30 in morning that it was not good news. Paul opened the front door to a young uniformed policeman. "Chief Sacco has sent a car to take you to his office."

Paul never asked why. He just told the cop to wait outside and he would be there in ten minutes. Later he told Millie that he knew Domenic would kill himself rather than have to face what he did.

When he returned from the morgue the boy gathered his sister and his parents into the parlor. "I'm not gonna lie to you," he said. "You need to know everything."

Momma and Poppa were inconsolable. For the Giannettis it was the final swing of the axe. All of them were so overburdened with confusion, sadness. And by now weary from grief.

Millie's heart ached for Momma and Poppa but it broke for her brother Paul. In their ignorance he was blamed because he was the messenger. He was the one they could blame for the final chaos.

"Why you all the time bringing me bad news?" his mother asked. "I never believe this from Domenic, maybe Tommy or Paul," Millie heard her father say.

"Why, why do they think like that?" she asked him. She was grateful he didn't have an answer. In reality she knew it was easier to attack a person, who was alive and always there, then to try and hate a ghost.

"Nothing could be more wrong than to lose a child," Momma had said. Now she had lost two.

And the girl didn't believe life could be worse for her family after Nina's passing. But she was to learn that after Domenic's death each day grew worse. Her world had been sad for a while but now it would change into turmoil. When a newspaper was tossed on the Giannettis' back porch the next morning they awoke to the headline: "Sex-driven homicidal priest commits suicide in the church tower."

The papers were relentless. They kept the family tied to the news every day. For a week they did a series about each of his victims with his picture posted next to the unfortunate women. One paper even showed a picture of Domenic saying the last rites at one of the funerals. They printed what information they had about Nina from her diaries and excerpted parts of her brother's letter. And they printed the words side by side on the front page.

Everyone was shattered followed by a mixture of pity and revulsion. With a definitive hatred as the neighborhood ostracized the Giannetti family. They were maligned and victimized over and over again.

People the Giannettis had grown up with passed them like vermin on the street. Their downstairs tenants were jeered and scoffed at, eventually they moved from the town. Merchants in the village where they had done business for years now refused them access to their stores. A simple grocery errand could turn into a fiasco that would leave Millie horrified and devastated.

The animosity traveled along the aisle of St. Bart's church. One night Monsignor sent the new pastor to visit the Giannettis.

"Come in," Momma welcomed. She thought he was there to give them comfort. Instead he sat down at the kitchen table and told her and Poppa that it would be appreciated if they didn't attend Sunday Mass at Saint Bart's any longer. "It would be better if you went to one of the other towns for Mass. Some place no one knows you."

"But why?" Poppa said. "I go here all my life."

"Monsignor is afraid for your safety," he said. "We do not want to be responsible."

"But my parents did nothing wrong," Paul said. "If you take the church away from Poppa it will kill him."

"I am very sorry," the priest said, "those are my orders."

Poppa didn't stop going to church. But week after week he would attend Mass and no one would sit next to him. One morning when he returned from Mass, he said, "I don't understand. They stand in the back of the church when my row is empty."

The Archdiocese tried to hide from the press but eventually cleared themselves by vilifying Domenic from the church pulpit. His burial was a sad affair for many reasons. There was not a funeral service in town that would allow a wake for him. And of course he had to be buried outside the Catholic cemetery in an unmarked plot without benefit or blessings from a priest. Even members of his family refused to attend.

Chief Sacco was the one that found a burial plot for the young priest in a municipal cemetery. And he volunteered to say a small prayer over the grave. After the ceremony he walked over to Paul and Millie.

"I found these on your brother the night he died," he said, then he handed the brown pouch to the boy. "I believe this was a way of repentance."

The two siblings looked inside and saw the money. Millie told Marty later that her and Paul had placed the coins in a catholic church a few towns away. They hoped that by doing that it would give Domenic a shove towards the gates of heaven.

At first the family wanted desperately not to believe what they were being told about their stepbrother. But as time went on they knew it was true. The other siblings tried to visit with their parents on a weekly basis, then monthly. Finally when the weight of Domenic's deed had taken its toll and the stigma began to attach itself to the Giannetti name, self-preservation became evident.

"We have children," Tommy explained. "We have to do this." And he changed their name.

While her brother and sisters agreed with the theory that Domenic's behavior stemmed from his mother's grip even in death, Millie saw her stepbrother's problem as going far beyond the grave. Even now they continued to ignore the issues by placing the blame on a young woman who had been dead for thirty years. Millie knew Domenic's problems went way beyond that sad perception. What caused Domenic to walk along the devil's floor would take more than her family's simple speculation.

As usual their remarks plundered not only Millie's perception of the family's beliefs but it vividly stomped on her sister's grave. She couldn't understand if they were masters of denial or if it was irresponsible acceptance of anything that a family member did. She was troubled and anxious by their defenses and she came to realize how truly dysfunctional her family was.

When she realized the close relationship that she believed existed had all but disappeared, she began to isolate herself from the rest of the Giannettis.

Not that Millie blamed them for not visiting. If it had been possible for her to shrink from the earth she would have. But unlike the others she was still too young to walk away. So she pleaded with her parents to sell the house and move.

"It's our home," Momma said. "You don't move away from your home not with all the memories that still live here, no matter what they are."

And so they stayed. Paul too.

Momma and Poppa continued to live in their home and abide by the same customs and habits for the remainder of their lives.

But the rest of the family moved on in a desperate attempt to put their world back together. In doing so they ignored the trauma of the past. Unable to handle the ordeal, Domenic was rarely mentioned.

Ironically the only friend Momma was left with was Grace Kerchak. She befriended the Giannettis for years and after George died her relationship with Momma became even more important to both of them. They had in some strange way learned to heal the wounds that had been allowed to fester too long.

Poppa was never the same after Domenic's death. He turned further inward. Her rarely spoke to anyone. Instead he preferred his own company. He neither worked in the garden nor went for walks. His days consisted of solitaire and old cowboy movies that prompted him to cry. Most nights he sat alone on the porch.

Momma's heart had been broken with Nina's death and for her Domenic just compounded the pain. She had lost the spark that Millie remembered while growing up. She no longer baked bread or made fresh pasta. It was an effort for her to change from the nightgown and slippers. There were days when she never ventured out of bed, choosing instead to stay locked up in her room to cry. Many nights as Millie passed by her room she could hear her mother pray, "Please, Jesu Christ. You let me die tonight?" And ironically it was in death that Millie finally saw her smile.

The threats from the town dwindled as old people died and new couples moved in. The town of Norwich did not prosper through the years. Instead the prettiness of the town became buried in unsightly strip malls and rows of brick apartment houses. Many of the local business people and community members sold out to developers who promised a seat to the future with higher revenues.

Chief Sacco and the small Norwich Police Department was changed when the town was declared a city because of its growing population. Millie heard that his wife died of breast cancer five years later.

The steeple that towered over the commons looks lost and a bit shabby today. The Christian values it represented have become compromised and weary. Now when Millie drives past the common it is overgrown with weeds and homeless people. The pretty section that housed Pearson's Hardware and Edna Kelly's Bridal Shop is nothing but empty stores with large "for rent" signs pasted against dirty windows.

Today Ethnic Village appears dismal and gloomy. The streets are scattered with people who wear torn clothing and rest in open doorways. Their glassy eyes follow Millie along the littered and dirty streets.

What she once knew, as a sharing of cultures and renewal of pride, is now nothing more than a habitat for the unemployed and drug infested.

A familiar man walks along the street, his thin body weary and he leans against a building. His empty eyes peer through the passenger side of Millie's car. In his lips he holds a cigarette.

It is in that one swift moment when Millie stares into his face that she is grateful. Although she let go of the past she never lost the memories. She still sees her sister in the flowers, and she smells the talcum powder they shared in the wind. The sounds of the footsteps and the slammed porch door are always in the back of her mind. It is the part of her life that has helped her realize who she is.

And the poor soul still visible from the rear view mirror, his timid smile makes it obvious to Millie that it is Josef Kerchak. Still lonely, alone and sad because he has never been able to escape from the memories of his past.

Printed in the United States
51527LVS00004B/190-213

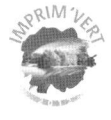 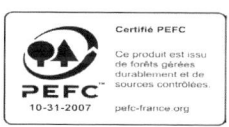

Imprimé en France par EMD S.A.S. en mai 2012
53110 Lassay-les-Châteaux
Dépôt légal : janvier 2011
N° d'imprimeur : 26698
N° 1309 (I) – GP 80°

Réalisation : Compo-Méca sarl
64990 Mouguerre

Gastrectomie 22, 46, 121, 141, 204, 266
Gastrite 46, 204, 248, 266
 – aiguë 22

H

Hémorragies digestives hautes 22
Hépatites 266
Hernie hiatale 204, 265
Hypercatabolisme 62, 88
 – (polytrauma) 269
Hypertension artérielle 72, 131, 151, 163, 166, 179, 269
Hyperuricémie 93
Hypoglycémies 131, 151
 – réactives fonctionnelles 268
Hypothyroïdie 72

I

Infarctus 163, 166
Infections aiguës 62, 269
Insuffisance
 – cardiaque 61, 163, 166, 169, 269
 – hépatique 111, 267
 – rénale 187
 – rénale aiguë 93, 164, 172, 267
 – rénale chronique 62, 93, 164, 169, 267
 – rénale terminale 179, 267
 – respiratoire chronique 62, 267
Intolérance aux protéines de lait de vache 268

L

Lavement baryté 237, 270
Leucinose 268
Lithiase 72
 – biliaire 266

M

Maladie
 – cardiovasculaire 72
 – cœliaque 87, 255, 270
 – de Crohn 87, 194, 204, 237, 266

O

Œsophagites 46, 265
Ostéomalacie 269
Ostéoporose 269

P

Pancréatectomie 204, 267
Pancréatite 111, 267
Pathologies
 – digestives chroniques 87
 – hypercatabolisantes 87
 – infectieuses 87
 – neurodégénératives/psychiatriques 269
 – neuropsychiatriques et neurodégénératives 62
Phénylcétonurie 268
Post-infarctus 101, 248, 269

R

Rectocolite hémorragique 87, 204, 237, 266
Reflux gastro-œsophagien 204, 265
Régime de sortie 11
Ruptures de varices œsophagiennes 22

S

Sténoses œsophagiennes 265
Surcharge pondérale 72, 88, 268
Syndrome néphrotique 88, 93, 169, 172, 267

T

Thrombose 163, 269
Troubles
 – de la déglutition 46
 – de la mastication 46
 – fonctionnels intestinaux 266
 – gastriques 46

U

Ulcère
 – gastrique 46
 – gastroduodénal 266

Index des pathologies

A

Anémies 88, 268
Ascite 121, 164, 169
Athéromatose 101
Athérosclérose 163, 269

C

Cancer 46, 61, 72, 204, 266, 267
   – de l'estomac 22, 265
   – de l'intestin grêle 204, 265
   – de l'œsophage 265
   – de la gorge 46
   – de la langue 46
   – du côlon 204
   – gastrique 46
Chirurgie
   – cardiaque 62, 269
   – digestive 33, 46
   – digestive haute 265, 266
Cholécystectomie 204, 267
Cirrhose 22, 88, 93, 164, 166, 169, 172, 204, 266
Coloscopie 237, 270
Constipation 193, 194, 200, 204, 266
Corticothérapie 88, 151, 164, 166, 169, 172, 269
Crises ulcéreuses gastriques 22

D

Dénutrition 22, 46, 61, 62, 63, 87, 268
Diabète 72, 121, 131, 151, 268
Diarrhées 18, 194, 200, 201, 204, 217, 237
   – aiguës et chroniques 266
Diverticules 194, 201
Diverticulites 266
Diverticulose 194
   – colique 266
Duodénopancréatectomie céphalique 204, 267
Dyslipidémies 72, 87, 268
Dysphagie 33, 46

E

Encéphalopathie hépatique 94, 267
Enquête alimentaire 7

F

Fistules 19, 237
   – digestives 266
Fracture 33
Fructosémie 268

G

Galactosémie 268

Pathologie	Prescription pouvant être proposée
Intolérance aux disaccharides (lactose et saccharose)	Suppression du lactose et du saccharose
Mucoviscidose	– Régime hyperprotidique – Régime hypolipidique – Régime hypersodique
Maladie cœliaque	– Régime sans gluten – Régime hyperprotidique – Régime hyperénergétique

7. *Les explorations spécialisées*

Coloscopie	– Régimes pauvres en résidus
Lavement baryté	– Régimes pauvres en résidus – Régimes pauvres en fibres

Collection « BTS diététique »
dirigée par Cristian Carip

Régimes

Émilie Fredot
Diététicienne – nutritionniste
Enseignante en science diététique
Institut de commerce et de gestion (ICOGES), Paris

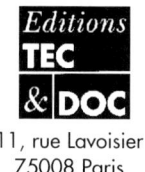

11, rue Lavoisier
75008 Paris

Dans la même collection

Préparer l'épreuve de biochimie-physiologie
O. Masson, 2e édition, 2011

Préparer l'épreuve de physiopathologie
C. Carip, F. Louet, S. Gendron, 3e édition, 2011

Microbiologie-hygiène – Bases microbiologiques de la diététique
C. Carip, 2008

Nutrition du bien-portant – Bases nutritionnelles de la diététique
É. Fredot, 2007

Biochimie – Bases biochimiques de la diététique
O. Masson, 2e édition, 2007

Physiologie – Bases physiologiques de la diététique
C. Carip, 2004

Physiopathologie – Bases physiopathologiques de la diététique
C. Carip, 2e édition, 2004

Économie-gestion – Bases économiques, financières et juridiques de la diététique
M. Camus, 2e édition, 2004

Techniques culinaires – Bases culinaires de la diététique
L. Cariel, V. Liégeois, M.-H. Salavert, 2002

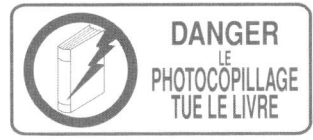

© **LAVOISIER, 2011**

ISBN : 978-2-7430-1309-7
ISSN : 1963-1987

Toute reproduction ou représentation intégrale ou partielle, par quelque procédé que ce soit, des pages publiées dans le présent ouvrage, faite sans l'autorisation de l'éditeur ou du Centre français d'exploitation du droit de copie (20, rue des Grands-Augustins, 75006 Paris), est illicite et constitue une contrefaçon. Seules sont autorisées, d'une part, les reproductions réservées à l'usage privé du copiste et non destinées à une utilisation collective, d'autre part, les analyses et courtes citations justifiées dans le caractère scientifique ou d'information de l'œuvre dans laquelle elles sont incorporées (loi du 1er juillet 1992 – art. L. 122-4 et L. 122-5 et Code pénal art. 425).

Table des matières

Introduction à l'alimentation thérapeutique 1
1. Présentation de la prise en charge diététique ou de la prescription diététique ... 1
2. Les différentes composantes de la prise en charge nutritionnelle 2

Chapitre 1

L'enquête alimentaire ou l'interrogatoire alimentaire ─────── 5
   Introduction 5
1. Données générales concernant le patient et son environnement 5
2. Histoire médicale du patient et données associées 6
3. Étude des besoins nutritionnels 6
4. Étude des apports alimentaires 7
   4.1. Questions préalables 7
   4.2. Mise en pratique de l'enquête alimentaire individuelle 7
5. Les objectifs particuliers de la prescription 10
6. Remise du régime de sortie
   (c'est-à-dire de la prescription diététique personnalisée) 11

Partie 1
Principaux types de prescriptions thérapeutiques

Section 1
Prescriptions nécessitant une modification de la texture

Chapitre 2

Les régimes à texture liquide — 17

Introduction 17
1. Le régime de la diète hydrique 17
   1.1. Définition et principe 17
   1.2. Les indications 18
   1.3. Couverture des besoins et apports nutritionnels conseillés 18
   1.4. Le choix des aliments 19
   1.5. En pratique 21
2. Le régime liquide lacté ou régime liquide froid 21
   2.1. Définition et principe 21
   2.2. Les indications 22
   2.3. Couverture des besoins et apports nutritionnels conseillés 22
   2.4. Le choix des aliments 24
   2.5. En pratique 29
   2.6. Exemple de ration, de répartition et de menu 31
3. Le régime liquide large 33
   3.1. Définition et principe 33
   3.2. Les indications 33
   3.3. Couverture des besoins et apports nutritionnels conseillés 33
   3.4. Le choix des aliments 35
   3.5. En pratique 41
   3.6. Exemple de ration, de répartition et de menu 41

Chapitre 3

Les régimes à texture molle — 45

1. Définition et principe 45
2. Les indications 46
   2.1. Les troubles de la mastication 46
   2.2. Les troubles de la déglutition (dysphagies) 46
   2.3. Les troubles gastriques nécessitant de ralentir la motilité de l'estomac
        (et par conséquence le péristaltisme) 46
   2.4. Autre chirurgie digestive en postopératoire 46
   2.5. Autres indications 46
3. Couverture des besoins et apports nutritionnels conseillés 47
   3.1. L'énergie 47
   3.2. Les protéines 47

3.3. Les lipides	47
3.4. Les glucides	47
3.5. Les fibres	48
3.6. Les vitamines	48
3.7. Les minéraux	48
3.8. L'eau	48
4. Le choix des aliments	48
5. En pratique	55
6. Exemple de ration, de répartition et de menu	56
6.1. Exemple de ration d'un régime de texture molle à 8 MJ/jour	56
6.2. Exemple de répartition d'un régime de texture molle à 8 MJ/jour	57
6.3. Exemple de menu d'un régime de texture molle à 8 MJ/jour	58

Section 2
Prescriptions nécessitant une modification des apports conseillés en énergie

Chapitre 4

Le régime hyperénergétique — 61

1. Définition et principe	61
2. Les indications	61
3. Objectifs nutritionnels	62
4. Couverture des besoins et apports nutritionnels conseillés	62
4.1. L'énergie	62
4.2. Les protéines	63
4.3. Les lipides	63
4.4. Les glucides	64
4.5. Les fibres, les vitamines, les minéraux et l'eau	64
5. Le choix des aliments	64
6. En pratique	65
7. Exemple de ration, de répartition et de menu	67
7.1. Exemple de ration d'un régime hyperénergétique-hyperprotidique à 12,3 MJ/jour	67
7.2. Exemple de répartition d'un régime hyperénergétique-hyperprotidique à 12,3 MJ/jour	68
7.3. Exemple de menu d'un régime hyperénergétique-hyperprotidique à 12,3 MJ/jour	69

Chapitre 5

Le régime hypoénergétique ou hypocalorique — 71

1. Définition et principe	71
2. Les indications	72
3. Couverture des besoins et apports nutritionnels conseillés	73
3.1. L'énergie	73

3.2. Les protéines	73
3.3. Les lipides	74
3.4. Les glucides	74
3.5. Les fibres	75
3.6. Les minéraux	75
3.7. Les vitamines	75
3.8. L'eau	76
4. Le choix des aliments	76
5. En pratique	80
6. Exemple de ration, de répartition et de menu	82
6.1. Exemple de ration d'un régime hypoénergétique à 5,5 MJ/jour	82
6.2. Exemple de répartition d'un régime hypoénergétique à 5,5 MJ/jour	83
6.3. Exemple de menu d'un régime hypoénergétique à 5,5 MJ/jour	84

Section 3
Prescriptions nécessitant une modification des apports conseillés en protéines

Chapitre 6

Le régime hyperprotidique — 87

1. Définition et principe	87
2. Les indications	87
3. Couverture des besoins et apports nutritionnels conseillés	88
3.1. L'énergie	88
3.2. Les protéines	88
3.3. Les lipides	88
3.4. Les glucides	89
3.5. Les fibres	89
3.6. Les vitamines	89
3.7. Les minéraux	89
3.8. L'eau	89
4. Le choix des aliments	90
5. En pratique	91
5.1. Exemples de recettes enrichies en protéines	92
6. Exemple de ration, de répartition et de menu	92

Chapitre 7

Le régime hypoprotidique — 93

1. Définition et principe	93
2. Les indications	93
3. Couverture des besoins et apports nutritionnels conseillés	94
3.1. L'énergie	94
3.2. Les protéines	94

	3.3. Les lipides	94
	3.4. Les glucides	94
	3.5. Les fibres	95
	3.6. Les vitamines et les minéraux	95
	3.7. L'eau	95
4.	Le choix des aliments	95
5.	En pratique	96
6.	Exemple de ration, de répartition et de menu	96
	6.1. Exemple de ration d'un régime hypoprotidique à 8,8 MJ/jour	96
	6.2. Exemple de répartition d'un régime hypoprotidique à 8,8 MJ/jour	97
	6.3. Exemple de menu d'un régime hypoprotidique à 8,8 MJ/jour	98

Section 4

Prescriptions nécessitant une modification des apports conseillés en lipides

Chapitre 8

Le régime normolipidique qualitatif — 101

1.	Définition et principe	101
2.	Les indications	101
3.	Couverture des besoins et apports nutritionnels conseillés	102
	3.1. L'énergie	102
	3.2. Les protéines	102
	3.3. Les lipides	102
	3.4. Les glucides	103
	3.5. Les fibres	103
	3.6. Les vitamines	103
	3.7. Les minéraux	103
	3.8. L'eau	103
4.	Le choix des aliments	104
5.	En pratique	108
6.	Exemple de ration, de répartition et de menu	108
	6.1. Exemple de ration d'un régime normolipidique qualitatif à 8,6 MJ/jour	108
	6.2. Exemple de répartition d'un régime normolipidique qualitatif à 8,6 MJ/jour	109
	6.3. Exemple de menu d'un régime normolipidique qualitatif à 8,6 MJ/jour	109

Chapitre 9

Le régime hypolipidique — 111

1.	Définition et principe	111
2.	Les indications	111
3.	Couverture des besoins et apports nutritionnels conseillés	112
	3.1. L'énergie	112
	3.2. Les protéines	112

3.3. Les lipides	112
3.4. Les glucides	112
3.5. Les fibres, les vitamines, les minéraux et l'eau	112
4. Le choix des aliments	112
5. En pratique	117
6. Exemple de ration, de répartition et de menu	118
6.1. Exemple de ration d'un régime hypolipidique à 8 MJ, 40 g de lipides par jour	118
6.2. Exemple de répartition d'un régime hypolipidique à 8 MJ, 40 g de lipides par jour	118
6.3. Exemple de menu d'un régime hypolipidique à 8 MJ, 40 g de lipides par jour	119

Chapitre 10

Le régime hypolipidique enrichi en triglycérides à chaîne moyenne — 121

1. Définition et principe	121
2. Les indications	121
3. Couverture des besoins et apports nutritionnels conseillés	122
3.1. L'énergie	122
3.2. Les protéines	122
3.3. Les lipides	122
3.4. Les glucides	122
3.5. Les fibres, les vitamines, les minéraux et l'eau	122
4. Le choix des aliments	123
5. En pratique	127

Section 5

Prescriptions nécessitant une modification des apports conseillés en glucides

Chapitre 11

Le régime contrôlé en glucides — 131

1. Définition et principe	131
2. Les indications	131
3. Couverture des besoins et apports nutritionnels conseillés	132
3.1. L'énergie	132
3.2. Les glucides	132
3.3. Les lipides	132
3.4. Les protéines	132
3.5. Les fibres	133
3.6. Les vitamines et les minéraux	133
3.7. L'eau	133
4. Le choix des aliments	133

5. En pratique	137
6. Exemple de ration, de répartition et de menu	138
6.1. Exemple de ration d'un régime contrôlé en glucides à 8,2 MJ, 250 g de glucides	138
6.2. Exemple de répartition d'un régime contrôlé en glucides à 8,2 MJ, 250 g de glucides	138
6.3. Exemple de menu d'un régime contrôlé en glucides à 8,2 MJ, 250 g de glucides	139

Chapitre 12

Le régime contrôlé en saccharose — 141

1. Définition et principe	141
2. Les indications	141
3. Couverture des besoins et apports nutritionnels conseillés	141
3.1. L'énergie	141
3.2. Les protéines	142
3.3. Les lipides	142
3.4. Les glucides	142
3.5. Les fibres	142
3.6. Les vitamines et les minéraux	142
3.7. L'eau	142
4. Le choix des aliments	143
5. En pratique	145
6. Exemple de ration, de répartition et de menu	146
6.1. Exemple de ration d'un régime contrôlé en saccharose à 8,9 MJ	146
6.2. Exemple de répartition d'un régime contrôlé en saccharose à 8,9 MJ	146
6.3. Exemple de menu d'un régime contrôlé en saccharose à 8,9 MJ	147

Section 6

Prescriptions nécessitant une modification des apports conseillés en lipides et en glucides

Chapitre 13

Le régime contrôlé en glucides et en lipides — 151

1. Définition et principe	151
2. Les indications	151
3. Couverture des besoins et apports nutritionnels conseillés	152
3.1. L'énergie	152
3.2. Les glucides	152
3.3. Les lipides	152
3.4. Les protéines	153
3.5. Les fibres	153
3.6. Les vitamines et les minéraux	153

3.7. L'eau	153
4. Le choix des aliments	153
5. En pratique	158
6. Exemple de ration, de répartition et de menu	158
6.1. Exemple de ration d'un régime contrôlé en lipides et en glucides à 8,3 MJ, 250 g de glucides	158
6.2. Exemple de répartition d'un régime contrôlé en lipides et en glucides à 8,3 MJ, 250 g de glucides	159
6.3. Exemple de menu d'un régime contrôlé en lipides et en glucides à 8,3 MJ, 250 g de glucides	160

Section 7

Prescriptions nécessitant une modification des apports conseillés en minéraux

Chapitre 14

Les régimes hyposodés — 163

1. Introduction	163
1.1. Définition et principe	163
1.2. Les indications	163
1.3. Couverture des besoins et apports nutritionnels conseillés	164
1.4. En pratique	164
2. Le régime hyposodé large	165
2.1. Définition et principe	165
2.2. Indications	166
2.3. Le choix des aliments	166
3. Le régime hyposodé standard	169
3.1. Définition et principe	169
3.2. Indications	169
3.3. Le choix des aliments	169
4. Le régime hyposodé strict	172
4.1. Définition et principe	172
4.2. Indications	172
4.3. Le choix des aliments	173
5. Exemple de ration, de répartition et de menu	175
5.1. Exemple de ration d'un régime hyposodé standard à 9 MJ/jour, 1 200 mg de sodium	175
5.2. Exemple de répartition d'un régime hyposodé standard à 9 MJ/jour, 1 200 mg de sodium	176
5.3. Exemple de menu d'un régime hyposodé standard à 9 MJ/jour, 1 200 mg de sodium	176

Chapitre 15

Le régime pauvre en potassium — 179
1. Définition et principe 179
2. Les indications.. 179
3. Couverture des besoins et apports nutritionnels conseillés 180
4. Le choix des aliments 180
5. En pratique 183
6. Exemple de ration, de répartition et de menu............................. 184
    6.1. Exemple de ration d'un régime hypopotassique à 11,1 MJ,
           3 g de potassium.. 184
    6.2. Exemple de répartition d'un régime hypopotassique à 11,1 MJ,
           3 g de potassium.. 185
    6.3. Exemple de menu d'un régime hypopotassique à 11,1 MJ,
           3 g de potassium.. 185

Chapitre 16

Le régime contrôlé en phosphore — 187
1. Définition et principe 187
2. Les indications.. 187
3. Couverture des besoins et apports nutritionnels conseillés 187
    3.1. L'énergie 187
    3.2. Les protéines 187
    3.3. Les lipides 188
    3.4. Les glucides 188
    3.5. Les fibres 188
    3.6. Les vitamines 188
    3.7. Les minéraux 188
    3.8. L'eau 188
4. Le choix des aliments 189
5. En pratique 190
6. Exemple de ration, répartition et menu 190

Section 8

Prescriptions nécessitant une modification des apports conseillés en fibres

Chapitre 17

Le régime riche en fibres — 193
1. Définition et principe 193
2. Les indications.. 193
3. Couverture des besoins, apports nutritionnels conseillés et choix des aliments 194
    3.1. Dans le cas d'une constipation primitive 194

3.2. Dans le cas d'une constipation secondaire	200
3.3. Dans le cas de diverticules	201
3.4. Dans le cas de diarrhées	201
4. Exemple de ration, de répartition et de menu	201
4.1. Exemple de ration d'un régime riche en fibres à 8,3 MJ, 30 g de fibres	201
4.2. Exemple de répartition d'un régime riche en fibres à 8,3 MJ, 30 g de fibres	202
4.3. Exemple de menu d'un régime riche en fibres à 8,3 MJ, 30 g de fibres	202

Chapitre 18

Les régimes pauvres en fibres — 203

1. Introduction	203
1.1. Définition et principe	203
1.2. Les indications	204
1.3. Étude des différents types de fibres alimentaires	205
1.4. Les différents facteurs à prendre en compte lors de la prescription de régimes pauvres en fibres	209
2. Le régime pauvre en fibres végétales, à fibres animales modifiées	211
2.1. Définition et principe	211
2.2. Les indications	211
2.3. Couverture des besoins et apports nutritionnels conseillés	211
2.4. Le choix des aliments	213
2.5. En pratique	216
3. Le régime pauvre en fibres végétales	217
3.1. Définition et principe	217
3.2. Les indications	217
3.3. Couverture des besoins et apports nutritionnels conseillés	217
3.4. Le choix des aliments	219
3.5. En pratique	223
4. Le régime d'épargne digestive	223
4.1. Définition et principe	223
4.2. Les indications	223
4.3. Couverture des besoins et apports nutritionnels conseillés	223
4.4. Le choix des aliments	225
4.5. En pratique	229
5. Exemple de ration, de répartition et de menu	230
5.1. Exemple de ration d'un régime pauvre en fibres à 6 MJ/jour	230
5.2. Exemple de répartition d'un régime pauvre en fibres à 6 MJ/jour	230
5.3. Exemple de menu d'un régime pauvre en fibres à 6 MJ/jour	231

Table des matières XIII

Section 9
Prescriptions nécessitant une modification qualitative globale de l'alimentation

Chapitre 19

Les régimes pauvres en résidus — 235

1. Introduction : les différents résidus.. 235
   1.1. Les fibres alimentaires végétales (FAV)... 235
   1.2. Les glucides incomplètement attaquables par le tube digestif 235
   1.3. Le lactose 236
   1.4. Les fibres animales... 236
2. Définition et principe 237
3. Les indications... 237
4. Couverture des besoins et apports nutritionnels conseillés...................... 238
   4.1. L'énergie 238
   4.2. Les protéines 238
   4.3. Les lipides 238
   4.4. Les glucides... 238
   4.5. Les fibres 239
   4.6. Les vitamines 239
   4.7. Les minéraux 239
   4.8. L'eau 239
5. Le choix des aliments.. 239
   5.1. Le choix des aliments du régime pauvre en résidus strict........... 240
   5.2. Le choix des aliments du régime pauvre en résidus large........... 242
6. En pratique 244
7. Exemple de ration, de répartition et de menu... 245
   7.1. Exemple de ration d'un régime pauvre en résidus strict à 8 MJ/jour 245
   7.2. Exemple de répartition d'un régime pauvre en résidus strict à 8 MJ/jour ... 245
   7.3. Exemple de menu d'un régime pauvre en résidus strict à 8 MJ/jour 246

Chapitre 20

Le régime normal léger — 247

1. Définition et principe 247
2. Les indications... 247
3. Couverture des besoins et apports nutritionnels conseillés...................... 248
   3.1. L'énergie 248
   3.2. Les protéines 248
   3.3. Les lipides 248
   3.4. Les glucides... 248
   3.5. Les fibres, les vitamines, les minéraux et l'eau 249
4. Le choix des aliments.. 249
5. En pratique 253

Chapitre 21

Le régime sans gluten — 255

1. Définition et principe 255
2. Les indications... 255
3. Couverture des besoins et apports nutritionnels conseillés............................ 255
   - 3.1. L'énergie 255
   - 3.2. Les protéines 256
   - 3.3. Les lipides 256
   - 3.4. Les glucides 256
   - 3.5. Les fibres 256
   - 3.6. Les vitamines 256
   - 3.7. Les minéraux 256
   - 3.8. L'eau 256
4. Le choix des aliments.. 257
5. En pratique 260
6. Exemple de ration, de répartition et de menu... 261
   - 6.1. Exemple de ration d'un régime sans gluten à 9,8 MJ/jour................. 261
   - 6.2. Exemple de répartition d'un régime sans gluten à 9,8 MJ/jour 261
   - 6.3. Exemple de menu d'un régime sans gluten 9,8 MJ/jour.................... 262

Partie 2

Prescriptions spécifiques à une pathologie

Chapitre 22

Les prescriptions selon les pathologies — 265

1. Les pathologies digestives et urinaires... 265
2. Les pathologies rénales (néphropathies) 267
3. Les pathologies respiratoires.. 267
4. Les pathologies de la nutrition ou métaboliques.. 268
5. Les pathologies cardiovasculaires ou MCV (maladies cardiovasculaires) 269
6. Autres pathologies.. 269
7. Les explorations spécialisées 270

Index des pathologies — 271

Introduction à l'alimentation thérapeutique

1. Présentation de la prise en charge diététique ou de la prescription diététique

Assurer la prise en charge nutritionnelle d'un patient consiste à :
- *définir le type d'alimentation* dont il a besoin selon sa pathologie et les caractéristiques qui lui sont propres (âge, sexe, taille, poids, état physiologique, mode de vie…) ;
- *préciser les éléments de cette prise en charge* (apports nutritionnels conseillés, choix des aliments, conseils généraux et spécifiques…) ;
- *assurer le suivi de son efficacité* à l'hôpital et/ou à domicile.

La prise en charge nutritionnelle doit donc suivre un cheminement cohérent afin d'assurer le maintien ou la récupération d'un état nutritionnel et métabolique aussi proche que possible de la normale.

> **Remarques**
> - À un nombre important de pathologies correspond un nombre moins important de prises en charge nutritionnelles (un même régime peut donc s'appliquer à différentes pathologies).
> - Les prises en charge peuvent être différentes ou modulées selon la sévérité, la forme clinique et/ou l'évolution de la pathologie.

2. Les différentes composantes de la prise en charge nutritionnelle

La prescription diététique est constituée de *sept composantes complémentaires*.

1. Connaître les objectifs de la prescription qui peuvent être les suivants :
- améliorer les paramètres du patient sachant qu'il en existe deux types :
  - paramètres cliniques (exemples : poids, appétit, fonction musculaire…),
  - paramètres biologiques (exemples : bilan lipidique, glycémie…) ;
- améliorer le pronostic suite à la découverte de la pathologie ;
- traiter la pathologie.

2. Connaître le type d'alimentation prescrit
La prescription diététique consiste à modifier les apports spontanés du patient en :
- les augmentant (« hyper ») ;
- les diminuant (« hypo ») ;
- les contrôlant (« contrôlé ») ;
- très rarement en les supprimant.

3. Maîtriser les apports conseillés du patient à savoir :
- connaître ses apports conseillés initiaux (c'est-à-dire « de forme ») en énergie, en fibres, en eau, en macronutriments et en micronutriments ;
- connaître ses apports adaptés selon sa pathologie ;
- évaluer un éventuel facteur d'activité et/ou facteur de stress :

Facteurs d'activité ou de stress

Facteur d'activité	Repos au lit	1,1
	Ambulatoire à l'hôpital	1,2
	Activité modérée	1,3
Facteur de stress	Chirurgie mineure	1,2
	Maladie chronique avec syndrome inflammatoire	1,2
	Polytraumatismes	1,2
Effet thermique	Fièvre	1,2

> **Remarque**
> En cas de situation mixte les facteurs se multiplient.

4. Maîtriser le choix des aliments adapté à la pathologie

Il importe de savoir quels aliments seront conseillés et déconseillés en vue de pouvoir assurer la prise en charge.

5. Connaître la voie d'administration

Au premier abord, il est toujours conseillé une *alimentation par voie orale* sachant qu'il est parfois nécessaire d'avoir recours à une alimentation hyperénergétique (et/ou hyperprotidique). Si la voie orale est impossible ou insuffisante, il convient de passer à une *nutrition entérale* (sonde nasale ou voie orale). Lorsque la voie digestive est impossible, contre-indiquée ou inefficace, il faut alors opter pour la *nutrition parentérale périphérique* (en cas de durée prévisible courte inférieure à deux semaines et d'un abord veineux suffisant). En dernier lieu, choisir la *nutrition parentérale par voie centrale* (cathéter ou chambre implantable) en cas de durée prévisible longue. À noter que cette technique est la plus coûteuse et la plus à risque.

6. Savoir évaluer des actions et ajuster la prescription

Lors du suivi d'un patient il est nécessaire de :
- réévaluer la prescription après sept jours d'hospitalisation si cela n'a pas été fait auparavant ;
- surveiller le poids, les paramètres cliniques et biologiques ;
- contrôler les ingesta spontanés ;
- contrôler l'acceptabilité et la tolérance du traitement diététique ;
- observer l'évolution de la pathologie.

7. Pratiquer une éducation nutritionnelle ou thérapeutique auprès du patient

Cette éducation peut se faire en individuel ou en groupe (pour des patients ayant une pathologie commune (exemple : patients diabétiques).

1

L'enquête alimentaire ou l'interrogatoire alimentaire

Introduction

Les objectifs de l'enquête alimentaire sont multiples à savoir :
1. Connaître le patient et son environnement.
2. Préciser son histoire médicale et les données associées.
3. Évaluer ses besoins nutritionnels.
4. Préciser ses apports alimentaires c'est-à-dire ses ingesta habituels.
5. Évaluer ses goûts individuels.
6. Déterminer des objectifs particuliers avec analyse de ses erreurs.
7. Établir son (ses) régime(s) lors de l'hospitalisation puis son régime de sortie c'est-à-dire sa prescription diététique personnalisée, adaptée à ses habitudes de consommation alimentaire.

> Permet de définir les écarts entre les apports théoriques et réels

1. *Données générales concernant le patient et son environnement*

Les premières questions pouvant être posées à un patient sont les suivantes :
– nom, prénom ;
– date de naissance ;
– nationalité (permet de cerner les facteurs religieux) ;
– adresse postale ;
– téléphone (fixe, portable)/e-mail ;
– situation familiale (célibataire, en couple, nombre d'enfants) ;

- pratique sportive (type et durée) ;
- horaires de travail : normales ou décalées (importance chez un diabétique par exemple) ;
- type de transport journalier et durée du trajet ;
- profession (pénible, debout, normale, sédentaire).

2. *Histoire médicale du patient et données associées*

Il est conseillé de connaître chez un patient :
- son poids actuel ;
- son poids habituel « de forme » ;
- son poids maximal et minimal atteint durant son existence ;
- la perte ou le gain de poids durant les deux derniers mois et la dernière année ;
- sa taille ;
- chez l'enfant : les courbes de taille et de poids du carnet de santé sont indispensables ;
- le(s) traitement(s) suivi(s) (contraception, médicaments) et la (les) pathologie(s) associée(s).

Remarque

Au mieux, on effectuera une courbe de poids retraçant précisément son histoire pondérale. D'autres renseignements associés peuvent être demandés tels que :
- le tour de taille, de fesse, de cuisse ;
- les antécédents de prescription diététique ;
- l'utilisation éventuelle de produits de diététique et de régimes ;
- les motivations pour entreprendre un régime (de santé, esthétiques, professionnelles, conditionnées par l'extérieur [médecin, famille, événement extérieur, arrêt du tabac…]) ;
- un éventuel tabagisme.

---

3. *Étude des besoins nutritionnels*

Afin de pouvoir prendre en charge un patient, il est nécessaire au préalable d'étudier ses besoins nutritionnels qui dépendent :
- de son sexe, de sa taille et de son poids de forme ;
- de son niveau d'activité physique qui varie selon sa profession, la pratique de sport et de ses activités de la vie journalière ;
- de ses antécédents médicaux ;
- des facteurs génétiques justifiant une étude des antécédents ;
- d'états physiologiques particuliers augmentant les besoins nutritionnels : grossesse, allaitement, croissance en particulier chez le nourrisson et au stade de la puberté.

Par la suite, il est donc nécessaire de chiffrer et/ou de déterminer :
- l'indice de masse corporelle ;

- le métabolisme de base ;
- le niveau d'activité physique (NAP) ;
- la dépense énergétique journalière (DEJ) ;
- le besoin énergétique (BE) ;
- les antécédents personnels et/ou familiaux en vue de les adapter au régime prescrit.

4. Étude des apports alimentaires

4.1. Questions préalables

Il faut en premier lieu rechercher l'existence d'un obstacle à une alimentation équilibrée à savoir :
- une anorexie globale ou sélective ;
- des allergies alimentaires et/ou des intolérances ;
- un trouble de la mastication, de la salivation, de la denture ;
- une dysphagie (trouble de la déglutition) ;
- des nausées, des vomissements, des troubles du transit (aérophagie, constipation, acidité gastrique…) ;
- la nécessité d'une tierce personne pour s'alimenter ;
- l'existence d'aversion(s) alimentaire(s) ;
- l'existence de restriction alimentaire religieuse ou personnelle (végétarisme, dissociation…) ;
- la présence de « préjugés » vis-à-vis de l'alimentation ;
- l'existence de compulsions alimentaires voire de tendance à la boulimie et/ou de grignotages réguliers ;
- les traitements médicamenteux parfois responsables d'inappétence (exemple : surdosage en digitaliques et vomissements – biguanides et diarrhées) ;
- un état morbide : réanimation post-chirurgicale ;
- si le sujet suit une prescription diététique ou consomme des compléments alimentaires.

4.2. Mise en pratique de l'enquête alimentaire individuelle

Parmi les méthodes d'enquête alimentaire individuelle, deux types de méthodes existent actuellement, à savoir celles recueillant les consommations sur des jours définis et celles recueillant des informations sur les consommations habituelles du sujet.

4.2.1. Méthodes de recueil des apports sur des jours définis

4.2.1.1. Méthode d'enregistrements alimentaires

On demande au patient de remplir un « journal alimentaire » sur 3 à 7 jours où il reporte le détail de ses consommations d'aliments et de boissons en y spécifiant le lieu, les horaires des repas et pour plus de précision en associant une pesée des aliments à l'aide d'une balance. La quantification en unités ménagères (cuillère, bol, verre…) ou la présentation de modèles de photographies sont d'autres moyens pour estimer les quantités consommées.

4.2.1.2. Méthode du rappel des 24 heures

Cette méthode est réalisée au cours d'un entretien pendant lequel on demande au patient de se remémorer et de décrire tous les aliments et boissons consommés pendant les précédentes 24 heures. Cet entretien peut se faire en face-à-face ou par téléphone.

4.2.2. Méthodes de recueil des apports habituels

4.2.2.1. Méthode de l'histoire alimentaire

Contrairement aux méthodes précédentes qui évaluent les apports alimentaires sur une période précise, l'histoire alimentaire cherche à évaluer les habitudes alimentaires typiques du patient. L'enquêteur interroge alors dans le détail celui-ci sur la répartition habituelle de son alimentation souvent retracée en fonction des repas.

4.2.2.2. Méthode avec questionnaires de fréquences de consommation

Ces questionnaires sont utilisés pour évaluer la consommation habituelle de certains aliments et ceux-ci sont constitués d'une liste d'aliments auxquels sont associés des catégories de fréquences de consommation (en nombre de fois par jours, par semaine, par mois, etc.). Il est ainsi demandé au patient de cocher, pour chaque aliment de la liste, la fréquence qui s'approche au mieux de sa consommation habituelle.

Il est important de noter que chacune de ces méthodes d'enquête présentent des avantages et des inconvénients tels que présentés dans le tableau suivant.

Principaux avantages et inconvénients pour les différentes méthodes d'enquêtes alimentaires

	Consommations sur des jours définis		Consommations habituelles	
	Enregistrements alimentaires	Rappels des 24 heures	Histoire alimentaire	Fréquences de consommations
Avantages	Informations précises sur les consommations Peu d'outils Méthode représentative	Rapidité Facilité Praticité Peu contraignant	Étude du profil alimentaire Répartition habituelle des consommations et des habitudes alimentaires	Pertinence du questionnaire Création de questionnaire spécifique aux besoins de l'enquête Méthode précise Simplicité et rapidité d'exploitation
Inconvénients/ limites	Méthode contraignante (coopération et investissement très important) Nécessité de savoir lire et écrire Risque d'influence des consommations pendant l'enregistrement Erreur quant à la description précise des aliments	Compétence primordiale de l'enquêteur Défauts de mémorisation Non représentatif de l'alimentation habituelle Estimation des portions difficile Manque de précisions	Erreurs d'estimation des apports Longueur de l'entretien Qualification de l'enquêteur Qualité des réponses très liée au patient	Gros travail de préparation en amont Non représentatif de la variabilité des choix alimentaires (modes de préparation, marques...) Nécessite l'association à une autre méthode d'enquête Erreurs dans l'estimation des apports

Par la suite, ces enquêtes permettront d'évaluer, selon chaque méthode utilisée et ce de manière plus ou moins précise :
- *l'apport calorique* quotidien du patient ;
- *des renseignements quantitatifs et qualitatifs* sur son alimentation tels que :
  - la répartition glucido-lipido-protidique,
  - la teneur de l'alimentation :
    - en protéines animales et végétales,
    - en acides gras saturés, acides gras monoinsaturés, acides gras polyinsaturés,
    - en glucides simples et complexes,
    - en produits sucrés,
    - en cholestérol,
    - en fer,
    - en calcium,
    - en magnésium,
    - en vitamines,
    - en fibres,
    - en eau...

- *la répartition de l'alimentation* dans la journée, le nombre de repas et de collations ;
- *les goûts alimentaires* permettant de personnaliser la prescription diététique proposée notamment lorsque l'enquête évalue des fréquences de consommation des aliments comme pour :
  - les charcuteries,
  - les fromages,
  - le sucre et ses dérivés,
  - les matières grasses,
  - l'alcool,
  - l'eau,
  - les viennoiseries, les pâtisseries,
  - les biscuits,
  - les boissons sucrées,
  - les fritures/panures…

> **Remarque**
> Il convient de ne pas oublier de demander au patient son attirance pour les aliments plutôt salés ou sucrés, ses modes de cuisson et les aliments qui lui paraissent « indispensables » quotidiennement, ainsi que ne pas oublier de préciser ses habitudes régionales (exemples : cuisine à la crème fraîche, utilisation de beurre salé…).
> Il est également important de savoir quelle est la personne qui prépare les repas du patient et où ses repas sont pris : travail, cantine, self-service, maison, restaurant, invitations, fast-food/sandwich…
> En situation de réanimation, les besoins nutritionnels sont évalués également en fonction de la fièvre et de la pathologie évolutive.

D'autres questions concernant le comportement alimentaire du patient pourront aussi être abordées telles que :
- son appétit (petit, moyen, gros) associé à ses besoins en volume ;
- s'il a pour habitude de se resservir ;
- s'il saute des repas ;
- l'ambiance, l'humeur dans laquelle il prend ses repas (calme/détendue, stressée/bousculée, variable, culpabilité/plaisir) ;
- le temps consacré aux repas (supérieur ou inférieur à 20 min) ;
- son goût pour la cuisine ;
- ses moyens financiers…

5. *Les objectifs particuliers de la prescription*

Ils peuvent être nombreux et sont différents en fonction des patients. En voici quelques exemples :
- amaigrissement/prise de poids ;
- gérer les repas à l'extérieur ;

Les régimes à texture liquide

1.3.5. L'eau

L'eau est à la base de ce type d'alimentation : il faut ainsi arriver à fournir au minimum 2 à 2,5 litres d'eau de boisson par jour. Ceci permet aussi la compensation des pertes souvent plus importantes (en cas de diarrhées, de fièvre…). L'eau de boisson doit ainsi être majorée de 200 mL par degré au-delà de 37 °C de température corporelle.

1.3.6. La vitamine C

D'une manière générale, la couverture en vitamine C ne peut être assurée. Elle pourra néanmoins être partiellement couverte lorsque la consommation de jus de fruits est rendue possible.

1.3.7. Le sodium et le potassium

En vue de maintenir l'équilibre hydroélectrolytique, leur apport par les aliments doit se faire selon les quantités suivantes :
– *pour le chlorure de sodium* (NaCl) : il doit être maintenu à 2 g de sel par jour (800 mg de sodium). Ceci permet de compenser les pertes en sodium souvent accentuées par des diarrhées, une transpiration excessive, d'éventuels vomissements, la présence de brûlures, de fistules (générant une exsudation très importante) ;
– *pour le chlorure de potassium* (KCl) : il est nécessaire d'en apporter au moins 1 g par jour (500 mg de potassium). En effet, tout comme pour le sodium, les pertes peuvent être augmentées en cas de diarrhées, de fistules, de troubles rénaux, de traitement diurétique et générer des troubles du rythme cardiaque dus à une dyskaliémie.

1.4. Le choix des aliments

Groupe d'aliments	Aliments conseillés	Aliments déconseillés
Légumes	*Dans le cas de troubles digestifs importants et d'interventions touchant le tube digestif ou avec une situation organique voisine (césarienne, hystérectomie…) :* **Bouillons de légumes filtrés** : bouillons clairs, passés, réalisés à partir de légumes non amylacés, peu fibreux, se digérant facilement (laitue, carottes, endives, courgettes, aubergines, blancs de poireaux…)	**Tous les autres légumes sous toute autre forme**

Groupe d'aliments	Aliments conseillés	Aliments déconseillés
Légumes	*Lorsque les troubles digestifs sont peu importants ou inexistants :* **Jus de légumes** : réalisés avec la pulpe de légumes peu acidulés, à goût peu prononcé (exemple : jus de carottes, de courgettes, d'aubergines). **Remarque :** les bouillons et les jus de légumes seront peu salés à savoir à 3 g/L seulement	
Fruits	*Dans le cas de troubles digestifs importants et d'interventions touchant le tube digestif ou avec une situation organique voisine (césarienne, hystérectomie…) :* **Bouillons de fruits filtrés** : bouillons clairs, passés, sucrés (à 5 % maximum) réalisés à partir de fruits peu fibreux, se digérant facilement (poire, abricot, pêche brugnon, nectarine…) *Lorsque tout problème digestif a été exclu (mycose buccale, plaies buccales ou œsophagienne…) :* **Jus de fruits** : peu sucrés (5 % maximum), réalisés avec la pulpe de fruits peu acidulés, à goût peu prononcé (poire, pêche, nectarines, abricot, brugnon…). Servir des petites quantités et les diluer éventuellement avec de l'eau	**Tous les autres fruits sous toute autre forme** *Remarque :* les jus d'orange, de raisins et de pommes sont particulièrement diarrhéiques et donnent des gaz
Boissons	**Eau de distribution publique** **Eaux** *plates non magnésiennes* **Infusions, tisanes** *tièdes* **Thé** *léger tiède* **Attention :** sucrer modérément les boissons tièdes	**Toutes les autres boissons**

- stabiliser les constantes sanguines ;
- gérer la prise d'alcool ;
- gérer les fringales ;
- stopper le grignotage ;
- intégrer un petit-déjeuner ;
- intégrer un groupe alimentaire non consommé habituellement ;
- adopter une hygiène alimentaire correcte ;
- organiser ses courses ;
- réaliser des menus équilibrés ;
- maîtriser les équivalences alimentaires ;
- modifier ou créer des rythmes concernant les repas ;
- augmenter l'activité physique ;
- intégrer un choix des aliments particulier (régime hyposodé, hypopotassique, pauvre/riche en fibres…) ;
- cuisiner équilibré ;
- comprendre les étiquetages…

6. Remise du régime de sortie (c'est-à-dire de la prescription diététique personnalisée)

Le régime de sortie correspond au document remis au patient en vue de son retour à domicile. Celui-ci doit obligatoirement contenir :
- des conseils nutritionnels généraux (modes de cuisson, assaisonnements, gestion des excès…) ;
- une répartition précise et quantitative ;
- des équivalences en unités ménagères et/ou en grammes ;
- un choix des aliments le plus détaillé possible et individualisé.

Partie 1

Principaux types de prescriptions thérapeutiques

Section 1

Prescriptions nécessitant une modification de la texture

2

Les régimes à texture liquide

Introduction

Les régimes à texture liquide s'adressent à des patients ne pouvant consommer que des *aliments sous forme liquide*.

La modification de cette alimentation est essentiellement qualitative de par le changement de texture mais elle entraîne aussi une diminution des apports nutritionnels recommandés notamment lorsqu'elle est préconisée lors d'une phase de réalimentation.

Les indications pour ce type de prescription sont diverses à savoir :
– asthénie (anorexie) ;
– rétrécissement des voies digestives hautes (exemple : sténose de l'œsophage) ;
– irritation des muqueuses digestives ;
– limitation du péristaltisme œsophagien et/ou gastrique.

1. Le régime de la diète hydrique

1.1. Définition et principe

Le régime de la diète hydrique est un régime à base de *boissons claires*, très souvent associé à une alimentation parentérale (intraveineuse). Il a pour but d'assurer les besoins nutritionnels les plus urgents.

1.2. Les indications

Les indications sont les suivantes :
- le dernier repas avant une anesthésie générale ;
- le premier stade lors d'une réalimentation postopératoire (la durée de la diète hydrique étant d'un repas à quelques jours). En effet, après une anesthésie générale, tous les systèmes organiques fonctionnent au ralenti notamment le tube digestif. Il faut donc attendre la reprise du transit (premiers gaz : 1 à 2 jours et premières selles : 2 à 3 jours) avant de réalimenter le patient en vue d'éviter tout désordre digestif (occlusion, diarrhées…) ;
- quand toute alimentation plus substantielle est impossible (par exemple lors de troubles digestifs et hépatiques sévères ne permettant plus une alimentation de texture normale) ;
- après un repas trop copieux ayant généré un état très nauséeux ou un gros embarras gastrique ;
- avant certains examens médicaux particuliers ;
- en cas de pathologies très graves (tels que les grands opérés ou les grands brûlés pour lesquels la diète hydrique est prolongée longuement).

1.3. Couverture des besoins et apports nutritionnels conseillés

1.3.1. L'énergie

Les besoins énergétiques ne sont pas satisfaits car c'est un régime apportant très peu de macronutriments puisque les protéines et les lipides sont quasi inexistants et que les glucides sont en très faible quantité.

L'apport énergétique étant très faible, une association à une alimentation parentérale est quasi obligatoire sauf si la diète hydrique est de très courte durée (une journée seulement).

1.3.2. Les protéines et les lipides

Les apports sont quasi inexistants.

1.3.3. Les glucides

Il est conseillé de maintenir un apport glucidique de 80 à 100 g par jour (au minimum 60 g) en vue d'éviter la formation de corps cétoniques, toxiques pour l'organisme.

1.3.4. Les fibres

La couverture en fibres est impossible de par le choix des aliments.

Groupe d'aliments	Aliments conseillés	Aliments déconseillés
Fromages	/	Tous déconseillés
Viandes	/	Toutes déconseillées
Charcuteries	/	Toutes déconseillées
Abats	/	Tous déconseillés
Produits de la pêche	/	Tous déconseillés
Œufs	Modes de consommation : intégrés dans les préparations *sous forme crue* Quantités : 3 œufs maximum par jour	*Pas de contre-indication*
Farines et dérivés	**Céréales fines** telles que : – *Farine de blé* : dosage à 5 % **Attention** : bien respecter les quantités afin de ne pas former d'empois d'amidon qui épaissirait fortement les préparations – *Farines infantiles (ou farines dextrinisées)* : celles-ci sont riches en fer, ne nécessitent pas de cuisson (car elles sont précuites par dextrinisation) et ne contiennent pas d'épaississant. Il est donc possible de majorer les doses de 15 % à 20 %	**Pains et dérivés**

Groupe d'aliments	Aliments conseillés	Aliments déconseillés
Farines et dérivés	– *Maïzena* : elle est plus facile d'utilisation, nécessite moins de cuisson et donne des préparations lisses. Il convient néanmoins que les quantités utilisées soient moins importantes car elle épaissit plus vite (ce qui engendre une diminution de l'énergie apportée et un dosage plus difficile). Elle doit de plus être utilisée à froid de par sa moins bonne dissolution Il est aussi possible de consommer (tout en étant attentif à chaque dosage) : – *fécule de pommes de terre* – *rizine* (farine de riz) – *poudre de tapioca*… – éventuellement de la *semoule fine de blé* Les quantités seront évaluées à environ 50-100 g par jour selon les recettes	
Féculents	/	**Tous déconseillés**
Légumes	*Dans le cas de troubles digestifs importants et d'interventions touchant le tube digestif ou avec une situation organique voisine (césarienne, hystérectomie…) :* **Bouillons de légumes filtrés** : bouillons clairs, passés, réalisés à partir de légumes non amylacés, peu fibreux, se digérant facilement (laitue, carottes, endives, courgettes, aubergines, blancs de poireaux…) *Lorsque les troubles digestifs sont peu importants ou inexistants :* **Jus de légumes** : réalisés avec la pulpe de légumes peu acidulés, à goût peu prononcé (exemple : jus de carottes, de courgettes, d'aubergines)	

Les régimes à texture liquide

Groupe d'aliments	Aliments conseillés	Aliments déconseillés
Légumes	**Remarque :** les bouillons et les jus de légumes seront peu salés à savoir à 3 g/L seulement	**Tous les autres légumes sous toute autre forme**
Fruits	*Dans le cas de troubles digestifs importants et d'interventions touchant le tube digestif ou avec une situation organique voisine (césarienne, hystérectomie…) :* **Bouillons de fruits filtrés :** bouillons clairs, passés, sucrés (à 5 % maximum) réalisés à partir de fruits peu fibreux, se digérant facilement (poire, abricot, nectarine, brugnon, pêche…) *Lorsque tout problème digestif a été exclu (mycose buccale, plaies buccales ou œsophagienne…) :* **Jus de fruits :** peu sucrés (5 % maximum), réalisés avec la pulpe de fruits peu acidulés, à goût peu prononcé (poire, pêche, nectarines, abricot, brugnon…). Servir des petites quantités et les diluer éventuellement avec de l'eau	**Tous les autres fruits sous toute autre forme** **Remarque :** les jus d'orange, de raisins et de pommes sont particulièrement diarrhéiques et donnent des gaz
Matières grasses	**Corps gras émulsionnés** – Beurre non allégé – Margarines non allégées (de préférence végétales) – Margarines diététiques (enrichies en acides gras essentiels, vitamines E et D) – Crème fraîche non allégée Mode de consommation : à introduire avant le refroidissement des préparations toujours sous forme crue Quantités : – beurre/margarine : 20 à 30 g par jour – crème fraîche : en équivalence avec le beurre	**Beurre, margarines et crème fraîche allégés** **Huiles** (leur utilisation est quasiment impossible de par les recettes autorisées)

Groupe d'aliments	Aliments conseillés	Aliments déconseillés
Sucres et produits sucrés	**Sucre** **Caramel liquide** **Gelées** **Miel** *(en petite quantité)* **Sirop d'érable** **Chocolat, poudre chocolatée** **Pâte à tartiner** **Produits glacés sans morceaux** **Sirops** **Crème de marron** Modes de consommation : – intégrés dans les préparations (desserts, laitages…) – sous forme fondue ou dilués dans du lait **Attention** aux préparations hypersucrées qui sont irritantes pour les muqueuses digestives et qui peuvent engendrer des diarrhées osmotiques Quantités : 80 g maximum par jour d'autant plus lorsque l'hygiène buccodentaire est moins bien assurée (notamment au niveau de la face interne des dents)	**Tous les autres produits sucrés**
Boissons	**Eaux plates non magnésiennes** **Thé léger tiède** **Tisanes, infusions tièdes** Il faut veiller à : – toujours vérifier les problèmes de fausse route et de plaies dans la bouche – contrôler la température qui doit être tiède de préférence – ne pas boire de trop grandes quantités de boisson avant les repas	**Eaux plates magnésiennes** **Eaux gazeuses** **Thé fort très chaud** **Café** (celui-ci empêche le resserrement des capillaires dans le cas d'hémorragies) **Boissons rafraîchissantes sans alcool** (autres que les éventuels jus de fruits et de légumes autorisés) **Alcools**

Les régimes à texture liquide 29

Groupe d'aliments	Aliments conseillés	Aliments déconseillés
Épices et aromates	**Aromates divers, sel, vanille, fleur d'oranger** Ils donnent du goût aux préparations souvent monotones de par la texture imposée Il convient cependant de faire attention à : – leur texture qui doit être sous forme de poudre ou liquide – aux préparations hyperconcentrées : il faut les utiliser en très petites quantités en vue d'éviter d'éventuels saignements et de favoriser les vasoconstrictions.	Épices
Produits diététiques et de régime	Il est possible d'utiliser des *dextrines maltoses* dont le pouvoir sucrant est deux fois moindre que celui du saccharose. Les quantités utilisées pourront ainsi être plus importantes permettant une augmentation de l'énergie De la *poudre de protéines* pourra être ajoutée aux recettes afin d'enrichir l'alimentation Des *produits de complémentation liquides hyperprotidiques et/ou hyperénergétiques* pourront être proposés notamment en cas de dénutrition avérée ou en cas de risque de dénutrition	

2.5. En pratique

La durée de la prescription est généralement de 5 jours maximum (cet état étant seulement transitoire). Il convient de bien surveiller le poids du patient car on est en période de réalimentation.

Pour ce qui est du volume des repas, celui-ci doit avoisiner :
– pour le petit-déjeuner : environ 300 à 400 mL ;
– pour les repas principaux : environ 400 mL avec un volume d'environ 200 à 300 mL pour les préparations salées et d'environ 100 à 200 mL pour les préparations sucrées ;

– pour les collations : environ 200 à 300 mL.

En effet, la pratique démontre que 3 bols de 250 mL est un maximum de volume qu'une personne peut ingérer à un même repas.

Il convient de :
- servir les préparations le plus souvent froides voire tièdes (c'est-à-dire à température ambiante) ;
- soigner les couleurs et les présentations afin de stimuler l'appétit des patients car l'alimentation proposée est plutôt fade) ;
- bien remuer les préparations avant consommation en vue de maintenir la texture liquide ;
- penser si nécessaire à enrichir les recettes avec : du jaune d'œuf (voire de l'œuf entier cru), de la poudre de lait, de la poudre de protéines, des matières grasses crues, des céréales fines, des produits sucrés.

Les idées de recettes pouvant être proposées pour ce type de prescription sont les suivantes :

Recettes sucrées

- Crème anglaise liquéfiée (chocolat, vanille, caramel, pistache…).
- Crème meunière à la pâte à tartiner liquéfiée.
- Crème pâtissière liquéfiée.
- Crème de riz chocolatée liquéfiée.
- Crème caramel liquéfiée.
- Œufs au lait liquéfiés sucrés.
- Lait de poule.
- Jus de fruits lactés.
- Compotes liquéfiées.
- Compote anglaise (compote + crème anglaise) liquéfiée.
- Bouillies aux fruits liquéfiés sucrés (gelées de fruits, sirop d'érable…).
- Desserts lactés lisses liquéfiés : laits gélifiés liquéfiés, crème renversée liquéfiée.
- Milk shake au sirop, aux fruits, à la pâte à tartiner, à la crème de marron, aux céréales fines liquéfiés.
- Chocolat tiède à la farine infantile.
- Laitages sucrés à la crème de marron, au miel liquéfiés.
- Yaourt à boire au sirop et aux céréales fines.
- Bouillons de fruits froids/tièdes.
- Glaces/sorbets liquéfiés…

Recettes salées

- Béchamel liquéfiée.
- Œufs au lait liquéfiés salés.
- Bouillons de légumes filtrés tièdes…

2.6. Exemple de ration, de répartition et de menu

2.6.1. Exemple de ration d'un régime liquide lacté à 4,5 MJ/jour

Aliments	Quantités (g ou mL)	Protéines g	Lipides g	Glucides g	Ca mg	Fer mg	Vit C mg	Fibres g
Lait demi-écrémé	600	21	9	30	720	0	0	0
Poudre de lait écrémé	60	21	0,5	30	780	0,3	0	0
Laitage demi-écrémé	50	3	1	2,5	68	0	0	0
Jaune d'œuf	20	3	6	0	27	1	0	0
Farine ou équivalent	10	1	0	7,2	1,5	0	0	0,4
Légumes bouillon	500	5	0	15	200	5	25	0
Beurre	10	0	8	0	0	0	0	0
Margarine	5	0	4	0	0	0	0	0
Sucre ou équivalent	60	0	0	60	0	0	0	0
Total (g)		55	29	145	1 796	7	25	0
Énergie (kJ)	4 492	928	1 105	2 459				
Pourcentages	100	21	25	55				

2.6.2. Exemple de répartition d'un régime liquide lacté à 4,5 MJ/jour

Aliments	Quantités (g ou mL)	Petit-déjeuner	Déjeuner	Collation	Dîner
		g	g	g	g
Lait demi-écrémé ou équivalent	600	200	150	150	100
Poudre de lait écrémé	60	10	20	10	20
Laitage demi-écrémé	50	0	0	0	50
Jaune d'œuf	20	0	20	0	0
Farine ou équivalent	10	10	0	0	0
Légumes bouillon	500	0	250	0	250
Beurre	10	10	0	0	0
Margarine	5	0	0	5	0
Sucre ou équivalent	60	20	20	15	5
Total (KJ)	4 500	1 486	1 552	1 248	1 861,0
%	100	33	34	28	41

2.6.3. Exemple d'un menu régime liquide lacté à 4,5 MJ/jour

Petit-déjeuner

Crème meunière au café enrichie liquéfiée (200 mL de lait demi-écrémé, 10 g de farine, 10 g de beurre, 20 g de sucre, 10 g de poudre de lait écrémé).

Déjeuner

Bouillon enrichi (250 mL de bouillon de légumes, 20 g de poudre de lait écrémé).

Crème anglaise liquéfiée enrichie (150 mL de lait demi-écrémé, 1 jaune d'œuf, 20 g de sucre).

Collation

Crème de riz au chocolat enrichie (150 mL de lait demi-écrémé, 5 g de crème de riz, 5 g de cacao, 10 g de sucre, 10 g de poudre de lait écrémé).

Dîner

Bouillon enrichi (250 mL de bouillon de légumes, 20 g de poudre de lait écrémé).

Fromage blanc liquéfié (50 g de fromage blanc, 100 mL de lait demi-écrémé, 10 g de gelée de groseille).

3. Le régime liquide large

3.1. Définition et principe

La texture est identique au régime liquide lacté (c'est-à-dire que les préparations doivent pouvoir être bues à la paille) mais cette prescription est :
- plus diversifiée car tous les groupes d'aliments sont introduits même si la texture impose un contrôle quantitatif et qualitatif de certains groupes (viandes, produits de la pêche, farines et dérivés, féculents…) ;
- plus équilibrée ;
- couplée au régime normal léger voire au régime pauvre en fibres ;
- parfois prescrit plus longtemps (plus de cinq jours).

3.2. Les indications

Les indications sont les mêmes que pour le régime de texture molle mais pour des patients ayant des problèmes de déglutition et de mastication accentués tels que :
- un blocage des maxillaires : après une chirurgie, un traumatisme facial, une fracture… ;
- une dysphagie prononcée avec rétrécissement œsophagien important ;
- une intervention au niveau de la bouche et/ou du larynx.

Parfois, le régime liquide large est aussi proposé quelques jours en début de réalimentation postopératoire après une chirurgie digestive. Il fait ainsi la transition entre la diète hydrique et le régime de texture molle.

3.3. Couverture des besoins et apports nutritionnels conseillés

3.3.1. L'énergie

Le niveau énergétique peut varier de 3 à 12 MJ par jour (500 à 2 200 kcal par jour). De même que pour le régime liquide lacté, le choix des aliments reste restreint et peu varié. La nécessité d'une complémentation dans le cas d'une dénutrition avérée est donc toujours recommandée (*cf.* régime hyperénergétique).

3.3.2. Les protéines

Le choix des aliments riches en produits laitiers et la réintroduction des viandes et des poissons rend le régime hyperprotidique soit de 1,2 à 1,5 g de protéines par kilo et par jour au minimum (ce qui représente environ 20 % de l'apport énergétique total).

Les protéines animales doivent être prépondérantes ce qui assure la couverture en acides aminés indispensables car les patients ont le plus souvent, de par leur pathologie, un besoin accru en protéines dû à la cicatrisation.

3.3.3. Les lipides

Les apports nutritionnels en lipides sont ceux de référence, à savoir de 30 à 35 % de l'apport énergétique total, et on constate une meilleure répartition des acides gras par rapport au régime liquide froid car il devient possible de cuire avec de petites quantités d'huile les viandes et les poissons réintroduits.

Il convient toutefois de rester vigilant quant à cette répartition puisqu'il est toujours impossible de proposer des vinaigrettes.

3.3.4. Les glucides

En tant que compléments énergétiques de la ration, les glucides représentent environ 45 à 50 % de l'apport énergétique total. Il est conseillé d'essayer de respecter le rapport de 50 à 55 % de glucides complexes et de 45 à 50 % de glucides simples, ceci étant rendu possible par l'élargissement du choix des aliments en farines et dérivés ainsi qu'en féculents.

Pour ce qui est des produits sucrés, ils ne doivent pas dépasser 10 % de l'apport énergétique total et il est, là encore, préconisé d'éviter toute préparation fortement concentrée.

3.3.5. Les fibres

Il est toujours très difficile d'atteindre les apports nutritionnels conseillés de par la texture liquide et le peu de fibres crues même si l'on constate leur légère augmentation due à la réintroduction de légumes et de fruits et à l'élargissement du groupe des denrées amylacées.

3.3.6. Les vitamines

On remarque une meilleure couverture en *vitamine C* mais il est toujours recommandé d'en surveiller les apports. En effet, les crudités ne sont représentées que par de petites quantités de fruits crus mixés liquéfiés.

3.3.7. Les minéraux

Sauf en cas de niveau énergétique très faible, le *calcium* est correctement couvert en raison de la forte proportion de lait et de produits laitiers.

On note une amélioration des apports en *fer* de bonne qualité (réintroduction des viandes et des poissons, principales sources de fer héminique) et du *magnésium* (élargissement du choix des aliments en produits amylacés).

3.3.8. L'eau

Les besoins en eau doivent être assurés selon les recommandations et augmentés en cas de fièvre et/ou de diarrhées.

3.4. Le choix des aliments

Groupe d'aliments	Aliments conseillés	Aliments déconseillés

Laits	**De préférence entiers voire demi-écrémés (en fonction de l'AET)**
	
	Quantités : 750 mL maximum soit 30-40 g maximum de lactose La quantité de lait est diminuée par rapport au régime liquide lacté car le choix des aliments est plus vaste
	
	Modes de consommation :
	– *liquide* (selon tolérance) :
	  - entier (augmente l'énergie)
	  - demi-écrémé
	– en *poudre ou concentré* : permet d'enrichir facilement les préparations en protéines, en glucides et en calcium
	– +/- *enrichi en fer*
	
	Le lait est essentiellement proposé au petit-déjeuner et en collation car il y a plus de choix dans les préparations salées
	
	Attention : si une réelle intolérance est constatée, il faut utiliser du lait sans lactose
		Lait écrémé liquide
		Lait écrémé concentré

Laitages	**De préférence entiers voire demi-écrémés (en fonction de l'AET)** Modes de consommation : – battus – liquéfiés c'est-à-dire dilués avec du lait – homogénéisés (si présence de morceaux)	**Laitages écrémés**
Desserts lactés	**Desserts lactés lisses et liquéfiés** (crème aux œufs liquéfiée, crème anglaise, laits gélifiés aromatisés liquéfiés…)	**Desserts lactés avec morceaux**

Groupe d'aliments	Aliments conseillés	Aliments déconseillés
Fromages	**Fromages fondus nature de préférence à base de pâte dure** **Fromages frais nature** Modes de consommation : intégrés dans les préparations tièdes et salées	**Fromages affinés**
Viandes	Les morceaux de viandes choisis seront de préférence : – **maigres** car ils présentent un meilleur rapport protéines sur lipides – **de première catégorie** (c'est-à-dire à fibres musculaires courtes) car ils sont plus faciles d'utilisation et sont dotés d'un rapport collagène sur protéines supérieur La liquéfaction se fait avec de la sauce ou du bouillon. Le mixage doit avoir lieu après la cuisson Modes de cuisson : au four, à l'eau, mijotés, papillote (sans grillage)…	**Viandes grasses, demi-grasses et/ou de deuxième et troisième catégorie**
Charcuteries	**Jambon blanc découenné/dégraissé** **Filets de bacon découennés/dégraissés** **Lardons découennés/dégraissés**	**Pâtés, mousses** **Rillettes, terrines** **Jambon blanc, filets de bacon, lardons non découennés/dégraissés** **Saucissons secs** **Jambon cru** **Saucisses, chair à saucisse** **Andouille, andouillette** **Boudin blanc** **Pâté en croûte** **Viande des grisons…** Ces charcuteries sont peu pratiques d'utilisation de par leur texture
Abats	/	**Tous déconseillés** (la texture empêche leur utilisation)

Groupe d'aliments	Aliments conseillés	Aliments déconseillés
Produits de la pêche	**Poissons maigres et demi-gras au goût peu prononcé** Car ils sont plus faciles d'utilisation Modes de cuisson conseillés : – court-bouillon – vapeur – papillotes – pochés… Modes de consommation : ils sont incorporés dans les préparations sous forme de filets sans arêtes et mixés après cuisson	**Poissons gras** **Poissons fumés/séchés** (car ils sont peu adaptés) **Mollusques/crustacés** (car ils sont peu adaptés) Modes de cuisson déconseillés : – fritures, – grillades…
Œufs	Modes de consommation : intégrés dans les préparations sous forme crue Quantités : 3 œufs maximum par jour	*Pas de contre-indication*
Farines et dérivés	On retrouve les mêmes aliments que pour le régime liquide lacté à savoir des céréales fines telles que : **Farine de blé :** – pour les préparations froides : dosage à 5 % – pour les préparations tièdes : dosage de 7 à 10 % **Farines infantiles** **Maïzena** **Fécule de pommes de terre** **Farine de riz** **Poudre de tapioca** **Semoule fine de blé…** **Attention :** bien respecter les quantités et la température afin de ne pas former d'empois d'amidon qui épaissirait fortement les préparations	**Pains et assimilés (pain de mie, pain brioché, pain viennois…)** **Pâtisseries, viennoiseries** **Céréales pour le petit-déjeuner** **Autres biscuits**

Groupe d'aliments	Aliments conseillés	Aliments déconseillés
Farines et dérivés	On peut aussi ajouter émiettés très finement et intégrés dans les préparations : **Chapelure Biscottes et assimilés, pains grillés et assimilés Biscuits secs type boudoirs, Biscuits « à thé » type Petit-beurre®**	
Féculents	**Semoule fine de blé (Floraline®) Pommes de terre Fruits amylacés** Il convient de bien respecter la texture lisse et de donner de petites quantités pour ne pas épaissir les préparations **Potages de légumes secs mixés très finement et liquéfiés** Attention à bien vérifier la tolérance du patient	**Pâtes Riz Semoule de blé moyenne et grosse Petits pois Maïs**
Légumes	**Légumes non amylacés, peu fibreux, se digérant facilement (laitue, jeunes carottes, endives, courgettes, aubergines, blancs de poireaux tomates sans peau, haricots verts extra-fins…)** Modes de consommation : – bouillons de légumes – jus de légumes – légumes cuits mixés, homogénéisés et liquéfiés	Tous les autres légumes sous toute autre forme
Fruits	**Fruits peu fibreux, se digérant facilement (poire, abricot, brugnon, nectarine, pêche, banane…)** Modes de consommation : – bouillons de fruits – jus de fruits – compotes liquéfiées	Tous les autres fruits sous toute autre forme

Les régimes à texture liquide

Groupe d'aliments	Aliments conseillés	Aliments déconseillés
Fruits	– fruits au sirop mixés et liquéfiés – fruits crus mixés, homogénéisés et liquéfiés – fruits pulpés liquéfiés	
Matières grasses	**Corps gras émulsionnés :** – beurre non allégé – margarines non allégées (de préférence végétales) – margarines diététiques (enrichies en acides gras essentiels, vitamines E et D) – crème fraîche non allégée Mode de consommation : à introduire avant le refroidissement des préparations toujours sous forme crue Quantités : – beurre/margarine : 10 à 20 g par jour – crème fraîche : en équivalence avec le beurre – **Huiles végétales** en petite quantité et utilisées pour la cuisson des viandes et des poissons	**Beurre, margarine et crème fraîche allégés**
Produits sucrés	**Sucre** **Caramel liquide** **Gelées** **Miel** *(en petite quantité)* **Sirop d'érable** **Chocolat, poudre chocolatée** **Pâte à tartiner** **Produits glacés sans morceaux** **Sirops** **Crème de marron** Modes de consommation : – intégrés dans les préparations (desserts, laitages…) – sous forme fondue ou dilués dans du lait	Confitures, marmelades Confiseries Produits glacés avec morceaux Fruits confits

Groupe d'aliments	Aliments conseillés	Aliments déconseillés
Produits sucrés	**Attention** aux préparations hypersucrées qui sont irritantes pour les muqueuses digestives et qui peuvent engendrer des diarrhées osmotiques Quantités : 80 g maximum par jour d'autant plus lorsque l'hygiène buccodentaire est moins bien assurée (notamment au niveau de la face interne des dents)	
Boissons	**Eaux plates non magnésiennes** **Thé et café léger tièdes** **Tisanes, infusions tièdes** Il faut veiller à : – toujours vérifier les problèmes de fausse route et de plaies dans la bouche – contrôler la température qui doit être de préférence tiède – ne pas boire de trop grandes quantités de boisson avant les repas	**Eaux plates magnésiennes** **Eaux gazeuses** **Thé fort et/ou très chaud** **Café fort et/ou très chaud** (celui-ci empêche le resserrement des capillaires dans le cas d'hémorragies) **Boissons rafraîchissantes sans alcool** (autres que les éventuels jus de fruits et de légumes autorisés) **Alcools**
Épices et aromates Épices et aromates	**Aromates divers, sel, vanille, fleur d'oranger, café soluble** Ils donnent du goût aux préparations souvent monotones de par la texture imposée Il convient cependant de faire attention à : – leur texture qui doit être sous forme de poudre ou liquide – aux préparations hyperconcentrées : il faut les utiliser en très petites quantités en vue d'éviter les éventuels saignements en favorisant les vasoconstrictions	Épices

Groupe d'aliments	Aliments conseillés	Aliments déconseillés
Produits diététiques et de régime	Il est possible d'utiliser des *dextrines maltoses* dont le pouvoir sucrant est deux fois moindre que celui du saccharose. Les quantités utilisées pourront ainsi être plus importantes permettant une augmentation de l'énergie De la *poudre de protéines* pourra être ajoutée aux recettes en vue d'enrichir l'alimentation Des *produits de complémentation liquides hyperprotidiques et/ou hyperénergétiques* pourront être proposés en cas de dénutrition	

3.5. En pratique

La répartition se fait en cinq à sept prises par jour en variant les préparations salées et sucrées.

Les volumes des repas sont identiques à ceux du régime liquide lacté.

D'autres recettes peuvent être servies telles que des veloutés de légumes, des purées de légumes liquéfiées, des potages crème liquéfiés, des milk-shake aux fruits liquéfiés…

3.6. Exemple de ration, de répartition et de menu

3.6.1. Exemple de ration d'un régime liquide large à 8 MJ/jour

Aliments	Quantités (g ou mL)	Protéines	Lipides	Glucides	Ca	Fer	Vit C	Fibres
		g	g	g	mg	mg	mg	g
Lait demi-écrémé	700	24,5	10,5	35	840	0	0	0
Poudre de lait écrémé	70	25	0,6	35	910	0,4	0	0
Laitage demi-écrémé	250	15	5	12,5	337,5	0	0	0
Fromage fondu 70 % pâte dure	20	1,6	6,7	0	100	0	0	0
Viande de catégorie 1 maigre	90	16	4,5	0	13,5	3	0	0
Jaune d'œuf	40	7	13	0	55	2	0	0

Aliments	Quantités (g ou mL)	Protéines g	Lipides g	Glucides g	Ca mg	Fer mg	Vit C mg	Fibres g
Farine ou équivalent	40	4	0	29	6	0	0	1
Biscottes ou équivalent	50	5	2	35	30	1	0	2
Légumes	350	3,5	0	17,5	140	3,5	35	0
Fruit homogénéisé	50	0	0	9	5	0	7,5	0
Margarine végétale	20	0	16	0	0	0	0	0
Sucre ou équivalent	70	0	0	70	0	0	0	0
Total (g)		101	58	242	2 437	10	43	4
Énergie (KJ)	8 058	1 724	2 214	4 120				
Pourcentages	100	21	27	51				

3.6.2. Exemple de répartition d'un régime liquide large à 8 MJ/jour

Aliments	Quantités (g ou mL)	Petit-déjeuner g	Déjeuner g	Collation g	Dîner g
Lait demi-écrémé ou équivalent	700	200	250	150	100
Poudre de lait écrémé	70	20	0	20	30
Laitage demi-écrémé	250	125	0	0	125
Fromage fondu 70 % pâte dure	20	0	0	0	20
Viande de catégorie 1 maigre	90	0	30	60	0
Jaune d'œuf	40	0	20	20	0
Farine ou équivalent	40	20	15	0	5
Biscottes ou équivalent	50	0	0	0	50
Légumes	350	0	100	150	100
Fruit homogénéisé	50	50	0	0	0
Margarine	20	0	10	0	10
Sucre ou équivalent	70	20	30	10	10
Total (KJ)	8 130	1 775	2 118	1 602	2 635,5
%	100	22	26	20	32

3.6.3. *Exemple de menu d'un régime liquide large à 8 MJ/jour*

Petit-déjeuner

Maïzena à la vanille enrichie liquéfiée (150 mL de lait demi-écrémé, 10 g de maïzena, 10 g de sucre, 10 g de Floraline®, 10 g de poudre de lait écrémé).

Yaourt liquéfié enrichi aux fruits homogénéisés (1 yaourt aux fruits dont 10 g de sucre, 50 mL de lait demi-écrémé, 50 g de fruits homogénéisés, 10 g de poudre de lait écrémé).

Déjeuner

Potage protidique à base de roux (200 mL d'eau, 100 g de carottes, 30 g de volaille cuite, 10 g de margarine, 5 g de farine).

Crème pâtissière liquéfiée (250 mL de lait demi-écrémé, 1 jaune d'œuf, 7 g de maïzena, 30 g de sucre).

Collation

Potage enrichi (200 mL d'eau, 150 g de courgettes, 60 g de jambon blanc découenné dégraissé, 10 g de poudre de lait écrémé).

Crème anglaise enrichie liquéfiée (150 mL de lait, 1 jaune d'œuf, 10 g de sucre, 10 g de poudre de lait écrémé).

Dîner

Potage à base de liaison glucidique enrichi (200 mL d'eau, 100 g de pulpe d'aubergine, 50 g de pommes de terre, 5 g de farine, 1 crème de gruyère, 10 g de margarine, 10 g de poudre de lait écrémé).

Petits suisses enrichis liquéfiés (100 mL de lait demi-écrémé, 2 petits suisses, 20 g de poudre de lait écrémé, 10 g de sucre).

3

Les régimes à texture molle

1. Définition et principe

Tous les aliments consommés doivent être de texture molle c'est-à-dire ne demandant pas d'effort de mastication ou de déglutition et n'entraînant pas de douleurs à la déglutition.

La texture doit être adaptée à chaque patient par des modifications mécaniques ou physicochimiques des aliments (cuisson, mixage, hachage…).

Ces textures particulières se déclinent alors par gradient :
- 1er gradient : *texture lisse ou semi-liquide* : la texture des aliments est fine et homogène. Les aliments protidiques et les accompagnements sont ou non mélangés ;
- 2e gradient : *texture mixée* : la texture de l'ensemble des aliments est homogène et de consistance plus épaisse ;
- 3e gradient : *texture moulinée* : la texture est granuleuse ; les éléments protidiques sont moulinés, les accompagnements sont très tendres et seulement écrasés ou moulinés. Les composantes sont séparées dans l'assiette ;
- 4e gradient : *texture normale hachée* : la viande seule est hachée ou l'élément protidique est tendre. La texture de l'accompagnement reste normale mais doit être tendre.

2. Les indications

2.1. Les troubles de la mastication
- Patients édentés (personnes âgées, nourrissons) ou ayant des problèmes dentaires (absence d'appareil dentaire, appareil non approprié…).
- Fractures des maxillaires.
- Inflammations de la bouche (glossite, stomatite [inflammation de la muqueuse buccale], muscite).
- Abcès (bouche, palais, fosses nasales).
- Extractions dentaires importantes.
- Chirurgie faciale (esthétique, suite à des brûlures).
- Paralysies faciales (suite d'hémiplégie).

Dans ces cas, la texture molle sera proposée en second car le premier régime prescrit est de consistance liquide.

2.2. Les troubles de la déglutition (dysphagies)
- Amygdalectomie.
- Fausse route.
- Œsophagites.
- Sténose de l'œsophage.
- Cancer de la langue.
- Angines, phlegmon (abcès de la gorge), cancer de la gorge.
- Oreillons (inflammation des glandes salivaires), hyposialie (diminution de la sécrétion de salive), asialie.
- Atteintes neurologiques (maladie de Parkinson, sclérose en plaques…).

2.3. Les troubles gastriques nécessitant de ralentir la motilité de l'estomac (et par conséquence le péristaltisme)
- Gastrectomie (en second).
- Gastrites.
- Ulcère gastrique.
- Cancer gastrique.

2.4. Autre chirurgie digestive en postopératoire
La texture molle est proposée en vue de ne pas léser les cicatrices.

2.5. Autres indications
- Altération de l'état général (pour démarrer la reprise de la consommation alimentaire mais il convient de ne pas maintenir cette texture trop longtemps à cause de son côté anorexigène).
- Sida, cancers, dénutrition, pontage carotidien, thyroïdectomie…

Les régimes à texture molle

3. Couverture des besoins et apports nutritionnels conseillés

3.1. L'énergie

Trois niveaux énergétiques sont possibles sachant qu'ils sont choisis en fonction de l'état du patient (fatigue, dénutrition…) et de ses activités journalières (alitement, déplacements…). On retrouve ainsi :
- premier cas : régime normoénergétique ;
- deuxième cas : régime hyperénergétique allant jusqu'à 10-15 MJ par jour (2 400 à 3 600 kcal par jour) ;
- troisième cas : lors d'une réalimentation, les apports énergétiques sont au départ très faibles, de l'ordre de 2 MJ par jour (500 kcal par jour) puis progressivement augmentés jusqu'à 8-10 MJ par jour (1 900 à 2 400 kcal par jour).

3.2. Les protéines

Le régime est hyperprotidique à savoir que l'apport protéique doit se situer au minimum entre 1,2 et 1,5 g par kilo et par jour (soit environ 20 % de l'apport énergétique total).

Les patients ayant de par leur pathologie un besoin accru en protéines (période de cicatrisation et/ou risque de dénutrition et/ou dénutrition avérée…), il est nécessaire d'assurer une couverture correcte en acides aminés indispensables en privilégiant les protéines d'origine animale.

> **Remarque**
> Dans le cas de dénutrition avérée et avancée, les protéines ne doivent pas représenter moins de 20 % de l'apport énergétique total et peuvent atteindre jusqu'à 25 % de l'énergie journalière.

3.3. Les lipides

Le régime est normolipidique soit 30 à 35 % de l'apport énergétique total. Il est conseillé de vérifier la répartition des acides gras en variant les matières grasses au sein des préparations chaudes. En effet, la non-consommation de crudités diminue la quantité d'acides gras indispensables ingérés (acides gras oméga 6 et oméga 3) ainsi que d'acides gras monoinsaturés due à l'absence de vinaigrettes.

3.4. Les glucides

Les glucides sont les compléments énergétiques de la ration. Il est parfois difficile de respecter le rapport glucides complexes (50 à 55 % des glucides totaux) sur glucides simples (45 à 50 % des glucides totaux) car la texture notamment lisse entraîne une sélection des types de pains et de ses dérivés ainsi que des féculents.

Les produits sucrés, quant à eux, ne devront pas dépasser 10 % de l'apport énergétique total.

3.5. Les fibres

Il est difficile d'atteindre systématiquement les apports conseillés d'autant plus que la texture modifie la structure des fibres ce qui altère leur efficacité.

3.6. Les vitamines

La couverture en *vitamine C* risque de ne pas être assurée de par l'absence de légumes crus (sauf éventuellement l'avocat, les soupes de tomates et de concombre) et qu'il n'y a pas voir peu de fruits crus. Une supplémentation médicamenteuse peut donc être proposée en cas de longue durée de la prescription.

3.7. Les minéraux

Les apports en *fer* ne peuvent être garantis car les aliments protidiques du groupe viandes/poissons/œufs sont souvent servis en petites quantités et faiblement appréciés des patients car ils semblent peu appétissants de par la texture.

Pour ce qui est du *calcium*, la quantité importante de lait et/ou de produits laitiers proposés assure facilement sa couverture.

3.8. L'eau

Il convient de respecter les besoins recommandés en eau en fonction de chaque patient. Ainsi, pour l'adulte ceux-ci s'évaluent à 0,25 mL/kJ dont la moitié d'eau de boisson au minimum.

4. Le choix des aliments

Attention : ce choix des aliments est valable uniquement si le tube digestif n'est pas fragilisé. Si c'est le cas, il doit être couplé au *régime normal léger* voire aux *régimes pauvres en fibres*.

Groupe d'aliments	Aliments conseillés	Aliments déconseillés
Laits	**Liquide, en poudre, concentré** **De préférence entier ou demi-écrémé** Modes de consommation : – tels quels – intégrés dans des préparations – poudre de lait de 10 à 20 g par recette	*Pas de contre-indication*

Les régimes à texture molle

Groupe d'aliments	Aliments conseillés	Aliments déconseillés
Laits	Attention à bien vérifier la tolérance au lait de chaque patient	
Laitages	**Yaourts** **Fromages blancs** **Petits suisses** **Faisselles** **De préférence entiers ou demi-écrémés** Modes de consommation : – tels quels – intégrés dans des préparations Les laitages sont souvent mieux tolérés que le lait et sont bien adaptés à la texture molle Si la texture souhaitée doit être homogène, il est nécessaire de mixer les laitages avec des morceaux de fruits	*Pas de contre-indication*
Desserts lactés	**Crèmes desserts** **Viennois/liégeois** **Mousses et assimilés** **Entremets** **Flans** Si la texture est lisse, il faut surveiller la présence d'éventuels morceaux (entremets céréaliers)	*Pas de contre-indication*
Fromages	**Fromages frais salés** **Fromages fondus** **Fromages affinés à pâte pressée** **Fromages affinés à pâte molle** **Fromages affinés à pâte persillée** Modes de consommation : – tels quels (surveiller la texture en fonction des gradients) – fondus dans des préparations (purées et potages uniquement)	**Fromages affinés à pâte pressée dure** Ces fromages sont déconseillés car ils donnent des fils quand ils sont utilisés chauds et peuvent être irritants s'ils sont sous forme de gratins. Toutefois, ils peuvent être éventuellement consommés crus râpés ou tout juste fondus (cas du parmesan par exemple)
Viandes	Les morceaux de viandes choisis sont de préférence : – **maigres** car ils présentent un meilleur rapport protéines sur lipides – **de première catégorie** (c'est-à-dire à fibres musculaires courtes) car ils sont plus faciles d'utilisation et sont dotés d'un rapport collagène sur protéines élevé	

Groupe d'aliments	Aliments conseillés	Aliments déconseillés
	Modes de consommation : Les textures possibles sont les suivantes : – normale hachée : la viande est hachée et souvent servie à part – moulinée : la viande est moulinée et servie à part – mixée : la viande est de consistance épaisse et servie à part ou non – lisse : la texture est fine et homogène et la viande est servie à part ou non Il existe différents modes d'obtention de la texture : – par mixage avant la cuisson (exemple : farces) – par mixage après la cuisson, ce qui évite de durcir la viande La viande peut aussi être mélangée avec un liant (de la sauce ou du bouillon) afin de rendre la préparation plus onctueuse et plus homogène Modes de cuisson : au four, à l'eau, mijotés, papillote (sans grillage)…	**Viandes demi-grasses et grasses et/ou de deuxième et de troisième catégorie**
Charcuteries	**Pâtés lisses, mousses** **Rillettes, terrines** *sauf pour la texture lisse* **Jambon blanc découenné/dégraissé** **Filets de bacon découennés/dégraissés** **Lardons découennés/dégraissés** **Saucissons peu secs sans la peau** *sauf pour la texture lisse* **Saucisses, chair à saucisse, andouille, andouillette sans la peau** **Boudin blanc sans la peau**	**Pâtés avec morceaux** **Jambon blanc, filets de bacon, lardons non découennés/dégraissés** **Saucissons secs** **Jambon cru** **Pâté en croûte** **Viande des grisons…** Ces charcuteries sont peu pratiques d'utilisation de par leur texture
Abats	/	**Tous déconseillés** (la texture limite leur utilisation)
Produits de la pêche	**Poissons maigres et demi-gras** Car ils sont plus faciles d'utilisation	**Poissons gras** **Poissons fumés/séchés** (car ils sont peu adaptés) **Mollusques/crustacés** (car ils sont peu adaptés)

Groupe d'aliments	Aliments conseillés	Aliments déconseillés
Produits de la pêche	Modes de cuisson conseillés : – court-bouillon – vapeur – papillotes – pochés… Modes de consommation : ils sont incorporés dans les préparations sous forme de filets sans arêtes ; mixés ou émiettés ou hachés (selon le gradient) après cuisson ; à part ou non, en fonction de la texture	Modes de cuisson déconseillés : – fritures – grillades…

Œufs	Modes de cuisson conseillés :
	– mixés
	– brouillés
	– mollets
	– coques
	– cocottes
	– pochés
	– au plat peu cuits
	– durs peu cuits
	– omelettes baveuses…
	
	Modes de consommation :
	– tels quels
	– intégrés à des préparations :
	  - comme liant (sauces, crème, entremets, mousses…)
	  - comme enrichissant : jaune d'œuf dans les potages, les purées… ; préparations contenant des blancs d'œufs (mousses, soufflés…)
	
	Attention : les œufs doivent être ajoutés hors du feu dans les préparations chaudes (afin d'éviter leur coagulation)
		Pas de contre-indication
		
		Modes de cuisson déconseillés :
		– au plat bien cuits
		– durs bien cuits
		– omelettes bien cuites…

Farines et dérivés	**Farine de blé** **Maïzena** **Tapioca** **Fécule de pommes de terre** **Fécule de riz** **Farines infantiles enrichies** (Si impossibilité de consommer les équivalents du pain)	

Groupe d'aliments	Aliments conseillés	Aliments déconseillés
Farines et dérivés	**Mie de pain (blanc, complet, seigle, son, brioché, viennois, au lait…)** *sauf si la texture est lisse* **Pain de mie sans croûte**	Pain aux céréales, pains fantaisies Pain de mie avec croûte
	Biscottes, pain grillé et assimilés trempées dans un liquide (lait, boissons chaudes) ou imbibés par la salive *sauf si la texture est lisse*	Petits pains grillés
	Viennoiseries molles : brioches, crêpes, pancakes, beignets… trempées ou imbibés par la salive *sauf si la texture est lisse*	Croissants, pains au chocolat, chaussons aux pommes, gaufres…
	Pâtisseries/gâteaux mous : charlottes, baba, tiramisu, gâteaux fondants/ moelleux, quatre-quarts peu cuit, biscuit de Savoie peu cuit, génoise peu cuite, bavarois, soufflés salés ou sucrés, madeleines trempées ou imbibés par la salive *sauf si la texture est lisse*	Pâtisseries/gâteaux dures type tartes, macarons, pain d'épice, crumble, feuilletés, à base de pâte à chou…
	Biscuits : boudoirs, petit beurre, biscuits à thé, biscuits secs fourrés… trempés ou imbibés par la salive *sauf si la texture est lisse*	Biscuits secs avec morceaux, biscuits à apéritif
	Céréales pour petit-déjeuner en pétales, flocons d'avoine trempées ou imbibés par la salive *sauf si la texture est lisse* Les quantités recommandées sont de ne pas dépasser 60 g de pain ou équivalents par jour	Céréales pour petit-déjeuner croustillantes (soufflées, éclatées), muesli, barres de céréales
Féculents	**Pâtes à potage (vermicelle) de petit calibre (nouilles, coquillettes…), pâtes fraîches** bien cuites *sauf si la texture est lisse*	Pâtes de gros calibre *al dente* (elles se mixent mal)
	Riz rond et riz Thaï bien cuits et collants, riz gluant *sauf si la texture est lisse*	Riz long et incollable
	Semoule fine de blé, polenta *sauf si la texture est lisse*	Semoule moyenne et grosse, boulgour, mil ou millet, blé dur précuit, quinoa, maïs…

Groupe d'aliments	Aliments conseillés	Aliments déconseillés
Féculents	**Petits pois, fruits amylacés, légumes secs** écrasés, en purée, en potage **Pommes de terre** cuites à l'eau ou à la vapeur en purée écrasées, potages **Mousses, soufflés salés et sucrés** **Quenelles**	**Petits pois, fruits amylacés, légumes secs entiers** **Pommes de terre** grillées, sautées, frites, chips… Autres préparations à base de féculents entiers
Légumes	**Légumes tendres sans la peau : pulpe d'aubergine, betterave, carottes jeunes, champignon, courgettes épépinées, tomates, navet, haricots verts extra-fins, épinards, salades sans côte, brocolis, endives, cœurs de fenouil, avocat, potirons, choux-fleur, choux romanesco, chou rave, céleri rave, poivrons, poireaux, concombres, fonds d'artichauts…** Modes de consommation conseillés : bouillons, jus, potages purées, écrasés *(selon le gradient)* Il convient de faire attention : – aux pépins si l'on constate des problèmes de déglutition – à ne pas proposer de crudités sauf éventuellement l'avocat, la soupe de tomates ou de concombre – à bien vérifier la tolérance de chaque patient (transit digestif, sensibilité à l'acidité…)	**Légumes à fibres dures : asperges, bettes, choux rouges, artichaut, céleri branche, salsifis, cœur de palmier, radis…** Modes de consommation déconseillés : les préparations gratinées, cuites au four, sautées formant une pellicule croustillante pouvant être difficile à mastiquer
Fruits	Fruits tendres, bien mûrs, sans la peau, plus ou moins épépinés : **pommes, poires, bananes, pêches, nectarines, abricots, cerises, prunes, pruneaux, ananas, fraises, agrumes, melon, pastèque, autres fruits rouges, kiwis, rhubarbe, coing, mangue…** Modes de consommation : jus, compotes, aux sirops mixés, frais mixés, écrasés, en purée… *(selon le gradient)*	Fruits difficiles à mixer, peu mûrs : **dates fraîches, fruits secs…**

Groupe d'aliments	Aliments conseillés	Aliments déconseillés
Fruits	Il convient de bien vérifier la tolérance de chaque patient (transit digestif, sensibilité à l'acidité…)	
Matières grasses	**Beurre** **Margarine** **Crème fraîche** **Huiles végétales** Les matières grasses donnent de l'onctuosité et de la palatabilité aux préparations Mode d'utilisation : de préférence crues Attention aux huiles qui sont plus difficiles d'utilisation (car il n'y a pas de vinaigrette)	*Pas de contre-indication*
Produits sucrés	**Sucre** **Caramel liquide** **Confitures lisses, gelées, miel** **Chocolat sans morceaux, poudre chocolatée** **Pâte à tartiner** **Confiseries molles (caramels, chamallow…)** **Produits glacés à consistance entièrement molle** **Crème de marron** **Sirops** **Pâtes de fruits** Modes de consommation : – tels quels – fondus dans les préparations (desserts, laitages…)	**Confitures avec morceaux** (sauf si mixée), **marmelades** **Chocolat avec morceaux, barres chocolatées** **Confiseries dures (bonbons, sucettes, nougats…)** **Produits glacés avec morceaux de consistance dure** **Fruits confits**
Boissons	**Eaux** **Thé, tisanes, cafés tièdes** **Jus de fruits, jus de légumes** **Autres boissons rafraîchissantes sans alcool** **Bouillons** **Eaux gélifiées** (si nécessaire) Il convient de toujours vérifier les éventuelles fausses routes ainsi que la présence de plaies dans la bouche	**Toutes les boissons alcoolisées**

Les régimes à texture molle   55

Groupe d'aliments	Aliments conseillés	Aliments déconseillés
Épices et aromates	**Sel, bouillons cube, épices** **Herbes aromatiques** crues ou cuites **(persil, ciboulette, basilic…)** ou éliminées après cuisson **(thym, laurier…)** **Vanille, cannelle, extrait de fleur d'oranger, café soluble…** Les épices et les aromates donnent du goût aux préparations souvent peu appétissantes et stimulent l'appétit Attention à bien vérifier la tolérance digestive de chaque patient et à éliminer les éventuels aromates (feuilles) restés entiers avant consommation	*Pas de contre-indication*
Produits diététiques et de régime	Différents types de produits peuvent être employés dans ce type de prescription selon leur utilité : **Préparations industrielles de 4ᵉ gamme (sous vide) et de 5ᵉ gamme (lyophilisées) de texture molle** Les avantages de ces préparations sont les suivantes : – elles sont variées – la texture est déjà adaptée – elles garantissent une qualité microbiologique – elles sont de longue conservation – elles sont faciles d'utilisation Cependant, notons que les qualités organoleptiques sont moindres Dans le cas de dénutrition, il est possible d'utiliser : **Des produits de complémentation orale (crèmes, boissons)** Ce sont des préparations hyperénergétiques et/ou hyperprotidiques Néanmoins, leur goût reste souvent peu agréable **Des produits modulaires riches en un nutriment particulier :** – les poudres de protéines très riches en protéines – les dextrines maltoses riches en glucides complexes à index glycémique bas modifiant peu la texture et le goût **Des poudres instantanées** Elles permettent d'épaissir les préparations	

5. *En pratique*

La répartition doit se faire sur au moins quatre repas par jour (dont une collation). Il est aussi nécessaire de :
- surveiller les volumes des préparations afin de ne pas surcharger le tube digestif ;

- bien tremper les aliments semi-durs ou les imbiber de suffisamment de salive ;
- éviter la monotonie concernant le choix des plats car la texture molle les rend souvent peu appétissants pouvant donc lasser le patient et lui couper l'appétit. Il est ainsi conseillé de varier les couleurs, les parfums, les présentations...

Si ce type de régime est prescrit à vie ou de manière très prolongée (exemple : cas de cancer) il faut penser à :
- stimuler le patient et son entourage ;
- donner une prescription la plus personnalisée possible (choix des aliments très ciblé en fonction des goûts, idées de menus, de recettes...) ;
- penser aux enrichissements.

Les recettes pouvant convenir à ce type de régime sont les suivantes :
- recettes sucrées :
  - crème renversée, crème anglaise, crème pâtissière,
  - île flottante, flans, mousses,
  - semoule au lait, riz au lait, tapioca au lait *sauf si la texture est lisse*,
  - gâteau de riz, gâteau de semoule *sauf si la texture est lisse* ;
- recettes salées :
  - potages, soupes avec du jambon mixé ;
  - sauce Béchamel et purées de légumes avec plus ou moins des œufs, du poisson, de la viande ;
  - sauce Mornay et purées de légumes avec plus ou moins des œufs, du poisson, de la viande ;
  - pain, mousse, quenelle de viande, de poisson, de légumes ;
  - flans, soufflés salés *sauf si la texture est lisse* ;
  - terrines de viande, de poisson, de légumes ;
  - hachis Parmentier *sauf si la texture est lisse* ;
  - brandade de poisson *sauf si la texture est lisse* ;
  - rillettes de poisson *sauf si la texture est lisse* ;
  - légumes farcis *sauf si la texture est lisse*.

6. *Exemple de ration, de répartition et de menu*

6.1. Exemple de ration d'un régime de texture molle à 8 MJ/jour

Aliments	Quantités (g ou mL)	Protéines	Lipides	Glucides	Ca	Fer	Vit C	Fibres
		g	g	g	mg	mg	mg	g
Lait demi-écrémé	450	16	7	22,5	540	0	0	0
Poudre de lait écrémé	10	4	0	5	130	0	0	0
Poudre de protéines	5	4,5	0	0	65	0	0	0
Laitage demi-écrémé	225	13,5	4,5	11	303,75	0	0	0

Les régimes à texture molle

Aliments	Quantités (g ou mL)	Protéines g	Lipides g	Glucides g	Ca mg	Fer mg	Vit C mg	Fibres g
Fromage fondu 70 % pâte dure	20	1,6	6,7	0	100	0	0	0
Viande de catégorie 1 maigre ou équivalent	140	37,8	7	0	21	4	0	0
Œuf	50	6	5	0	0	1	0	0
Jaune d'œuf	20	3	6	0	0	1,1	0	0
PC cuits ou équivalent	200	4	0	40	12	1	20	4
Farine ou équivalent	15	1,5	0	11	2	0,2	0	0,5
Pain ou équivalent	60	5	0	30	15	1,2	0	3
Légumes cuits	250	2,5	0	12,5	100	2,5	25	4
Fruits ou équivalent	300	0	0	36	90	1,5	90	3
Huile	10	0	10	0	0	0	0	0
Beurre ou équivalent	10	0	8,2	0	0	0	0	0
Margarine	10	0	8,2	0	0	0	0	0
Sucre ou équivalent	60	0	0	60	0	0	0	0
Total (g)		99	63	228	1 379	12	135	14
Énergie (kJ)	7 956	1 684	2 396	3 876				
Pourcentages	100	21	30	49				

6.2. Exemple de répartition d'un régime de texture molle à 8 MJ/jour

Aliments	Quantités (g ou mL)	Petit-déjeuner g	Déjeuner g	Collation g	Dîner g
Lait demi-écrémé ou équivalent	450	200	50	0	200
Poudre de lait écrémé	10	0	0	0	10
Poudre de protéines	5	5	0	0	0
Laitage demi-écrémé	225	0	100	125	0
Fromage fondu 70 % pâte dure	20	0	20	0	0
Viande de catégorie 1 maigre ou équivalent	140	0	80	0	60

Aliments	Quantités (g ou mL)	Petit-déjeuner	Déjeuner	Collation	Dîner
		g	g	g	g
Œuf	50	0	50	0	0
Jaune d'œuf	20	0	20	0	0
PC cuits ou équivalent	200	0	100	0	100
Farine ou équivalent	15	10	0	0	5
Pain ou équivalent	60	40	20	0	0
Légumes cuits	250	0	150	0	100
Fruits ou équivalent	300	150	0	0	150
Huile	10	0	5	0	5
Beurre	10	10	0	0	0
Margarine	10	0	10	0	0
Sucre ou équivalent	60	20	10	10	20
Total (kJ)	**7 956**	**1 969**	**3 163**	**501**	**2 323**
%	100	25	40	6	29

6.3. Exemple de menu d'un régime de texture molle à 8 MJ/jour

Petit-déjeuner

Thé léger nature.

Crème meunière enrichie (200 mL de lait demi-écrémé, 10 g de farine, 10 g de beurre, 20 g de sucre, 30 g de petits beurres émiettés finement, 5 g de poudre de protéines).

Une compote de pomme.

Déjeuner

Pain de poisson-coulis de tomates (80 g de filet de poisson, 50 g de tomates appertisées, 10 g d'oignon jaune, 1 tranche de pain de mie, 5 g d'huile d'olive, 1 œuf, 50 mL de lait demi-écrémé).

Purée de carottes enrichie (100 g de carottes, 100 g de pommes de terre, 1 jaune d'œuf, 20 g de fromage fondu, 10 g de margarine).

Un fromage blanc sucré.

Collation

Un yaourt à la pêche (dont 10 g de sucre).

Dîner

Jambon blanc mixé.

Purée de haricots verts (100 g de haricots verts, 100 g de pommes de terre, 5 g d'huile de noix).

Bouillie à la banane enrichie (1 petite banane, 200 mL de lait demi-écrémé, 5 g de farine, 20 g de sucre, 10 g de poudre de lait écrémé).

Section 2

Prescriptions nécessitant une modification des apports conseillés en énergie

4

Le régime hyperénergétique

1. Définition et principe

Le régime hyperénergétique correspond à une alimentation au cours de laquelle l'apport global en énergie est augmenté.

Notons aussi qu'une hausse de l'apport énergétique conduit à augmenter en valeur absolue (c'est-à-dire par rapport aux besoins réels du patient) la quantité de protéines : l'alimentation hyperénergétique est donc également hyperprotidique.

2. Les indications

Le régime hyperénergétique est prescrit dans le cas de pathologies pour lesquelles il existe :
- un catabolisme excessif ;
- et/ou un anabolisme augmenté ;
- et/ou des pertes durables ;
- et/ou des apports énergétiques insuffisants par rapport aux besoins.

Il s'agit :
- des cas de dénutritions avérées ;
- des situations à risque de dénutrition progressive :
  - affections malignes (cancers, hémopathies),
  - pathologies infectieuses chroniques (VIH, tuberculose…),
  - maladies chroniques du tube digestif,
  - hépatopathies évoluées,
  - insuffisance cardiaque,

- insuffisance respiratoire chronique,
- insuffisance rénale chronique (dialysée ou non),
- pathologies neuropsychiatriques et neurodégénératives,
- escarres ;
– des situations à risque de dénutrition aiguë :
  - hypercatabolisme,
  - situations postopératoires : chirurgie viscérale majeure, chirurgie cardiaque, greffes d'organes…,
  - polytraumatismes,
  - blessures multiples,
  - brûlures étendues,
  - pathologies médicales : infections aiguës curables (pneumopathie, septicémie…) ;
– des sujets âgés de plus de 75 ans et hospitalisés depuis plus de 3 jours.

3. Objectifs nutritionnels

Les buts du régime hyperénergétique sont les suivants :
– prévenir ou corriger une dénutrition ;
– obtenir selon les cas :
  - un poids stable,
  - une stabilisation de la perte de poids,
  - le retour à un poids de forme.

4. Couverture des besoins et apports nutritionnels conseillés

4.1. L'énergie

Le niveau énergétique dépend de différents cas.

4.1.1. *Cas d'une dénutrition avérée ou progressive et des personnes âgées de plus de 75 ans*

L'apport énergétique doit tout d'abord représenter 150 kJ par kilogramme de poids de forme et par jour (soit 35 kcal/kg/jour). Les apports sont ensuite augmentés progressivement d'environ 20 % tous les jours ou tous les deux jours.

Remarque
Chez l'adulte, le poids de forme est calculé pour un IMC compris entre 18,5 et 24,9 kg/m^2 tandis que chez les personnes âgées l'IMC de forme doit être d'au minimum 21 kg/m^2.

4.1.2. Cas d'une dénutrition aiguë

Les apports énergétiques sont compris entre 100 et 150 kJ par kilogramme de poids de forme et par jour (soit 25 à 35 kcal/kg/jour) avec :
- plutôt 100 kJ/kg/jour (soit 25 kcal/kg/jour) lors de la phase aiguë de la maladie ou lors d'une agression ;
- plutôt 125 à 150 kJ/kg (soit 30 à 35 kcal/kg/j) lors de la phase de convalescence ou lors de l'amélioration d'une affection catabolisante.

> **Remarques**
> Les besoins en énergie peuvent éventuellement être exprimés en pourcentage de l'apport énergétique total (exemple : 130 % de l'AET).
> Les modes d'administration doivent être précisés (voie orale et/ou entérale et/ou parentérale).

4.2. Les protéines

Comme nous l'avons vu précédemment, le régime hyperénergétique est aussi hyperprotidique en valeur absolue en vue de lutter contre l'hypercatabolisme.

Le rapport calorico-azoté doit ainsi être surveillé à savoir qu'il doit être de 1 g d'azote pour 650 à 850 de kJ glucidolipidique (150 à 200 kcal) de telle sorte que l'utilisation protéique soit maximisée.

Si la dénutrition est progressive, l'apport calorique et protidique doit permettre d'obtenir progressivement un bilan azoté positif (c'est-à-dire que les entrées doivent être plus élevées que les sorties), correspondant à un flux de synthèse protéique supérieur au catabolisme.

Si l'on constate un hypercatabolisme (deuxième phase d'une situation d'agression aiguë), les pertes urinaires d'azote deviennent élevées. L'apport de calories et d'azote doit donc permettre de limiter l'utilisation par l'organisme des protéines musculaires et viscérales, même si le bilan azoté reste souvent négatif (c'est-à-dire que les sorties sont supérieures aux entrées).

> **Remarque**
> En cas d'obésité associée à une dénutrition, il faut veiller à un apport protéique d'au moins 0,8 à 1 g par kg de poids de forme et par jour afin de maintenir la masse maigre et d'éviter l'aggravation de la dénutrition.

4.3. Les lipides

Le régime est normolipidique, soit 30 à 35 % de l'apport énergétique total avec une répartition en acides gras correspondant aux recommandations.

4.4. Les glucides

D'une manière générale, le régime est normoglucidique voire légèrement hypoglucidique (selon l'apport protidique établi), les glucides étant les compléments énergétiques de la ration.

4.5. Les fibres, les vitamines, les minéraux et l'eau

Les apports en ces différents nutriments doivent correspondre aux besoins de chaque individu selon son âge, son état physiologique et son niveau d'activité physique.

En cas de régime hyperprotidique réellement associé, il convient d'être vigilant vis-à-vis de certains micronutriments (*cf.* régime hyperprotidique).

5. *Le choix des aliments*

Groupe d'aliments	Aliments conseillés	Aliments déconseillés
Laits	Laits entiers (voire demi-écrémés) sous toutes leurs formes Poudre de lait écrémé	Laits écrémés liquides et concentrés
Laitages	Laitages entiers (voire demi-écrémés) sous toutes leurs formes Poudre de lait écrémé	Laitages écrémés sous toutes leurs formes
Desserts lactés	Desserts lactés non allégés	Desserts lactés allégés
Fromages	Fromages non allégés **Remarque :** privilégier les pâtes dures	Fromages allégés
V/P/O	Pas de contre-indications Respecter les quantités et les fréquences de consommation recommandées	Plats cuisinés du commerce allégés
Farines et dérivés/féculents	Pas de contre-indications Respecter les quantités et les fréquences de consommation recommandées	Plats cuisinés du commerce allégés
Légumes	Pas de contre-indications Respecter les quantités et les fréquences de consommation recommandées	Plats cuisinés du commerce allégés
Fruits	Pas de contre-indications Respecter les quantités et les fréquences de consommation recommandées	Produits du commerce à base de fruits allégés

Groupe d'aliments	Aliments conseillés	Aliments déconseillés
Matières grasses et équivalents	**Matières grasses non allégées** En équivalence : **Graines oléagineuses** **Fruits oléagineux**	**Matières grasses allégées**
Sucre et produits sucrés	**Tous les produits sucrés non allégés**	**Produits sucrés allégés**
Boissons	**Toutes les boissons non allégées** Respecter les quantités et les fréquences de consommation recommandées pour les boissons sucrées	**Boissons alcoolisées** **Boissons allégées**
Épices et aromates	**Pas de contre-indications**	
Produits diététiques et de régime	**Produits de complémentation orale hyperénergétiques et/ou hyperprotidiques** **Poudre de protéines** **Poudre de maltodextrines**	**Produits à base d'édulcorants de synthèse**

6. *En pratique*

Afin de s'assurer du bon suivi de la prescription, il est nécessaire de surveiller les éléments cliniques et biologiques du patient en particulier :
– l'évolution du poids ;
– l'indice de masse corporelle (IMC) ;
– l'albuminémie ;
– la préalbuminémie (transthyrétinémie) ;
– la protéine C réactive ;
– la tolérance digestive et les capacités d'alimentation ;
– le bilan azoté (natrémie).

En pratique, la nature de l'alimentation peut être modifiée en ayant recours :

1. À un enrichissement de l'alimentation normale en énergie et/ou en protéines :
– avec de la poudre de lait (sachant que 3 cuillères à soupe correspond à environ 120 mL de lait liquide) ou du lait concentré ou du jaune d'œuf ou de la poudre de protéines (à intégrer dans du lait, des laitages, des desserts lactés, des compotes, des gâteaux, des pâtisseries, des omelettes, des purées, des potages, des sauces…) ;

- en utilisant de préférence du lait entier ;
- en rajoutant des matières grasses dans les préparations de base ;
- en additionnant : du sucre, du miel, de la confiture, de la gelée, du sirop d'érable, du caramel, des graines oléagineuses en poudre, du chocolat râpé, du chocolat en poudre, de la pâte à tartiner, du beurre de cacahuète, des fruits confits, du sirop, de la crème de marron, des fruits secs… dans les préparations sucrées ;
- en ajoutant des morceaux d'œuf dur, de fromage, de viande hachée, de jambon, de lardon, de poulet, de thon, des crevettes, du maïs, des croûtons, du vermicelle, des olives, des graines oléagineuses… dans les entrées, les potages, les purées… ;
- en servant les plats de viandes avec de la sauce (de préférence à base d'huiles insaturées) ;
- en servant les légumes en gratin et/ou avec une sauce enrichie type béchamel enrichie ;
- en utilisant au besoin des poudres à base de maltodextrines permettant d'enrichir la ration glucidique. Elles ont l'avantage d'être bien tolérées par l'organisme et de ne pas entraîner d'inconfort digestif et intestinal comme avec les mélanges de sucres simples (dextrose, fructose).

2. À la prescription de collations (apports plus fréquents dans la journée d'aliments standard tels que des laitages, des biscuits, des desserts lactés plus ou moins enrichis).

3. À une adaptation de la texture selon l'appétit du patient. Ainsi, une texture molle voire liquide peut être plus facilement ingérée.

4. À des suppléments diététiques oraux industriels (notamment en cas d'échec de l'optimisation de l'alimentation « normale ») qui doivent être adaptés à la situation ; ils peuvent être selon les cas :
- hyperénergétiques, hyperprotidiques ;
- hyperénergétiques, normoprotidiques ;
- normoénergétiques, hyperprotidiques.

Ces produits diététiques de complémentation sont des préparations complexes qui apportent des protéines, des glucides et des lipides, répartis selon les apports recommandés, ainsi que des vitamines et des oligo-éléments. Ils apportent de 1 à 1,5 kcal/mL et entre 8 et 20 g de protéines par portion. Ils sont en général dépourvus de gluten et la plupart de lactose. Les grandes variétés d'arômes et de goûts permettent de les adapter aux préférences des patients.

Tout comme pour la supplémentation orale par l'alimentation, ils ne sont efficaces que si leur mode de consommation respecte certaines règles :
- expliquer au patient l'objectif thérapeutique de leur intégration, le rassurer sur leur tolérance digestive, l'encourager à les ingérer en cas d'anorexie ;
- servir le supplément frais et à distance des repas (au moins 2 heures) ;

Le régime hyperénergétique

- adapter les arômes et les goûts en fonction de chaque patient ;
- insister pour que le complément soit consommé au moment où il est servi ;
- aider éventuellement à sa consommation (ouverture…) ;
- contrôler leur réelle consommation et en analyser les raisons.

5. Une modification du mode d'administration des nutriments en raison de l'impossibilité d'une alimentation orale. Il sera ainsi décidé d'une nutrition entérale voire parentérale si le tube digestif est non fonctionnel ou non accessible. C'est le cas des patients dont les ingesta réels sont très diminués (inférieurs à 50 % des apports conseillés) et que la dénutrition est considérée comme sévère.

Lors de la prescription de sortie, il est possible de proposer :
- des suppléments nutritionnels diététiques adaptés aux besoins et acceptés par le patient ;
- une alimentation entérale à domicile ;
- des idées d'enrichissement des plats ;
- des équivalences caloriques ;
- des équivalences protéiques.

7. Exemple de ration, de répartition et de menu

7.1. Exemple de ration d'un régime hyperénergétique-hyperprotidique à 12,3 MJ/jour

Aliments	Quantités (g ou mL)	Protéines g	Lipides g	Glucides g	Ca mg	Fer mg	Vit C mg	Fibres g
Lait demi-écrémé ou équivalent	275	10	4	14	330	0	0	0
Poudre de lait écrémé	20	7	0	10	300	0	0	0
Fromage	60	12	13	0	300	0	0	0
Fromage fondu pâte dure	20	2	7	0	100	0	0	0
VPO	200	36	20	0	30	4	0	0
Œufs	50	6	5	0	0	1	0	0
Jaune d'œuf	20	3	6	0	0	1	0	0
Pain ou équivalent	200	16	0	100	50	4	0	10
PC crus ou équivalent	80	8	0	60	20	0,8	0	1
Légumes	500	5	0	25	200	5	100	15
Fruits	300	0	0	36	90	1,5	90	6

Aliments	Quantités (g ou mL)	Protéines g	Lipides g	Glucides g	Ca mg	Fer mg	Vit C mg	Fibres g
Huile	25	0	25	0	0	0	0	0
Beurre/Margarine	25	0	20,5	0	0	0	0	0
Sucre ou équivalent	80	0	0	80	0	0	0	0
Poudre de protéines	10	9	0,2	0	140	0	0	0
Complément oral	200	20	5	25	500	0	0	0
Total (g)		134	106	350	2 060	17	190	32
Énergie (kJ)	12 270	2 274	4 044	5 953				
Pourcentages	100	19	33	49				

7.2. Exemple de répartition d'un régime hyperénergétique-hyperprotidique à 12,3 MJ/jour

Aliments	Quantités (g ou mL)	Petit-déjeuner g	Déjeuner g	Collation g	Dîner g
Lait demi-écrémé ou équivalent	275	150	125	0	0
Poudre de lait écrémé	20	10	10	0	0
Fromage	60	0	20	0	40
Fromage fondu pâte dure	20	0	0	0	20
VPO	200	0	100	0	100
Œuf	50	0	50	0	0
Jaune d'œuf	20	0	20	0	0
Pain ou équivalent	200	100	0	0	100
PC crus ou équivalent	80	0	80	0	0
Légumes	500	0	100	0	400
Fruits	300	150	0	0	150
Huile	25	0	15	0	10
Beurre/Margarine	25	15	10	0	0
Sucre ou équivalent	80	45	25	0	10

Aliments	Quantités (g ou mL)	Petit-déjeuner	Déjeuner	Collation	Dîner
		g	g	g	g
Poudre de protéines	10	10	0	0	0
Complément oral	200	0	0	200	0
Total (kJ)	**12 272**	3 137	4 490	956	3 690
Pourcentages	100	26	37	8	30

7.3. Exemple de menu d'un régime hyperénergétique-hyperprotidique à 12,3 MJ/jour

Petit-déjeuner
Café au lait sucré enrichi (3 morceaux de sucre, 10 g de poudre de lait écrémé).
Baguette beurrée et miel d'accacia (50 g).
Une compote d'abricot enrichie (10 g de poudre de protéines).

Déjeuner
Tomates au basilic (10 mL d'huile d'olive).
Sauté de porc au curry (30 g de crème fraîche).
Gratin de pennes au parmesan (dont 5 mL d'huile de colza).
Crème caramel enrichie (125 mL de lait demi-écrémé, 1 œuf, 25 g de sucre dont 15 g pour le caramel, 10 g de poudre de lait écrémé, 1 jaune d'œuf).

Collation
Un complément oral hyperénergétique-hyperprotidique (200 mL).

Dîner
Potage au potiron enrichi (150 g de potiron, 1 crème de gruyère).
Darne de saumon en papillote.
Courgettes braisées (250 g de courgettes, 10 mL d'huile de tournesol).
Comté fruité.
Pain aux céréales.
Une petite banane.

5

Le régime hypoénergétique ou hypocalorique

1. Définition et principe

Le régime hypoénergétique est un régime dont l'apport calorique journalier est contrôlé en vue de déséquilibrer la balance énergétique, le but étant d'obtenir une fonte progressive et durable du tissu adipeux tout en préservant la masse maigre.

Les objectifs nutritionnels du régime hypocalorique sont donc d'obtenir un amaigrissement qui doit être :

– *progressif,* c'est-à-dire de 2 à 4 kg par mois (ce qui représente en moyenne 0,5 à 1 kg par semaine) ce qui a pour effet d'éviter l'effet « yoyo » par la suite. Notons que lors de la première semaine de prescription, la perte de poids enregistrée est généralement assez rapide due à un début de perte de masse grasse associé à une légère fonte de masse maigre (celle-ci étant riche en eau et servant de substrat en glycogène). Les semaines suivantes, on assiste à un ralentissement progressif de la perte de poids car il est plus difficile pour l'organisme de puiser de l'énergie essentiellement au sein du tissu adipeux ;

– *durable* : la perte de poids fait partie intégrante du traitement du surpoids et/ou de l'obésité d'autant plus qu'elle permet la prévention de nombreuses pathologies associées (pathologies digestives et/ou métaboliques, dérèglements hormonaux, troubles psychologiques…) ;

– *sans fatigue* : une asthénie pourrait signifier que les quantités d'aliments ingérées sont insuffisantes par rapport aux besoins et donc engendrer une déficience en certains micronutriments. De plus, il est nécessaire que l'organisme puisse maintenir sa masse maigre ;

– *sans fringale* : ne pas avoir faim entre les repas assure un suivi du régime sur du long terme et limite les risques de frustrations ;

– *permettant de stabiliser les constantes sanguines* : de nombreux patients suivant un régime hypoénergétique présentent des bilans sanguins anormaux avec le plus souvent une hypercholestérolémie et/ou une hypertriglycéridémie et/ou une hyperglycémie et/ou une hypertension artérielle... Le choix des aliments du régime hypocalorique permet par conséquent de participer à une amélioration de leur santé.

2. *Les indications*

Les indications du régime hypoénergétique sont les suivantes :
- patients en surpoids (c'est-à-dire dont l'indice de masse corporelle est supérieur ou égal à 25) ;
- patients obèses (c'est-à-dire dont l'indice de masse corporelle est supérieur ou égal à 30) ;
- patients présentant d'autres pathologies liées au surpoids et/ou à l'obésité telles que :
  - le diabète non insulinodépendant : au moins 60 % des patients sont en surpoids ou obèses et le régime hypoénergétique participe au rééquilibre de la glycémie,
  - les lithiases : la perte de poids fait partie intégrante du traitement d'autant plus que le régime hypoénergétique permet de limiter les crises,
  - l'hypertension artérielle,
  - les dyslipidémies (hypercholestérolémies, hypertriglycéridémies),
  - d'autres maladies cardiovasculaires (insuffisance coronarienne, troubles du rythme à l'effort...),
  - des perturbations hormonales ayant engendré une prise de poids (ménopause, hypothyroïdie...).

Il existe néanmoins des contre-indications au régime hypoénergétique à savoir :
- les personnes âgées de plus de 80 ans (sauf si le traitement d'une maladie associée justifie réellement une réduction de l'excès de poids) ; les apports contrôlés en énergie pouvant engendrer des déficiences voire des carences chez cette population particulièrement fragile ;
- les femmes enceintes et les femmes allaitantes : les apports doivent être suffisants afin de répondre aux besoins durant ces périodes spécifiques ;
- les maladies évolutives (cancers, pathologies chroniques du tube digestif...) pouvant être aggravées par une restriction calorique ;
- les nourrissons et les enfants de par le fait que leurs besoins sont extrêmement particuliers et variables.

3. Couverture des besoins et apports nutritionnels conseillés

3.1. L'énergie

On se base sur les apports énergétiques spontanés du patient que l'on diminue par paliers de 30 % en vue de permettre une diminution progressive et durable de la perte de poids. On distingue alors deux cas de figure pour atteindre l'objectif de poids :
- cas n° 1 : patients ayant peu de poids à perdre (moins de 5 kg) : on revient à une alimentation normo-équilibrée en tentant de ne pas descendre en dessous de la dépense énergétique journalière ;
- cas n° 2 : patients nécessitant une perte de poids plus importante (au minimum 5 kg) : on atteint progressivement un apport calorique égal à la dépense énergétique journalière et on descend en dessous de celle-ci uniquement lorsque l'objectif de poids n'est pas atteint à ce stade. Une stabilisation sera alors nécessaire par la suite.

Le niveau énergétique est donc variable en fonction de la perte de poids de chaque patient puisque la réduction des apports énergétiques est réalisée chaque fois que la perte de poids se ralentit ou se stabilise.

Notons qu'afin d'atteindre l'objectif de poids, il est parfois nécessaire de passer par un AET inférieur aux recommandations (et donc inférieur à la dépense énergétique journalière). Il convient dans ce cas de ne pas descendre en dessous de 5 MJ (1 200 kcal) pour une femme et de 5,8 MJ (1 400 kcal) pour un homme en vue d'éviter la perte de masse maigre et d'éventuelles déficiences en micronutriments (voire en macronutriments).

Remarque

En milieu hospitalier, certains régimes hypoénergétiques prescrits sont nettement plus stricts, le but étant d'obtenir des résultats rapides car il y a urgence pour le traitement du patient. On atteint ainsi parfois jusqu'à 3,5 MJ par jour (800 kcal par jour) chez une femme et jusqu'à 5 MJ par jour (1 200 kcal par jour) chez un homme.

3.2. Les protéines

Le taux protéique est fixé selon l'apport énergétique. On distingue ainsi deux possibilités :
- le régime est normoprotidique lorsque l'apport énergétique est supérieur à la dépense énergétique journalière ;
- le régime est hyperprotidique (soit 1,2 à 1,5 g/kg/j/kg de poids de forme) lorsque l'apport énergétique est inférieur à la dépense énergétique journalière. En effet, une ration restrictive en protéines pourrait provoquer une perte accrue de masse maigre et négativer la balance azotée.

Outre leur rôle dans le maintien de la masse maigre aux dépens du tissu adipeux, les protéines sont aussi satiétantes ce qui explique que leurs quantités doivent être importantes. De plus, il conviendra de privilégier les protéines d'origine animale celles-ci étant de meilleure qualité et donc plus efficaces pour lutter contre une éventuelle sarcopénie.

3.3. Les lipides

Les lipides étant les nutriments les plus énergétiques et les plus rapidement mis en réserve dans le tissu adipeux, le régime peut être légèrement hypolipidique soit 25 à 30 % de l'AET. De plus, les lipides retardent le rassasiement en augmentant le contenu énergétique des repas et il a même été démontré qu'ils stimuleraient moins la leptine que les glucides ce qui réduirait leur effet satiétant à long terme.

La répartition des acides gras (cas de l'adulte) peut alors se faire de la manière suivante :
- AGS : 6,5 % AET ;
- AGMI : 16,5 % AET ;
- AGPI : 4 % AET avec 3 % d'oméga 6 et 1 % d'oméga 3 dont 0,05 % de DHA.

Remarque

Il est fortement déconseillé de réduire l'apport lipidique à moins de 25 % de l'AET car :
- les lipides participent à la palatabilité des repas ;
- ils assurent la couverture en acides gras essentiels et en vitamines liposolubles ;
- ils aident au maintien de l'élasticité de la peau (notamment lors d'une importante perte de poids).

3.4. Les glucides

En tant que compléments énergétiques de la ration, les glucides représentent :
- 55 à 65 % de l'AET lorsque le régime est normoprotidique ;
- 50 à 60 % de l'AET lorsque le régime est hyperprotidique.

Pour ce qui est de la répartition des glucides, il est recommandé d'atteindre 55 % de glucides complexes et 45 % de glucides simples (même si en pratique cela peut être difficile de par le choix des aliments).

Les produits sucrés ne doivent pas dépasser 5 % de l'AET mais ils restent des aliments plaisir facilitant l'acceptabilité du régime. Ils peuvent, dans le cas d'un régime hypoénergétique strict, être totalement supprimés en les considérant seulement en tant que calories vides (d'autant plus à faible volume, forte valeur énergétique et index glycémique souvent élevé).

Il est également conseillé de privilégier les aliments à index glycémique bas et de ne pas consommer d'aliments à index glycémique élevé en prise isolée en vue d'éviter les pics d'hyperinsulinisme pouvant être responsables d'hypoglycémies réactionnelles (d'où de fringales).

Enfin, il est préconisé de ne jamais donner moins de 100 g de glucides par jour pour empêcher tout risque d'hypoglycémie, de souffrance des tissus glucodépendants et un éventuel effet « rebond » lors de la phase de stabilisation (engendré par la reconstitution d'un stock glucidique plus important suite à une privation de l'organisme).

3.5. Les fibres

Les apports conseillés en fibres ne sont pas modifiés, soit pour l'adulte bien portant 25 à 30 g par jour dont 10 à 15 g de fibres solubles. Celles-ci jouent des rôles essentiels lors de la prescription d'un régime hypocalorique car :
- elles sont satiétantes en retardant la vidange gastrique (elles participent à la gestion des fringales) ;
- elles sont hypocholestérolémiantes et diminuent la glycémie postprandiale (elles aident donc à l'amélioration des perturbations des constantes sanguines d'autant plus lorsqu'elles sont solubles).

Notons que la plupart des patients en surpoids ou obèses sont de petits consommateurs de végétaux dont les apports spontanés en fibres sont peu élevés. Leur réintroduction doit donc se faire de manière progressive pour éviter tout risque d'irritation du côlon.

3.6. Les minéraux

Une déficience en *fer* peut provoquer une anémie ferriprive et donc une asthénie ce qui perturberait l'observance du régime notamment à long terme.

Il est donc judicieux de proposer régulièrement des aliments riches en fer héminique (mieux absorbé) adaptés tels que du foie et d'autres abats peu gras, des viandes maigres, des crustacés, des poissons…

De par son pouvoir sédatif (dû à ses effets myorelaxants), le *magnésium* intervient dans la gestion du stress, facteur dont il est important de tenir compte lors de régimes restrictifs. Sa consommation doit par conséquent être contrôlée voire accentuée par des aliments qui en sont riches : céréales pour petit-déjeuner au son, mollusques, pains complets, crustacés, riz complet, poissons, légumes feuilles, eaux magnésiennes…

3.7. Les vitamines

La *vitamine C* aidant à lutter contre l'asthénie, les apports conseillés doivent être couverts. C'est pourquoi, les légumes et les fruits, notamment sous forme de crudités, sont des aliments de choix du régime hypoénergétique.

De plus, on peut constater un risque de déficience en *vitamines B_1, B_3, B_5 et B_6* lors de régime assez restrictif de par les petites quantités de pain ou équivalents et/ou de féculents servies. Une complémentation par de la levure de bière peut alors être proposée.

La réduction des apports lipidiques peut aussi engendrer un manque de *vitamines liposolubles* (notamment A, D et E). Il est donc conseillé de consommer des aliments qui en sont riches, adaptés au choix des aliments proposés.

3.8. L'eau

En raison de leur effet « coupe-faim », les apports en eau de boisson doivent être correctement couverts et bien répartis tout au long de la journée. Ils assurent également l'évacuation suffisante des déchets azotés et limitent la mise à contribution trop importante des reins d'autant plus si le régime est hyperprotidique.

4. *Le choix des aliments*

Groupe d'aliments	Aliments conseillés	Aliments déconseillés
Laits	Lait liquide demi-écrémé, écrémé Lait concentré, en poudre demi-écrémé, écrémé nature reconstitué	Lait liquide entier Lait concentré entier et/ou sucré Lait en poudre entier Laits aromatisés
Laitages	Yaourts ordinaires et/ou édulcorés Yaourts 0 % MG et/ou édulcorés Fromages frais 0 % et 10 % MG nature ou édulcorés	Yaourts au lait entier et/ou sucrés Fromages frais au lait entier (20 % MG), 30 % MG et 40 % MG et/ou sucrés Laitages « crémeux »
Desserts lactés	Desserts lactés allégés en matières grasses et en sucre Attention : il convient de les décomposer en équivalences (lait, matières grasses et sucre) si nécessaire	Desserts lactés non allégés en matières grasses et/ou contenant des matières sucrantes
Fromages	Fromages les moins riches en lipides : Camembert 40 %/MS Camembert 45 %/MS	Fromages les plus riches en lipides : Beaufort Bleu

Le régime hypoénergétique ou hypocalorique

Groupe d'aliments	Aliments conseillés	Aliments déconseillés
Fromages	Camembert 25 %/MS Chèvre frais Carré de l'est Coulommiers Édam Emmental peu affiné Fromages allégés 25 % MG/MS Fromages fondus à base de pâte dure Fromages fondus 45 %/MS Fromage type Babybel® Fromage type Carré frais® Fromage type Chaource® Pont-l'évêque Raclette Reblochon Roquefort Saint Marcellin Sainte Maure Saint Nectaire Saint Paulin Selle sur Cher Tomme **Attention :** la quantité et les étiquetages des fromages doivent être bien contrôlés	Camembert 50 %, 60 %/MS Cantal Cheddar Chèvre mi-secs et secs Comté Emmental très affiné Fromages fondus 65 %, 70 %/MS Fromage type Boursin® Gruyère Gouda Maroilles Munster Mimolette Morbier Neuchâtel Parmesan Pyrénées Vacherin
Viandes	**Viandes de boucherie maigres Volailles maigres sans la peau Gibiers Abats maigres** Modes de cuisson : sans ou avec peu de matières grasses, sauces dégraissées, papillotes, four (rôtis), grillées, brochettes…	**Viandes de boucherie grasses et demi-grasses Volailles grasses et/ou les morceaux riches en peau Abats riches en lipides Autres :** paupiettes de viande, viandes panées, beignets, plats cuisinés à base de viandes…
Charcuteries	**Charcuteries maigres**	**Charcuteries grasses**
Produits de la pêche	**Poissons maigres, demi-gras et gras *en équivalence*** Modes de consommation conseillés : – frais – surgelés non cuisinés – en conserve au naturel	*Pas de contre-indication* Modes de consommation déconseillés : – en conserve à l'huile ou en sauce

Groupe d'aliments	Aliments conseillés	Aliments déconseillés
Produits de la pêche	Modes de cuisson : de préférence sans ou avec peu de matières grasses : grillés, court-bouillon, four, vapeur, papillote, brochettes…	– préparations du commerce : poissons panés, en beignet, rillettes, mousses, pâtés, terrines… – plats cuisinés à base de poisson
Œufs	Modes de cuisson : de préférence sans ou avec peu de matières grasses Modes de consommation : omelettes, pochés, à la coque, au plat (poêle antiadhésive), cocotte, durs, mollets, brouillés…	*Pas de contre-indication*
Farines et dérivés	**Farines (de blé, de sarrasin, complète), fécules, maïzena, tapioca…** **Pains : blanc (type baguette), campagne, complet, seigle, son, aux céréales, précuit, azyme, pain de mie… nature** **Biscottes, pains grillés, petits pains grillés, cracottes, galettes de blé ou de riz type Wasa®… nature** **Biscuits secs nature** Les recettes doivent être avec le moins de lipides et de glucides simples possibles et ils doivent être décomposés en farine, matières grasses et sucre si nécessaire **Céréales pour petit-déjeuner non fourrées, non chocolatées (de préférence pétales de maïs soufflées et grains de riz soufflés), mueslis, flocons d'avoine nature** Mode de consommation : privilégier les aliments complets	**Pain brioché, pain viennois, pain au lait, pain pour hamburger, pains fantaisies…** **Produits de biscotterie fourrés Viennoiseries** **Biscuits à apéritif Autres biscuits Pâtisseries et autres gâteaux** **Céréales pour petit-déjeuner fourrées, chocolatées, barres de céréales…**
Féculents	**Féculents non cuisinés** Mode de consommation : privilégier les féculents complets	**Plats cuisinés à base de féculents**

Le régime hypoénergétique ou hypocalorique

Groupe d'aliments	Aliments conseillés	Aliments déconseillés
Légumes	Légumes frais Légumes surgelés non cuisinés Légumes en conserve non cuisinés Potages maison et du commerce (à moins de 1 % de lipides) Modes de cuisson : de préférence sans ou avec peu de matières grasses (à l'eau, à la vapeur, au four, à l'étouffée, au grill…) Mode de consommation : privilégier les crudités (riches en antioxydants)	Légumes cuisinés du commerce Potages du commerce à plus de 1 % de lipides
Fruits	Fruits frais Fruits surgelés non sucrés Coulis de fruits non sucrés Compotes de fruits du commerce non sucrées ou édulcorés Compotes de fruits maison nature ou aux édulcorants Jus de fruits maison ou du commerce non sucrés *En équivalence :* Fruits secs, fruits au sirop **Attention :** faire des équivalences en fonction du pourcentage glucidique de chaque type de fruits	Fruits surgelés sucrés Coulis de fruits sucrés Compotes sucrées Jus de fruits sucrés
Matières grasses et équivalents	**En quantité très contrôlée :** **Toutes les huiles** (de préférence sources d'acides gras insaturés) Margarines et margarines allégées Beurre et beurre allégé Crème fraîche et crème fraîche allégée Vinaigrette et vinaigrette allégée *En équivalence :* graines et fruits oléagineux	Sauces du commerce et/ou sauces riches en lipides Fritures, panures

Groupe d'aliments	Aliments conseillés	Aliments déconseillés
Sucre et produits sucrés	Édulcorants de synthèse Une unité ou une cuillère à soupe équivaut au pouvoir sucrant d'un morceau de sucre	Sucre **Confitures, gelées, marmelades, miels** **Confiseries** **Sorbets** **Crème de marron** **Fruits confits** **Pâtes de fruits** **Chocolats et dérivés** **Pâtes à tartiner** **Crèmes glacées, glaces**
Boissons	**Eaux du robinet, minérales plates ou gazeuses, de source** **Eaux minérales aromatisées non sucrées et/ou édulcorées** **Thé, café, infusions, tisanes non sucrés** **Boissons rafraîchissantes non sucrées et/ou édulcorées** Sirops édulcorés Jus de légumes **Attention : concernant les boissons édulcorées :** bien vérifier la non-présence de sucre et en contrôler les quantités ingérées	Eaux minérales aromatisées sucrées Préparations à base de thé, café sucrées Boissons rafraîchissantes sucrées Sirops sucrés Toutes les boissons alcoolisées
Épices et aromates	Pour les préparations salées : **toutes les fines herbes et épices, bouillons cubes dégraissés et/ou aux légumes** Pour les préparations sucrées : **vanille, extrait de café, extrait d'amande, fleur d'oranger, menthe...**	Bouillons cubes non dégraissés

5. *En pratique*

En pratique, il est recommandé de :
- veiller à la qualité de l'interrogatoire alimentaire indispensable au succès de la perte de poids ;
- proposer un choix des aliments le plus large possible, très détaillé et adapté avec un grand nombre d'équivalences ;

- tenter d'obtenir un apport énergétique le plus élevé possible ;
- penser à associer le régime avec un soutien psychologique si nécessaire ;
- gérer la phase de stabilisation dont la durée totale est à peu près identique à celle de l'amaigrissement (remonter par paliers de 500 à 1 000 kJ par jour (150 à 250 kcal par jour) en maintenant le nouveau niveau énergétique pendant environ 2 à 3 semaines.

Pour ce qui est de l'alimentation journalière :
- donner au moins 150 g de VPO par jour (pour leurs protéines animales de bonne qualité et satiétantes) ;
- les légumes (non cuisinés) peuvent être proposés à volonté (de par leur faible valeur énergétique, leur volume élevé, leur richesse en eau, en fibres…) ;
- les aliments amylacés sont obligatoires au petit-déjeuner, au minimum au déjeuner ou au dîner (apport de glucides complexes, vitamines du groupe B, fibres…) ;
- les portions de fruits sont fixées à 2-3 par jour environ (apports de glucides simples à index glycémique bas) ;
- veiller à la consommation d'un aliment riche en vitamine C par jour (de par ses rôles importants).

Certains conseils généraux peuvent être donnés aux patients tels que :
- manger lentement, en mastiquant bien chaque bouchée (au minimum 20 minutes par repas), dans le calme (éviter la télévision, les lieux bruyants…) ;
- manger à heures régulières (le rassasiement se fait alors sur du plus long terme) ;
- ne pas sauter de repas (le risque de fringale et de fatigue s'accentuerait associé à une possible mise en réserve énergétique excessive le repas suivant suite à la privation de l'organisme) ;
- se peser régulièrement c'est-à-dire une fois par semaine ou deux (mais pas deux fois par jour !), sur la même balance et dans les mêmes conditions ;
- apprendre à bien faire ses courses ;
- ne pas grignoter (prévoir des solutions anti-fringales) ;
- s'autoriser jusqu'à 2 écarts par semaine et apprendre à les compenser (prévoir les aliments nécessaires) ;
- éventuellement, faire l'acquisition d'une balance alimentaire ;
- apprendre à cuisiner ;
- consommer du poisson au minimum 3 fois par semaine ;
- prévoir une crudité (légume ou fruit cru) par repas ;
- éviter de « goûter » systématiquement les aliments pendant la préparation des repas ;
- ne pas trop saler les préparations (en excès, le sel a tendance à stimuler l'appétit) ;
- utiliser les fines herbes et les épices qui donnent du goût aux préparations tout en étant acaloriques ;

- bien respecter les quantités indiquées en contrôlant précisément les portions de chaque groupe ;
- penser aux matières grasses allégées qui augmentent le confort des plats mais bien en respecter les équivalences ;
- varier le plus possible entre les différents types de matières grasses (les quantités proposées étant peu élevées) ;
- assurer des quantités importantes de légumes à chaque repas (au moins 300 g) ;
- utiliser des assiettes de taille moyenne ;
- varier les couleurs des préparations pour obtenir des repas les plus attrayants possibles ;
- ne pas se resservir ;
- boire 1,5 à 2 L d'eau par jour (environ 8 grands verres) et bien la répartir tout au long de la journée ;
- pratiquer une activité physique régulière (l'équivalent d'une demi-heure de marche chaque jour ou de 3 heures de sport par semaine au minimum).

6. *Exemple de ration, de répartition et de menu*

6.1. Exemple de ration d'un régime hypoénergétique à 5,5 MJ/jour

Aliments	Quantités (g ou mL)	Protéines g	Lipides g	Glucides g	Ca mg	Fer mg	Vit C mg	Fibres g
Lait écrémé ou équivalent	450	16	0	22,5	540	0	0	0
Fromage	30	6	7	0	150	0	0	0
VPO maigres	150	27	7,5	0	22,5	3	0	0
Pain ou équivalent	100	8	0	50	25	2	0	5
PC crus ou équivalent	50	5	0	37,5	12,5	0,5	0	0,75
Légumes	400	4	0	20	160	4	80	12
Fruits	300	0	0	36	90	1,5	90	6
Huile	20	0	20	0	0	0	0	0

Le régime hypoénergétique ou hypocalorique

Aliments	Quantités (g ou mL)	Protéines g	Lipides g	Glucides g	Ca mg	Fer mg	Vit C mg	Fibres g
Beurre/margarine allégé	15	0	6	0	0	0	0	0
Total (g)		66	40	166	1 000	11	170	24
Énergie (kJ)	5 469	1 118	1 530	2 822				
Pourcentages	100	20	28	52				

6.2. Exemple de répartition d'un régime hypoénergétique à 5,5 MJ/jour

Aliments	Quantités (g ou mL)	Petit-déjeuner g	Déjeuner g	Collation g	Dîner g
Lait écrémé ou équivalent	450	150	150	150	0
Fromage	30	0	0	0	30
VPO maigres	150	0	100	0	50
Pain ou équivalent	100	50	0	0	50
PC crus ou équivalent	50	0	50	0	0
Légumes	400	0	100	0	300
Fruits	300	150	0	0	150
Huile	20	0	15	0	5
Beurre/margarine allégé	15	10	0	0	5
Total (kJ)	5 458	1 172	2 098	218	1 970
Pourcentages	100	21	38	4	36

6.3. Exemple de menu d'un régime hypoénergétique à 5,5 MJ/jour

Petit-déjeuner
Thé édulcoré.
Baguette grillée au beurre allégé.
Une compote d'abricot sans sucre ajouté.

Déjeuner
Tomates au basilic à la vinaigrette allégée (5 mL d'huile d'olive).
Cabillaud poché au court-bouillon.
Riz complet (10 mL d'huile de tournesol).
Un yaourt nature écrémé édulcoré.

Collation
Un fromage blanc écrémé édulcoré.

Dîner
Radis au beurre allégé.
Une tranche de rôti de bœuf au four.
Courgettes braisées (200 g de courgettes, 5 mL d'huile d'olive).
Fromage frais salé.
Pain de seigle.
Une pomme golden.

Section 3

Prescriptions nécessitant une modification des apports conseillés en protéines

6

Le régime hyperprotidique

1. Définition et principe

Le régime hyperprotidique correspond à une alimentation au cours de laquelle l'apport global de protéines peut être augmenté selon deux solutions à savoir :
- *un enrichissement traditionnel* par consommation d'aliments courants riches en protéines animales (de meilleure qualité) et/ou ;
- *un enrichissement industriel* par consommation de produits de complémentation orale hyperprotidiques.

2. Les indications

Le régime hyperprotidique est prescrit en vue d'assurer une reconstruction tissulaire (cas de cicatrisation) et/ou une compensation des pertes lorsque celles-ci sont considérées comme excessives.

Les indications sont alors les suivantes :
- *dénutritions* (quelle qu'en soit la cause et notamment en cas de malnutrition protéinoénergétique : Marasme, Kwashiorkor) ;
- *pathologies hypercatabolisantes* : cancers, VIH… ;
- *pathologies infectieuses* (tuberculose) ou *virales* (grippes, septicémie) ;
- pathologies nécessitant *une cicatrisation très importante* (grands brûlés) ;
- pathologies avec *une chirurgie et une perte de sang importante* ;
- certaines *pathologies digestives chroniques* nécessitant une cicatrisation de la muqueuse associées à une fuite protéique (rectocolite hémorragique, maladie de Crohn, maladie cœliaque…) ;
- certaines *dyslipidémies* (IIa, IIb, III, IV, V) ;

- *cirrhose* (dénutrition alcoolique) ;
- *anémies* ;
- *obésité* (quand l'apport énergétique prescrit devient inférieur à la dépense énergétique journalière) ;
- pour des *corticothérapies prolongées* (c'est-à-dire de plus de 3 mois à des doses supérieures à 0,5 mg/kg) ;
- *avant une intervention chirurgicale* afin de positiver le bilan azoté en vue d'une cicatrisation future ;
- *après une intervention chirurgicale* pour restaurer le pool d'acides aminés, favoriser la cicatrisation et lutter contre l'hypercatabolisme ;
- *lors de fuites protéiques rénales* (syndrome néphrotique) ;
- *en cas de post-transplantation rénale* (lors des 1ers mois pour éviter de négativer la balance azotée face à l'augmentation du catabolisme protéique).

3. Couverture des besoins et apports nutritionnels conseillés

3.1. L'énergie

Le régime hyperprotidique est quasiment toujours associé à un régime hyperénergétique (sauf cas d'obésité, de dyslipidémies…).

3.2. Les protéines

Les protéines étant les nutriments de choix, celles-ci doivent représenter de 1,2 à 1,5 gramme par kilo de poids et par jour au minimum (ce qui fait selon le contexte : 120 à 150 % des apports nutritionnels conseillés) soit environ 16 à 22 % de l'apport énergétique total.

> **Remarque**
>
> Dans le cas de dénutrition, le poids utilisé est le poids réel tandis que lors d'une surcharge pondérale, le poids utilisé correspond au poids de forme.
>
> Il convient de privilégier les protéines animales (en s'assurant du rapport protéines animales sur protéines végétales) de par leur qualité supérieure associée à leur richesse en acides aminés indispensables. Elles positivent ainsi le bilan azoté ou favorisent son retour à l'équilibre.
>
> Il est de plus nécessaire d'assurer une bonne répartition des protéines sur la journée en vue de limiter leur effet satiétant (d'autant plus que les patients sont souvent innapétants).
>
> Il est néanmoins préconisé de ne pas surcharger l'organisme en protéines afin d'éviter la production excessive de déchets azotés toxiques (sans compter que cela va à l'encontre des objectifs recherchés).

3.3. Les lipides

Il est recommandé de proposer 30 % de l'apport énergétique total en lipides car :
- ils représentent la principale réserve énergétique de l'organisme ;

Le régime hyperprotidique 89

- ils permettent de maintenir un apport suffisant en glucides.

Il en découle la répartition en acides gras suivante (cas de l'adulte) :
- acides gras saturés = 7,3 % de l'AET ;
- acides gras monoinsaturés = 18,2 % de l'AET ;
- acides gras polyinsaturés = 4,5 % de l'AET avec :
   - 3,6 % de l'AET en oméga 6 et,
   - 0,9 % de l'AET en oméga 3.

3.4. Les glucides

En tant que compléments énergétiques, les glucides doivent représenter en moyenne 48 à 54 % de l'apport énergétique total. Pour ce qui est de leur répartition qualitative, les glucides complexes doivent être le plus proche possible de 55 % des glucides totaux et les glucides simples de 45 % des glucides totaux.

Les produits sucrés ne doivent, en théorie, pas dépasser 10 % de l'apport énergétique total. En cas d'inappétence, cette valeur peut être légèrement plus élevée (jusqu'à 15 % de l'AET) afin de stimuler l'appétit du patient.

3.5. Les fibres

Les apports en fibres doivent suivre les recommandations fixées selon la tranche d'âge au sein de laquelle se situe le patient.

3.6. Les vitamines

Les apports suivants doivent être vérifiés :
- *la vitamine C* notamment car elle stimule le système immunitaire (d'autant plus si le patient présente une anémie quel qu'en soit le type) ;
- *les vitamines du groupe B* qui, d'une manière générale, sont indispensables à la synthèse tissulaire ;
- *la vitamine B_6* en particulier de par son intervention dans les réactions de transamination (indispensables au métabolisme des acides aminés) ;
- *la vitamine D* en relation avec l'importance de surveiller les apports calciques.

3.7. Les minéraux

La couverture en *calcium* doit être contrôlée surtout quand le niveau d'activité physique est très faible (NAP de 1,1 à 1,3), celui-ci jouant un rôle primordial dans la contraction musculaire et donc dans la préservation de la masse maigre.

Une anémie ferriprive étant souvent constatée, la couverture en *fer* doit aussi être assurée.

3.8. L'eau

Les apports en eau doivent correspondre aux besoins de chaque individu selon son âge, son état physiologique et son niveau d'activité physique.

4. Le choix des aliments

Attention : le choix des aliments proposé ne convient pas lorsque les régimes hypocaloriques et/ou contrôlés en lipides et en glucides sont associés.

Groupe d'aliments	
Laits	*Pas de contre-indication* Consommer de préférence du lait entier ou demi-écrémé. Attention à bien tester la tolérance au lactose (pas plus de 40 g par jour) de chaque patient notamment lorsque la quantité de lait est importante
Laitages	*Pas de contre-indication* Consommer de préférence des laitages entiers ou demi-écrémés
Desserts lactés	*Pas de contre-indication* Les fréquences de consommation recommandées peuvent être légèrement augmentées
Fromages	*Pas de contre-indication* Il est conseillé de privilégier les fromages les plus riches en protéines (pâtes dures et demi-dures) Les fromages affinés présentent l'avantage d'un apport protéique élevé sous un faible volume
Viandes	*Pas de contre-indication* Les viandes les plus riches sont les morceaux de bœuf de 1re catégorie et les volailles (27 % de protéines une fois cuites) Les viandes de 2e et de 3e catégorie sont donc à limiter car le rapport protéines sur collagène est moins intéressant
Charcuteries	*Pas de contre-indication* Les charcuteries les plus riches en protéines sont les charcuteries… maigres [viande des grisons (40 %), jambon blanc (20 %), jambon sec (27 %)] Il est nécessaire de respecter les fréquences conseillées pour les charcuteries grasses
Abats	*Pas de contre-indication* Les abats les plus riches en protéines sont les ris de veau (32 %) Penser cependant à vérifier l'appétence du patient pour ces aliments
Produits de la pêche	*Pas de contre-indication* À noter que le poisson le plus riche en protéine est le thon (teneur de 24 %)

Le régime hyperprotidique

Groupe d'aliments	
Œufs	*Pas de contre-indication* Les œufs (notamment le jaune d'œuf) peuvent facilement être intégrés dans les préparations en tant qu'enrichissement (entremets, purées, potages…) Il est possible d'en consommer tous les jours
Farines, dérivés et féculents	*Pas de contre-indication* Ils permettent d'apporter des glucides complexes et représentent ainsi de l'énergie à long terme Les quantités sont à adapter selon chaque patient
Légumes et fruits	*Pas de contre-indication* Les apports doivent correspondre aux fréquences et aux quantités de consommation recommandées
Matières grasses et équivalents	*Pas de contre-indication* Elles stimulent l'appétence des patients pour les préparations salées
Sucre et produits sucrés	*Pas de contre-indication* Ils stimulent l'appétence des patients pour les préparations sucrées
Boissons	*Pas de contre-indication* Privilégier les boissons de bonne qualité
Épices et aromates	*Pas de contre-indication* Ils aident le patient à manger
Produits diététiques et de régime	Il est possible d'utiliser pour les enrichissements : – de la poudre de lait (dosage de 10 %) – du lait concentré – de la poudre de protéines (90 % de protéines) – des produits de complémentation orale hyperprotidiques (*cf.* régime hyperénergétique)

5. *En pratique*

D'un point de vue biologique, il faut :
– tenter de maintenir une albuminémie supérieure à 30-35 g/L ;
– surveiller attentivement la reprise de poids et l'indice de masse corporelle traduisant l'efficacité du régime.

Les repas doivent être bien répartis sur la journée et servis sous de petits volumes. En cas de réelle anorexie, une partie des glucides peut être remplacée par des dextrines maltoses (*cf.* régime hyperénergétique).

Les préparations peuvent être enrichies en protéines grâce à :
– de la poudre de lait ou du lait concentré entier à raison de 10 à 20 g (4 à 8 g de protéines) : laitages enrichis, desserts lactés enrichis, crèmes enrichies,

compotes enrichies, potages enrichis, purées enrichies, terrines enrichies, sauces enrichies... ;
- du fromage râpé à raison de 20 g (6 g de protéines) : gratins, purées, tartes, sauces, potages enrichis... ;
- des morceaux de jambon (une tranche = 10 g de protéines) : entrées, soupes enrichies... ;
- des crèmes de gruyère (2 unités = 8 g de protéines) : soupes, sauces enrichies... ;
- des œufs durs en morceaux (1 unité = 6,5 g de protéines) dans les entrées ou des jaunes d'œufs (1 jaune = 3,5 g de protéines) dans les desserts lactés ;
- des poudres de protéines (même utilisation que le lait en poudre) à raison d'une à trois cuillères à soupe (soit 5 à 15 g de protéines) dans 150 mL de liquide ou d'aliments.

5.1. Exemples de recettes enrichies en protéines

Recettes/Composition	P (g)	L (g)	G (g)	kJ/kcal
Fromage blanc fruité enrichi : 100 g de fromage blanc 20 % MG 10 g de sucre en poudre 10 g de poudre de lait écrémé 15 g de confiture	11	6	24	850/200
Crème pâtissière au caramel enrichie : 100 mL de crème pâtissière 10 g de poudre de protéines 10 mL de caramel	14	5,5	32	1 000/250
Entremet crémeux : 100 mL de lait demi-écrémé 10 g de lait entier en poudre 10 g de poudre à entremet 5 g de poudre de protéines 5 g de crème fraîche	12	6,5	19	750/180
Fromage blanc biscuité : 50 g de fromage blanc à 20 % de MG 1 biscuit type petit beurre 50 mL de lait demi-écrémé 10 g de sucre 10 g de poudre de lait entier	9	6,5	25,5	850/200

6. *Exemple de ration, de répartition et de menu*

Voir régime hyperénergétique.

7

Le régime hypoprotidique

1. Définition et principe

Le régime hypoprotidique correspond à une alimentation au cours de laquelle on limite l'apport protéique en définissant une quantité maximale de protéines exprimée en grammes par jour.

Il a ainsi pour but de diminuer la production urinaire de déchets du catabolisme azoté (ammoniac, urée, acide urique) dont le taux plasmatique est trop élevé en limitant le catabolisme protéique.

2. Les indications

Les indications se basent sur les constantes sanguines :
– pathologies rénales :
  - insuffisance rénale aiguë : la quantité de protéines dépendra de la fréquence des séances d'épuration (hémodialyse ou dialyse péritonéale),
  - insuffisance rénale chronique : le régime permet de ralentir l'évolution de la maladie et de retarder la mise sous dialyse. L'apport protéique est fixé en fonction de la clairance de la créatinine,
  - syndrome néphrotique : le régime est hypoprotidique lorsque le syndrome est associé à une insuffisance rénale chronique ;
– hyperuricémie ;
– pathologies digestives :
  - cirrhose décompensée avec hyperamoniémie,

- anastomose porto-cave : une réalimentation progressive en protéines doit avoir lieu car les variations de l'amoniémie accentuent les risques d'encéphalopathie hépatique.

> **Remarque**
> De par ses indications, le régime hypoprotidique est souvent associé aux régimes hyposodés et/ou hypopotassiques.

3. Couverture des besoins et apports nutritionnels conseillés

3.1. L'énergie

L'alimentation étant peu restrictive, on peut essayer de s'approcher d'un apport énergétique normal selon les besoins physiques et physiologiques de chaque patient.

3.2. Les protéines

Le taux de protéines est fixé selon l'urémie (c'est-à-dire l'azotémie) et/ou la créatininémie et/ou la clairance de la créatinine de chaque patient.

Il varie en général de 8 à 10,5 % de l'apport énergétique total.

Le rapport protéines animales/protéines végétales doit être particulièrement surveillé, les aliments contenant des protéines animales étant riches en ces nutriments (essentiellement les fromages et les VPO ceux-ci étant donnés en très faible quantité).

> **Remarque**
> Le procédé de complémentation entre des aliments végétaux peut s'avérer utile lors d'un régime hypoprotidique.

3.3. Les lipides

Le régime peut être normolipidique sachant qu'étant donné le choix des aliments (pauvreté en produits d'origine animale), les lipides de bonne qualité sont plus facilement privilégiés. La répartition en acides gras se fait selon les recommandations.

3.4. Les glucides

En tant que compléments énergétiques et à raison de 8 à 10,5 % de protéines, les glucides représentent 54,5 à 62 % de l'apport énergétique total.

La répartition en glucides complexes et simples peut se faire selon les recommandations (tendre vers 55 % des glucides totaux pour les glucides complexes et 45 % pour les glucides simples).

Les produits sucrés seront normalement limités à 10 % maximum de l'AET.

Le régime hypoprotidique

3.5. Les fibres

La couverture des apports en fibres peut être assurée étant donné la prescription.

3.6. Les vitamines et les minéraux

La réduction de la consommation des produits laitiers peut amener à vérifier la couverture en *vitamines A, D, B_2, B_{12}* et en *calcium*.

Quant aux conséquences de la diminution des quantités d'aliments du groupe VPO, on retrouve aussi un risque de déficiences en *vitamines A et D* mais aussi en *vitamines B_3, B_5, B_6 et B_8*. À ceci s'ajoute le *fer héminique* peu représenté (d'autant plus s'il s'agit d'une femme réglée).

3.7. L'eau

Les besoins en eau sont facilement atteignables et calculés en fonction de chaque individu.

À noter que dans les cas de pathologies rénales, les apports en eau de boisson peuvent être contrôlés.

4. *Le choix des aliments*

Groupe d'aliments	Choix des aliments selon leur teneur en protéines
Laits/Laitages	Les laits et les laitages sont **sources de protéines**, les quantités seront donc bien contrôlées : – lait : environ 100 à 300 mL par jour – laitages : éventuellement une portion par jour
Fromages	Les fromages **sont riches en protéines**, les quantités seront donc très contrôlées avec une portion par jour si possible
VPO	Les VPO sont **riches en protéines**, les quantités seront donc très contrôlées : une portion (50 à 70 g maximum par repas) par jour si possible Mode de consommation : les intégrer à des préparations pour limiter la frustration (légumes farcis, hachis…)
Farines et équivalents/féculents	La plupart des aliments amylacés sont **sources de protéines**, les quantités seront bien contrôlées : – pain ou équivalents : environ 100 à 150 g par jour si possible – féculents : essayer de maintenir des quantités normales
Légumes et fruits	Les légumes et les fruits sont de **faibles sources de protéines** mais de par les quantités de consommation recommandées, ils devront être contrôlés.
Matières grasses ou équivalents	D'une manière générale, ce sont des aliments **pauvres voire sans protéines**

Groupe d'aliments	Choix des aliments selon leur teneur en protéines
Produits sucrés ou équivalents	D'une manière générale, ce sont des aliments **pauvres voire sans protéines**
Boissons	D'une manière générale, ce sont des aliments **pauvres voire sans protéines.**
Produits diététiques et de régime	Il existe différents types d'aliments hypoprotidiques (dont la teneur est inférieure à 1 % de protéines) tels que des boissons et des desserts type lactés, des substituts d'œufs, des farines, des pains, des féculents, des biscuits, des préparations pour sauces, des confiseries…

5. En pratique

- Bien vérifier les paramètres sanguins nécessaires pour fixer le taux maximum de protéines.
- Surveiller tout risque de dénutrition en particulier protéique.
- Penser à proposer des produits de régime hypoprotidiques.
- Privilégier dès que possible les aliments les plus restreints quantitativement.

6. Exemple de ration, de répartition et de menu

6.1. Exemple de ration d'un régime hypoprotidique à 8,8 MJ/jour

Aliments	Quantités (g ou mL)	Protéines g	Lipides g	Glucides g	Ca mg	Fer mg	Vit C mg	Fibres g
Lait demi-écrémé ou équivalent	300	10,5	4,5	15	360	0	0	0
Fromage	40	8	9	0	200	0	0	0
VPO	70	12,6	7	0	10,5	1,4	0	0
Pain hypoprotidique	150	1,05	7,5	82,5	45	3	0	4,5
PC crus hypoprotidiques	90	0,315	0	76,5	22,5	0,9	0	1,35
Légumes	500	5	0	25	200	5	100	15

Le régime hypoprotidique

Aliments	Quantités (g ou mL)	Protéines g	Lipides g	Glucides g	Ca mg	Fer mg	Vit C mg	Fibres g
Fruits	450	2,25	0	54	135	2,25	135	9
Huile	30	0	30	0	0	0	0	0
Beurre/Margarine	25	0	20,5	0	0	0	0	0
Sucre ou équivalent	50	0	0	50	0	0	0	0
Total (g)		40	78	303	973	13	235	30
Énergie (kJ)	8 802	675	2 975	5 151				
Pourcentages	100	8	34	59				

6.2. Exemple de répartition d'un régime hypoprotidique à 8,8 MJ/jour

Aliments	Quantités (g ou mL)	Petit-déjeuner g	Déjeuner g	Dîner g
Lait demi-écrémé ou équivalent	300	150	0	150
Fromage	40	0	40	0
VPO	70	0	0	70
Pain hypoprotidique	150	60	30	60
PC crus hypoprotidique	90	0	90	0
Légumes	500	0	100	400
Fruits	450	150	150	150
Huile	30	0	10	20
Beurre/Margarine	25	10	15	0

Aliments	Quantités (g ou mL)	Petit-déjeuner	Déjeuner	Dîner
		g	g	g
Sucre ou équivalent	50	30	10	10
Total (kJ)	**8 763**	**2 111**	**3 544**	**3 107,9**
Pourcentages	100	24	40	35

6.3. Exemple de menu d'un régime hypoprotidique à 8,8 MJ/jour

Petit-déjeuner
Thé vert sucré (2 morceaux de sucre).
Un pain individuel hypoprotidique beurré et au miel (30 g).
Un verre de jus de pomme (150 mL).
Déjeuner
Betterave vinaigrette (10 mL d'huile de noix).
Gratin de pâtes hypoprotidiques au chèvre frais et à l'estragon (dont 15 g de beurre).
Fraises au sucre.
Dîner
Carottes et choux râpés à la coriandre (10 mL d'huile de soja).
Une tranche de rôti de porc aux herbes.
Aubergines sautées (250 g d'aubergines, 10 mL d'huile d'olive).
Un pain individuel hypoprotidique.
Poires au sirop (dont 10 g de sucre).

Section 4

Prescriptions nécessitant une modification des apports conseillés en lipides

8

Le régime normolipidique qualitatif

1. Définition et principe

Le régime normolipidique qualitatif correspond à une alimentation visant à normaliser le taux de LDL-cholestérol et donc la cholestérolémie grâce à :
– une diminution des apports en graisses saturées au profit des graisses insaturées ;
– une réduction des apports en cholestérol alimentaire.

2. Les indications

Les indications sont les suivantes :
– prévention primaire de l'athéromatose :
  - hypercholestérolémie à LDL (IIa) ou secondaires (IIb, III),
  - traitement aux immunosuppresseurs (notamment chez les transplantés rénaux ou cardiaques) ;
– prévention secondaire de l'athéromatose :
  - post-infarctus du myocarde,
  - certains cas de post-accident vasculaire cérébral ischémique ;
– patients présentant des facteurs de risque cardiovasculaires :
  - tabagiques,
  - hypertendus,
  - obèses,
  - sédentaires,
  - diabétiques,

- hypoHDLémie à moins de 35 g/L,
- hommes de plus de 45 ans,
- femmes de plus de 55 ans.

> **Remarque**
> Il faut donc tenir compte de tous les facteurs de risque et les associer à la prescription.
> À noter que ce régime est à proscrire chez les patients très âgés et/ou en fin de vie.

3. Couverture des besoins et apports nutritionnels conseillés

3.1. L'énergie

Dans la plupart des cas, il s'agit d'un régime normoénergétique sauf lorsque l'indice de masse corporelle se situe en dehors des fourchettes de référence.

3.2. Les protéines

L'apport en protéines est normal soit 11 à 15 % de l'apport énergétique total.

3.3. Les lipides

Les lipides doivent représenter 30 à 35 % de l'apport énergétique total. Il s'agit donc d'un régime normolipidique.

Néanmoins, la répartition qualitative des acides gras (exprimée en % des acides gras totaux) chez l'adulte se fait de la manière suivante :
- 25 % d'acides gras saturés car en excès ils sont athérogènes et thrombogènes ;
- 50 % d'acides gras monoinsaturés : ils sont anti-athérogènes, anti-thrombogènes et hypocholestérolémiants ;
- 25 % d'acides gras polyinsaturés avec :
  - 80 % d'acides gras oméga 6 car ils aident à la fluidité sanguine et sont hypocholestérolémiants,
  - 20 % d'acides gras oméga 3 de par leurs propriétés hypotriglycéridémiantes et leur participation au bon fonctionnement cardiaque.

Le rapport entre les acides gras oméga 6 et les oméga 3 doit tendre vers 5 en vue d'assurer la synthèse de l'ensemble des acides gras essentiels.

Les apports en cholestérol alimentaire (source exogène) doivent être limités à 300 mg maximum par jour.

3.4. Les glucides

Les glucides sont les compléments énergétiques de la ration. Les glucides complexes et les glucides simples doivent être correctement répartis (l'idéal étant de 55 % de glucides complexes et de 45 % de glucides simples). Les produits sucrés sont, comme habituellement, limités à 10 % de l'AET.

3.5. Les fibres

Les apports en fibres sont fixés selon la tranche d'âge de chaque patient. Celles-ci aident activement à la stabilisation des constantes lipidiques :
- les fibres solubles (fibres les plus représentées au sein des fruits et des légumes) sont les plus intéressantes de par leur effet hypocholestérolémiant dû à plusieurs mécanismes :
  - elles augmentent l'élimination des sels biliaires d'où une diminution de la réabsorption du cholestérol,
  - elles sont fermentées au niveau du côlon et produisent des acides gras volatils qui auraient la propriété de réduire le LDL-cholestérol ;
- les fibres insolubles (essentiellement dans les céréales et les légumes secs), quant à elles, accélèrent le transit et diminuent ainsi l'assimilation des lipides dont le cholestérol, en augmentant l'excrétion fécale des sels biliaires.

3.6. Les vitamines

Les apports en *vitamines antioxydantes* (vitamine C, bêta carotène et vitamine E) doivent être surveillés car elles limitent l'oxydation du LDL-cholestérol.

3.7. Les minéraux

De même que pour les vitamines, la couverture des minéraux à propriété antioxydante *(zinc, sélénium)* doit être vérifiée.

3.8. L'eau

Les besoins en eau doivent correspondre aux recommandations d'autant plus que l'eau de boisson assure une hydratation des fibres leur permettant d'exercer correctement leurs effets bénéfiques.

4. Le choix des aliments

Groupe d'aliments	Aliments conseillés	Aliments déconseillés
Laits	Lait liquide demi-écrémé, écrémé Lait concentré demi-écrémé, écrémé reconstitué Lait en poudre demi-écrémé, écrémé reconstitué	Lait liquide entier Lait concentré entier Lait en poudre entier
Laitages	Yaourts ordinaires Yaourts 0 % MG Fromages frais 0 % et 10 % MG	Yaourts au lait entier Fromages frais au lait entier (20 % MG), 30 % MG et 40 % MG Laitages « crémeux »
Desserts lactés	Desserts lactés allégés en matières grasses et/ou sans œufs et/ou sans crème	Desserts lactés non allégés en matières grasses et/ou contenant des œufs et/ou de la crème
Fromages	Fromages les moins riches en lipides (AGS et cholestérol) : Camembert 40 %/MS Camembert 45 %/MS Camembert 25 %/MS Chèvre frais Carré de l'est Coulommiers Édam Emmental peu affiné Fromages allégés 25 % MG/MS Fromages fondus à base de pâte dure Fromages fondus 45 %/MS Fromage type Babybel® Fromage type Carré frais® Fromage type Chaource® Pont-l'évêque Raclette Reblochon Roquefort Saint Marcellin Sainte Maure	Fromages les plus riches en lipides (AGS et cholestérol) : Beaufort Bleu Camembert 50 %, 60 %/MS Cantal Cheddar Chèvres mi-secs et secs Comté Emmental très affiné Fromages fondus 65 %, 70 %/MS Fromage type Boursin® Gruyère Gouda Maroilles Munster Mimolette Morbier Neuchâtel Parmesan Pyrénées Vacherin

Le régime normolipidique qualitatif

Groupe d'aliments	Aliments conseillés	Aliments déconseillés
Fromages	**Saint Nectaire** **Saint Paulin** **Selle sur Cher** **Tomme** La quantité et les étiquetages des fromages doivent être bien contrôlés	
Viandes	**Viandes de boucherie maigres** **Volailles maigres sans la peau** **Gibiers** Mode de cuisson : sans ou avec peu de matières grasses, sauces dégraissées, papillotes, four (rôtis), grillées, brochettes…	**Viandes de boucherie grasses et demi-grasses** **Volailles grasses et/ou les morceaux riches en peau** **Autres : paupiettes de viande, viandes panées, beignets, plats cuisinés à base de viandes**
Charcuteries	**Charcuteries maigres**	**Charcuteries grasses**
Abats	**Foie** (une fois par mois) **Cœur** **Ris de veau** **Rognons** **Tripes**	**Langue** **Moelle** **Boudin noir** **Cervelle**
Produits de la pêche	**Poissons maigres, demi-gras et gras en équivalence** Modes de consommation conseillés : – frais – en conserve à l'huile – surgelés non cuisinés – en conserve au naturel	*Pas de contre-indication* Modes de consommation déconseillés : – en conserve en sauce – préparations du commerce : poissons panés, en beignet, rillettes, mousses, pâtés, terrines… – plats cuisinés à base de poisson
Œufs	**4 œufs entiers maximum par semaine** Modes de consommation : omelettes, pochés, à la coque, au plat (poêle antiadhésive), cocotte, dur, mollets, brouillés…	*Pas de contre-indication*

Groupe d'aliments	Aliments conseillés	Aliments déconseillés
Farines et dérivés	Farines (de blé, de sarrasin, complète), fécules, maïzena, tapioca…	
	Pains : blanc (baguette), campagne, complet, seigle, son, aux céréales, précuit, azyme, pain de mie… nature	Pain brioché, pain viennois, pain au lait, pain pour hamburger, pains fantaisies…
	Biscottes, pains grillés, petits pains grillés, cracottes, galettes de blé ou de riz type Wasa®… nature	Produits de biscotterie fourrés Viennoiseries
	Biscuits secs type boudoirs, biscuits à la cuillère, pain d'épice, génoises… Les recettes doivent être sans beurre ou à base de margarine végétale	Biscuits à apéritif Autres biscuits sucrés Pâtisseries et autres gâteaux
	Céréales pour petit-déjeuner non fourrées, non chocolatées (de préférence pétales de maïs soufflées et grains de riz soufflés), mueslis, flocons d'avoine nature	Céréales pour petit-déjeuner fourrées, chocolatées, barres de céréales…
	Mode de consommation : privilégier les aliments complets	
Féculents	Féculents non cuisinés	Plats cuisinés à base de féculents
	Mode de consommation : privilégier les féculents complets	
Légumes	Légumes frais Légumes surgelés non cuisinés Légumes en conserve non cuisinés Potages maison et du commerce (à moins de 1 % de lipides)	Légumes cuisinés du commerce Potages du commerce à plus de 1 % de lipides
	Mode de consommation : privilégier les crudités (riches en antioxydants)	

Le régime normolipidique qualitatif 107

Groupe d'aliments	Aliments conseillés	Aliments déconseillés
Fruits	**Fruits frais** **Fruits surgelés** **Compotes de fruits** **Fruits au sirop** **Fruits secs** **Attention :** faire des équivalences en fonction du pourcentage glucidique de chaque type de fruits	*Pas de contre-indication*
Matières grasses et équivalents	**Huiles d'arachide, d'olive, de colza, de noisette, de sésame, de maïs, de tournesol, de germes de blé, de pépins de raisins, de noix, de soja, huiles mélangées (variété des acides gras insaturés) Margarines végétales, margarines diététiques, matières grasses à tartiner exclusivement d'origine végétale Graisses de canard, graisse d'oie Sauces maison sans beurre ni œufs ni crème fraîche** *En équivalence* : **graines et fruits oléagineux sauf noix de coco**	Huiles de palme et de coprah Sauces du commerce Beurre même allégé Margarines standard (en emballage papier) Crème fraîche même allégée Noix de coco et dérivés Végétaline® Préparations industrielles contenant des graisses hydrogénées
Sucre et produits sucrés	**Sucre Confitures, gelées, marmelades, miels Confiseries Sorbets Crème de marron Fruits confits Pâtes de fruits**	Chocolats et dérivés Pâtes à tartiner Crèmes glacées, glaces
Boissons	**Eaux du robinet, minérales plates ou gazeuses, de source Thé, café, infusions, tisanes Boissons rafraîchissantes sans alcool Jus de légumes**	Toutes les boissons alcoolisées
Épices et aromates	**Toutes les épices et tous les aromates**	*Pas de contre-indication*

5. *En pratique*

- Le LDL-cholestérol doit être surveillé et un traitement médicamenteux peut être mis en place si le régime hypocholestérolémiant s'avère insuffisant à lui seul.
- Penser à donner l'ensemble des conseils relatifs à la prévention des maladies cardiovasculaires en apprenant notamment au patient à maîtriser les sources et apports de lipides.
- Vérifier systématiquement les ingestions quantitatives d'acides gras saturés et de cholestérol alimentaire.

6. *Exemple de ration, de répartition et de menu*

6.1. Exemple de ration d'un régime normolipidique qualitatif à 8,6 MJ/jour

Aliments	Quantités (g ou mL)	Protéines	Lipides	Glucides	Ca	Fer	Vit C	Fibres	Cholestérol
		g	g	g	mg	mg	mg	g	mg
Lait demi-écrémé ou équivalent	300	10,5	4,5	15	360	0	0	0	16,5
Fromage	30	6	6,6	0	150	0	0	0	24
Viandes/poissons	200	36	20	0	30	4	0	0	150
Pain ou équivalent	150	12	0	75	37,5	3	0	7,5	0
PC crus ou équivalent	70	7	0	52,5	17,5	0,7	0	1,05	0
Légumes	500	5	0	25	200	5	100	15	0
Fruits	450	0	0	54	135	2,25	135	9	0
Huile	25	0	25	0	0	0	0	0	0
Margarine végétale	20	0	16,6	0	0	0	0	0	0
Sucre ou équivalent	45	0	0	45	0	0	0	0	0
Total (g)		77	73	266,5	930	15	235	33	191
Énergie (kJ)	8 594	1 301	2 763	4 530,5					
Pourcentages	100	15	32	53					

6.2. Exemple de répartition d'un régime normolipidique qualitatif à 8,6 MJ/jour

Aliments	Quantités (g ou mL)	Petit-déjeuner	Déjeuner	Collation	Dîner
		g	g	g	g
Lait demi-écrémé ou équivalent	300	150	150	0	0
Fromage	30	0	0	0	30
Viandes/Poissons	200	0	100	0	100
Pain ou équivalent	150	100	0	0	50
Pc crus ou équivalent	70	0	70	0	0
Légumes	500	0	100	0	400
Fruits	450	0	150	150	150
Huile	25	0	10	0	15
Margarine végétale	20	15	5	0	0
Sucre ou équivalent	45	20	10	15	0
Total (kJ)	8 595	2 101	3 115	561	2 817
Pourcentages	100	24	36	7	33

6.3. Exemple de menu d'un régime normolipidique qualitatif à 8,6 MJ/jour

Petit-déjeuner
Café nature.
Pain aux céréales et margarine végétale.
Un yaourt demi-écrémé à la confiture de fraise (30 g).

Déjeuner
Champignons de Paris vinaigrette (10 mL d'huile d'olive).
Escalope de veau grillée.
Blé dur précuit à la sauce tomate (dont 5 g de margarine végétale).
Une faisselle demi-écrémée au miel (15 g).
Deux kiwis.

Collation
Une compote de rhubarbe (dont 15 g de sucre).
Dîner
Artichaut vinaigrette à la moutarde (10 mL d'huile de tournesol).
Deux tranches de jambon blanc découenné dégraissé.
Brocolis persillés (5 mL d'huile de colza).
Edam.
Un pain individuel.
Une poire comice.

9

Le régime hypolipidique

1. Définition et principe

Le régime hypolipidique est une alimentation au cours de laquelle la quantité de lipides est très limitée. C'est par conséquent un régime hyperglucidique et riche en protéines.

Le but de cette prescription est de solliciter au minimum la sécrétion biliaire et pancréatique en vue de ramener la triglycéridémie à une valeur normale.

> **Remarque**
> Cette prescription reste de courte durée à savoir de 10 à 14 jours maximum.

2. Les indications

Les indications sont les suivantes :
– pancréatite aiguë en phase de reprise de l'alimentation orale ;
– hypertriglycéridémie supérieure à 10 g/L (car il y a un risque de pancréatite aiguë) ;
– insuffisance hépatique sévère ;
– colecystopathies ;
– interventions sur les voies biliaires ;
– stéatorrhée.

3. Couverture des besoins et apports nutritionnels conseillés

3.1. L'énergie

Les apports énergétiques doivent correspondre aux besoins réels du patient le plus rapidement possible (sachant qu'en début de réalimentation ils ne peuvent être qu'inférieurs aux recommandations).

3.2. Les protéines

Il en est de même pour les protéines avec tout d'abord un régime hyperprotidique qui tend à se normaliser par la suite.

3.3. Les lipides

Les lipides doivent représenter 30 % de l'apport énergétique total au maximum.
Le taux lipidique est, en premier lieu, fixé à 5 % de l'AET puis progressivement élargi jusqu'à 30 % selon la tolérance de chaque patient. Ainsi, les sécrétions biliaires et pancréatiques sont minimisées.

3.4. Les glucides

Au regard de la réduction des lipides, le régime est hyperglucidique (jusqu'à normoglucidique). On associe de plus un contrôle du saccharose et du fructose en vue de limiter la triglycéridémie. Les produits sucrés ou équivalents doivent ainsi représenter moins de 5 % de l'apport énergétique total et la quantité de fruits limitée à deux portions maximum par jour.

3.5. Les fibres, les vitamines, les minéraux et l'eau

Il convient dans la mesure du possible de respecter les besoins en ces différents nutriments selon les spécificités de chaque patient.

4. Le choix des aliments

Groupe d'aliments	Aliments conseillés	Aliments déconseillés
Laits	Lait liquide demi-écrémé, écrémé Lait concentré, en poudre demi-écrémé, écrémé nature reconstitué	Lait liquide entier Lait concentré entier et/ou sucré Lait en poudre entier Laits aromatisés

Le régime hypolipidique

Groupe d'aliments	Aliments conseillés	Aliments déconseillés
Laitages	**Yaourts ordinaires et/ou édulcorés** **Yaourts 0 % MG et/ou édulcorés** **Fromages frais 0 % et 10 % MG nature ou édulcorés**	**Yaourts au lait entier et/ou sucrés** **Fromages frais au lait entier (20 % MG), 30 % MG et 40 % MG et/ou sucrés** **Laitages « crémeux »**
Desserts lactés	Desserts lactés allégés en matières grasses et en sucre **Attention :** il convient de les décomposer en équivalences (lait, matières grasses et sucre) si nécessaire	Desserts lactés non allégés en matières grasses et/ou contenant des matières sucrantes
Fromages	Fromages les moins riches en lipides : Camembert 40 %/MS Camembert 45 %/MS Camembert 25 %/MS Chèvre frais Carré de l'est Coulommiers Édam Emmental peu affiné Fromages allégés 25 % MG/MS Fromages fondus à base de pâte dure Fromages fondus 45 %/MS Fromage type Babybel® Fromage type Carré frais® Fromage type Chaource® Pont-l'évêque Raclette Reblochon Roquefort Saint Marcellin Sainte Maure Saint Nectaire Saint Paulin Selle sur Cher Tomme	Fromages les plus riches en lipides : Beaufort Bleu Camembert 50 %, 60 % /MS Cantal Cheddar Chèvres mi-secs et secs Comté Emmental très affiné Fromages fondus 65 %, 70 %/MS Fromage type Boursin® Gruyère Gouda Maroilles Munster Mimolette Morbier Neuchâtel Parmesan Pyrénées Vacherin

Groupe d'aliments	Aliments conseillés	Aliments déconseillés
Fromages	**Attention :** la quantité et les étiquetages des fromages doivent être bien contrôlés	
Viandes	**Viandes de boucherie maigres Volailles maigres sans la peau Gibiers Abats maigres** Modes de cuisson : sans ou avec peu de matières grasses, sauces dégraissées : papillotes, four (rôtis), grillées, brochettes…	**Viandes de boucherie grasses et demi-grasses Volailles grasses et/ou les morceaux riches en peau Abats riches en lipides Autres : paupiettes de viande, viandes panées, beignets, plats cuisinés à base de viandes**
Charcuteries	**Charcuteries maigres**	**Charcuteries grasses**
Produits de la pêche	**Poissons maigres** Modes de consommation conseillés : – frais – surgelés non cuisinés – en conserve au naturel Modes de cuisson : – de préférence sans ou avec peu de matières grasses : grillés, court-bouillon, four, vapeur, papillote, brochettes…	**Poissons demi-gras et gras** Modes de consommation déconseillés : – en conserve à l'huile ou en sauce – préparations du commerce : poissons panés, en beignet, rillettes, mousses, pâtés, terrines… – plats cuisinés à base de poisson
Œufs	Modes de cuisson : de préférence sans ou avec peu de matières grasses Modes de consommation : omelettes, pochés, à la coque, au plat (poêle antiadhésive), cocotte, dur, mollets, brouillés…	*Pas de contre-indication*
Farines et dérivés	**Farines (de blé, de sarrasin, complète), fécules, maïzena, tapioca…** **Pains : blanc (type baguette), campagne, complet, seigle, son, aux céréales, précuit, azyme, pain de mie… nature**	**Pain brioché, pain viennois, pain au lait, pain pour hamburger, pains fantaisies…**

Groupe d'aliments	Aliments conseillés	Aliments déconseillés
Farines et dérivés	Biscottes, pains grillés, petits pains grillés, cracottes, galettes de blé ou de riz type Wasa®… nature	Produits de biscotterie fourrés Viennoiseries
	Biscuits secs nature Les recettes doivent être avec le moins de lipides et de glucides simples possibles et ils doivent être décomposés en farine, matières grasses et sucre si nécessaire	Autres biscuits sucrés Pâtisseries et autres gâteaux Biscuits à apéritif
	Céréales pour petit-déjeuner non fourrées, non chocolatées (de préférence pétales de maïs soufflées et grains de riz soufflés), mueslis, flocons d'avoine nature Mode de consommation : privilégier les aliments complets	Céréales pour petit-déjeuner fourrées, chocolatées, barres de céréales…
Féculents	Féculents non cuisinés Mode de consommation : privilégier les féculents complets	Plats cuisinés à base de féculents
Légumes	Légumes frais Légumes surgelés non cuisinés Légumes en conserve non cuisinés Potages maison et du commerce (à moins de 1 % de lipides) Modes de cuisson : de préférence sans ou avec peu de matières grasses (à l'eau, à la vapeur, au four, à l'étouffée, au grill…) Mode de consommation : privilégier les crudités (riches en antioxydants)	Légumes cuisinés du commerce Potages du commerce à plus de 1 % de lipides
Fruits	**En quantité très contrôlée :** (pas plus de 2 portions de fruits par jour)	

Groupe d'aliments	Aliments conseillés	Aliments déconseillés
Fruits	Fruits frais Fruits surgelés non sucrés Coulis de fruits non sucrés Compotes de fruits du commerce non sucrées ou édulcorées Compotes de fruits maison nature Jus de fruits maison ou du commerce non sucrés ou édulcorées En équivalence : Fruits secs, fruits au sirop Attention : faire des équivalences en fonction du pourcentage glucidique de chaque type de fruits	Fruits surgelés sucrés Coulis de fruits sucrés Compotes sucrées Jus de fruits sucrés
Matières grasses et équivalents	En quantité très contrôlée : Toutes les huiles (de préférence sources d'acides gras insaturés) Margarines et margarines allégées Beurre et beurre allégé Crème fraîche et crème fraîche allégée Vinaigrette et vinaigrette allégée En équivalence : graines et fruits oléagineux	Sauces du commerce et/ou sauces maison riches en lipides Fritures, panures
Sucre et produits sucrés	Édulcorants de synthèse Une unité ou une cuillère à soupe équivaut au pouvoir sucrant d'un morceau de sucre	Sucre Confitures, gelées, marmelades, miels Confiseries Crème de marron Fruits confits Pâtes de fruits Chocolats et dérivés Pâtes à tartiner Produits glacés
Boissons	Eaux du robinet, minérales plates ou gazeuses, de source Eaux minérales aromatisées non sucrées et/ou édulcorées	Eaux minérales aromatisées sucrées

Groupe d'aliments	Aliments conseillés	Aliments déconseillés
Boissons	Thé, café, infusions, tisanes non sucrés **Boissons rafraîchissantes non sucrées et/ou édulcorées** **Sirops édulcorés** **Jus de légumes** **Attention :** concernant les boissons édulcorées : bien vérifier la non-présence de sucre et en contrôler les quantités ingérées	Préparations à base de thé, café sucrées **Boissons rafraîchissantes sucrées** **Sirops sucrés** **Toutes les boissons alcoolisées**
Épices et aromates	Pour les préparations salées : **toutes les fines herbes et épices, bouillons cube dégraissés et/ou aux légumes** Pour les préparations sucrées : **vanille, extrait de café, extrait d'amande, fleur d'oranger, menthe…**	**Bouillons cube non dégraissés**

5. *En pratique*

Il convient d'apprendre au patient :
- à supprimer les aliments riches en lipides et à privilégier les aliments maigres ;
- à choisir ses matières grasses ;
- à reconnaître les graisses visibles et invisibles ;
- à limiter les acides gras saturés ;
- à supprimer l'alcool ;
- à contrôler son apport en glucides simples (saccharose et fructose) ;
- à apprendre à cuisiner avec peu ou pas de matières grasses (selon la sévérité de la prescription).

6. *Exemple de ration, de répartition et de menu*

6.1. Exemple de ration d'un régime hypolipidique à 8 MJ, 40 g de lipides par jour

Aliments	Quantités (g ou mL)	Protéines g	Lipides g	Glucides g	Ca mg	Fer mg	Vit C mg	Fibres g
Lait écrémé	500	17,5	0	25	600	0	0	0
Fromage allégé	30	6	4,5	0	150	0	0	0
VPO maigres	200	36	10	0	30	4	0	0
Pain ou équivalent	250	20	0	125	62,5	5	0	12,5
PC crus ou équivalent	80	8	0	60	20	0,8	0	1,2
Légumes frais	400	4	0	20	160	4	80	12
Fruits frais	300	0	0	36	90	1,5	90	6
Huile	15	0	15	0	0	0	0	0
Margarine	15	0	12	0	0	0	0	0
Sucre ou équivalent	20	0	0	20	0	0	0	0
Total (g)		92	41	286	1 113	15	170	32
Énergie (kJ)	8 006	1 556	1 588	4 862				
Pourcentages	100	19	20	61				

6.2. Exemple de répartition d'un régime hypolipidique à 8 MJ, 40 g de lipides par jour

Aliments	Quantités (g ou mL)	Petit-déjeuner g	Déjeuner g	Dîner g
Lait écrémé	500	200	150	150
Fromage allégé	30	0	30	0
VPO maigres	200	0	100	100
Pain ou équivalent	250	125	125	0
PC crus ou équivalent	80	0	0	80
Légumes frais	400	0	300	100
Fruits frais	300	0	150	150

Aliments	Quantités (g ou mL)	Petit-déjeuner g	Déjeuner g	Dîner g
Huile	15	0	10	5
Margarine	15	15	0	0
Sucre ou équivalent	20	5	5	10
Total (kJ)	**8 014**	2 074	3 299	2 640,8
Pourcentages	100	**26**	**41**	**33**

6.3. Exemple de menu d'un régime hypolipidique à 8 MJ, 40 g de lipides par jour

Petit-déjeuner
Thé sucré (1 morceau) avec un nuage de lait écrémé (50 mL).
Une demi-baguette et margarine végétale.
Un yaourt écrémé édulcoré.

Déjeuner
Carottes râpées vinaigrette allégée (5 mL d'huile de noix).
Steak haché 5 % grillé.
Ratatouille niçoise (dont 5 mL d'huile d'olive).
Camembert allégé.
Pain de campagne.
Un fromage blanc écrémé sucré et morceaux de pêche (dont 5 g de sucre).

Dîner
Asperges vinaigrette allégée (5 mL d'huile de sésame).
Filet de sole en papillotte au citron.
Purée de patate douce.
Une faisselle écrémée au coulis de fruits rouges (dont 10 g de sucre).

10

Le régime hypolipidique enrichi en triglycérides à chaîne moyenne

1. Définition et principe

Le régime hypolipidique enrichi en triglycérides à chaîne moyenne est une alimentation au cours de laquelle la quantité de triglycérides à chaîne longue (TCL) est limitée avec un apport compensatoire de triglycérides à chaîne moyenne (TCM).

Le but de cette prescription est de fournir un apport lipidique rapidement hydrolysé et absorbé, empruntant le système porte et non la voie lymphatique.

2. Les indications

Les indications sont les suivantes :
- hyperchylomicronémie (hypertriglycéridémie de type exogène : type I) ou hypertriglycéridémie mixte (type V) ;
- épanchement chyleux (pleurésie, ascite…) ;
- certains cas de stéatorrhée (suite à une résection iléale étendue, une gastrectomie) ;
- entéropathie exsudative ;
- obstruction des voies lymphatiques (cholestase).

Néanmoins il existe des contre-indications :
- certaines dyslipoprotéinémies ;
- diabète mal équilibré ;
- cirrhotiques porteurs d'une anastomose porto-cave.

3. *Couverture des besoins et apports nutritionnels conseillés*

3.1. L'énergie

Les apports énergétiques doivent correspondre aux besoins réels du patient.

3.2. Les protéines

Il en est de même pour les protéines qui doivent correspondre aux apports conseillés à savoir de 11 à 15 % de l'apport énergétique total.

3.3. Les lipides

Les lipides doivent représenter 30 % maximum de l'apport énergétique total en diminuant l'apport en triglycérides à chaîne longue c'est-à-dire en les remplaçant totalement ou partiellement par des triglycérides à chaîne moyenne. En effet, les triglycérides à chaîne longue étant absorbés par le système lymphatique, ceux-ci ont tendance à augmenter la triglycéridémie tandis que les triglycérides à chaîne moyenne sont de demi-vie brève.

La répartition des acides gras se fait alors de la manière suivante (cas de l'adulte) :
– acides gras saturés : 6,5 % de l'AET ;
– acides gras monoinsaturés : 16,5 % de l'AET ;
– acides gras polyinsaturés : 4 % de l'AET avec 3 % d'acide gras oméga 6 et 1 % d'acide gras oméga 3 dont 0,05 % de DHA.

3.4. Les glucides

En tant que compléments énergétiques, les glucides doivent représenter de 55 à 59 % de l'apport énergétique total.

Cependant, dans le cas d'une hypertriglycéridémie mixte (type V), on applique aussi une alimentation contrôlée en glucides.

3.5. Les fibres, les vitamines, les minéraux et l'eau

Il convient dans la mesure du possible de respecter les besoins en ces différents nutriments selon les spécificités de chaque patient.

On constate toutefois un risque de déficience en *vitamines liposolubles* (A, D, E, K) de par la diminution voire la suppression des aliments riches en lipides associé à la réduction de leur absorption.

4. Le choix des aliments

Groupe d'aliments	Aliments conseillés	Aliments déconseillés
Laits	Lait liquide demi-écrémé, écrémé Lait concentré, en poudre demi-écrémé, écrémé reconstitué	Lait liquide entier Lait concentré entier Lait en poudre entier
Laitages	Yaourts ordinaires Yaourts 0 % MG Fromages frais 0 % et 10 % MG	Yaourts au lait entier Fromages frais au lait entier (20 % MG), 30 % MG et 40 % MG Laitages « crémeux »
Desserts lactés	Desserts lactés allégés en matières grasses **Attention :** il convient de les décomposer en équivalences (lait, matières grasses) si nécessaire	Desserts lactés non allégés en matières grasses
Fromages	Fromages les moins riches en lipides : Camembert 40 %/MS Camembert 45 %/MS Camembert 25 %/MS Chèvre frais Carré de l'est Coulommiers Edam Emmental peu affiné Fromages allégés 25 % MG/MS Fromages fondus à base de pâte dure Fromages fondus 45 %/MS Fromage type Babybel® Fromage type Carré frais® Fromage type Chaource® Pont-l'évêque Raclette Reblochon Roquefort Saint Marcellin Sainte Maure Saint Nectaire Saint Paulin	Fromages les plus riches en lipides : Beaufort Bleu Camembert 50 %, 60 % /MS Cantal Cheddar Chèvres mi-secs et secs Comté Emmental très affiné Fromages fondus 65 %, 70 %/MS Fromage type Boursin® Gruyère Gouda Maroilles Munster Mimolette Morbier Neuchâtel Parmesan Pyrénées Vacherin

Groupe d'aliments	Aliments conseillés	Aliments déconseillés
Fromages	Selle sur Cher Tomme **Attention :** la quantité et les étiquetages des fromages doivent être bien contrôlés	
Viandes	**Viandes de boucherie maigres** **Volailles maigres sans la peau** **Gibiers** **Abats maigres** Modes de cuisson : sans ou avec peu de matières grasses, sauces dégraissées : papillotes, four (rôtis), grillées, brochettes…	**Viandes de boucherie grasses et demi-grasses** **Volailles grasses et/ou les morceaux riches en peau** **Abats riches en lipides** **Autres : paupiettes de viande, viandes panées, beignets, plats cuisinés à base de viandes**
Charcuteries	**Charcuteries maigres**	**Charcuteries grasses**
Produits de la pêche	**Poissons maigres** Modes de consommation conseillés : – frais – surgelés non cuisinés – en conserve au naturel Modes de cuisson : de préférence sans ou avec peu de matières grasses : grillés, court-bouillon, four, vapeur, papillote, brochettes…	**Poissons demi-gras et gras** Modes de consommation déconseillés : – en conserve à l'huile ou en sauce – préparations du commerce : poissons panés, en beignet, rillettes, mousses, pâtés, terrines… – plats cuisinés à base de poisson
Œufs	Modes de cuisson : de préférence sans ou avec peu de matières grasses Modes de consommation : omelettes, pochés, à la coque, au plat (poêle antiadhésive), cocotte, dur, mollets, brouillés…	*Pas de contre-indication*
Farines et dérivés	**Farines (de blé, de sarrasin, complète), fécules, maïzena, tapioca…** **Pains : blanc (type baguette), campagne, complet, seigle, son, aux céréales, précuit, azyme, pain de mie… nature**	**Pain brioché, pain viennois, pain au lait, pain pour hamburger, pains fantaisies…**

Groupe d'aliments	Aliments conseillés	Aliments déconseillés
Farines et dérivés	**Biscottes, pains grillés, petits pains grillés, cracottes, galettes de blé ou de riz type Wasa®… nature**	**Produits de biscotterie fourrés Viennoiseries**
	Biscuits secs pauvres en lipides Les recettes doivent être avec le moins de lipides possibles et ils doivent être décomposés en farine, matières grasses si nécessaire	**Autres biscuits sucrés Pâtisseries et autres gâteaux Biscuits à apéritif**
	Céréales pour petit-déjeuner pauvres en lipides (de préférence pétales de maïs soufflées et grains de riz soufflés), mueslis pauvres en lipides, flocons d'avoine Mode de consommation : privilégier les aliments complets	**Céréales pour petit-déjeuner riches en lipides, mueslis riches en lipides, barres de céréales…**
Féculents	**Féculents non cuisinés** Mode de consommation : privilégier les féculents complets	**Plats cuisinés à base de féculents**
Légumes	**Légumes frais Légumes surgelés non cuisinés Légumes en conserve non cuisinés Potages maison et du commerce (à moins de 1 % de lipides)** Modes de cuisson : de préférence sans ou avec peu de matières grasses (à l'eau, à la vapeur, au four, à l'étouffée, au grill…) Mode de consommation : privilégier les crudités (riches en antioxydants)	**Légumes cuisinés du commerce Potages du commerce à plus de 1 % de lipides**
Fruits	**Fruits frais Fruits surgelés Coulis de fruits Compotes de fruits Jus de fruits maison ou du commerce**	*Pas de contre-indication*

Groupe d'aliments	Aliments conseillés	Aliments déconseillés
Fruits	**En équivalence :** **Fruits secs, fruits au sirop** **Attention :** faire des équivalences en fonction du pourcentage glucidique de chaque type de fruits	
Matières grasses et équivalents	**Matières grasses enrichies en TCM : huiles et margarines spéciales** Exemples : *Huiles :* Tricèm (100 % TCM), Liprocil (67 % TCM), Triceryl (67 % TCM), Liprogram 20 (80 % TCM), Ceres (67 % TCM) *Margarines :* Ceres (67 % TCM) **Attention :** – quantités inférieures à 50 g/jour (risques de nausées) – pas de cuisson possible : utilisation sous forme de vinaigrettes, mayonnaises… SAUF le Liprocil qui peut être chauffé jusqu'à 130 °C	Toutes déconseillées **Huiles** **Beurres** **Margarines** **Crèmes fraîches** **Sauces** **Graines oléagineuses**
Sucre et produits sucrés	**En quantité contrôlée :** **Sucre** **Confiture, gelée, marmelade, miel** **Confiseries** **Sorbets** **Crème de marron** **Fruits confits**	Chocolats et dérivés Pâtes à tartiner Crèmes glacées, glaces
Boissons	**Eaux du robinet, minérales plates ou gazeuses, de source** **Thé, café, infusions, tisanes** **Boissons rafraîchissantes sans alcool** **Sirops** **Jus de légumes** **Attention :** faire des équivalences avec les produits sucrés pour toutes les boissons contenant du sucre	Toutes les boissons alcoolisées

Groupe d'aliments	Aliments conseillés	Aliments déconseillés
Épices et aromates	Pour les préparations salées : **toutes les fines herbes et épices, bouillons cube dégraissés et/ou aux légumes** Pour les préparations sucrées : vanille, **extrait de café, extrait d'amande, fleur d'oranger, menthe…**	**Bouillons cube non dégraissés**

5. *En pratique*

Il convient d'apprendre au patient :
– à supprimer les aliments riches en lipides et à privilégier les aliments maigres ;
– à choisir ses matières grasses ;
– à reconnaître les graisses visibles et invisibles ;
– à limiter les acides gras saturés ;
– à supprimer l'alcool ;
– à contrôler son apport en glucides simples (saccharose et fructose) ;
– à apprendre à cuisiner avec peu ou pas de matières grasses (selon la sévérité de la prescription) ;
– à maîtriser l'utilisation des matières grasses enrichies en triglycérides à chaîne moyenne.

Section 5

Prescriptions nécessitant une modification des apports conseillés en glucides

11

Le régime contrôlé en glucides

1. Définition et principe

Le régime contrôlé en glucides correspond à une alimentation équilibrée au cours de laquelle l'apport total, la répartition et la nature des glucides sont contrôlés.

Les objectifs nutritionnels de ce régime sont les suivants :
- atteindre les objectifs glycémiques ;
- prévenir et/ou traiter les hypoglycémies ;
- prévenir la survenue des complications micro- et macroangiopathiques ;
- prendre en charge les divers facteurs de risques cardiovasculaires (normaliser le bilan lipidique, traiter l'hypertension artérielle, arrêt du tabac…) ;
- apprendre à fractionner la prise alimentaire en particulier chez les femmes enceintes.

2. Les indications

Les indications sont les suivantes :
1. diabète de type 1 (diabète insulinodépendant),
2. diabète gestationnel.

3. Couverture des besoins et apports nutritionnels conseillés

3.1. L'énergie

Le régime est normoénergétique et l'apport calorique est fixé en fonction des besoins de chaque individu.

3.2. Les glucides

Le régime étant contrôlé en glucides, ils représentent les nutriments de choix et doivent être généralement compris entre 50 et 55 % de l'apport énergétique total. Le taux de glucides autorisé est fixé de manière précise et exprimé en grammes par jour.

La répartition qualitative des glucides se fait de la manière suivante :
– 55 % de glucides complexes ;
– 45 % de glucides simples.

Les aliments présentant un index glycémique bas sont privilégiés car ils induisent une augmentation modérée de la glycémie et réduisent donc ainsi la résistance à l'insuline.

Les produits sucrés ne sont pas systématiquement limités (ils peuvent alors atteindre jusqu'à 10 % maximum de l'AET) mais ceux présentant un index glycémique haut sont à éviter et ne peuvent en aucun cas être consommés de manière isolée.

3.3. Les lipides

Le régime est normolipidique (30 à 35 % de l'AET) avec une répartition des acides gras réalisée selon les références (cas de l'adulte) :
– acides gras saturés : 8 % de l'AET ;
– acides gras monoinsaturés : 20 % de l'AET ;
– acides gras polyinsaturés : 5 % de l'AET avec :
  - acides gras oméga 6 : 4 % de l'AET,
  - acides gras oméga 3 : 0,8 % de l'AET,
  - acides gras polyinsaturés à longue chaîne : 0,2 % de l'AET dont 0,05 % de DHA.

Pour les patients suivant ce type de régime et présentant des risques de maladies cardiovasculaires accentués, la qualité des matières grasses est particulièrement surveillée notamment en ce qui concerne l'apport en acides gras saturés.

3.4. Les protéines

Les protéines représentent dans ce cas le complément de la ration à savoir de 10 à 20 % de l'AET.

D'un point de vue qualitatif, le rapport entre les protéines animales et végétales doit être respecté.

3.5. Les fibres

Les apports en fibres doivent correspondre aux besoins de chaque individu en particulier ceux en fibres solubles (évalués à 10-15 g par jour chez l'adulte) puisque celles-ci ont tendance à diminuer la glycémie postprandiale en formant des complexes avec les glucides ingérés réduisant alors l'action des enzymes digestives.

3.6. Les vitamines et les minéraux

L'alimentation étant normo-équilibrée, l'ensemble des vitamines et des minéraux peuvent être correctement couverts.

3.7. L'eau

Les quantités d'eau sont déterminées selon les recommandations.

4. *Le choix des aliments*

Groupe d'aliments	Aliments conseillés	Aliments déconseillés
Laits	Lait liquide demi-écrémé, écrémé Lait concentré, en poudre demi-écrémé, écrémé reconstitués	Lait liquide entier Lait concentré entier Lait en poudre entier
Laitages	Yaourts ordinaires Yaourts 0 % MG Fromages frais 0 % et 10 % MG	Yaourts au lait entier Fromages frais au lait entier (20 % MG), 30 % MG et 40 % MG Laitages « crémeux »
Desserts lactés	Desserts lactés allégés en sucre et en matières grasses (faire si nécessaire des équivalences en lait, matières grasses et/ou sucre)	Desserts lactés non allégés en sucre et en matières grasses
Fromages	Fromages les moins riches en lipides et en acides gras saturés : Camembert 40 %/MS Camembert 45 %/MS Camembert 25 %/MS Chèvre frais Carré de l'est Coulommiers	Fromages les plus riches en lipides et en acides gras saturés : Beaufort Bleu Camembert 50 %, 60 %/MS Cantal Cheddar Chèvres mi-secs et secs Comté

Groupe d'aliments	Aliments conseillés	Aliments déconseillés
Fromages	Edam Emmental peu affiné Fromages allégés 25 % MG/MS Fromages fondus à base de pâte dure Fromages fondus 45 %/MS Fromage type Babybel® Fromage type Carré frais® Fromage type Chaource® Pont-l'évêque Raclette Reblochon Roquefort Saint Marcellin Sainte Maure Saint Nectaire Saint Paulin Selle sur Cher Tomme La quantité et les étiquetages des fromages doivent être bien contrôlés	Emmental très affiné Fromages fondus 65 %, 70 %/MS Fromage type Boursin® Gruyère Gouda Maroilles Munster Mimolette Morbier Neuchâtel Parmesan Pyrénées Vacherin
Viandes	**Viandes de boucherie maigres** **Volailles maigres sans la peau** **Gibiers**	**Viandes de boucherie grasses et demi-grasses** **Volailles grasses et/ou les morceaux riches en peau** **Autres : paupiettes de viande, viandes panées, beignets, plats cuisinés à base de viandes**
Charcuteries	**Charcuteries maigres**	**Charcuteries grasses**
Abats	**Abats maigres**	**Abats riches en lipides**
Produits de la pêche	**Poissons maigres, demi-gras et gras *en équivalence*** Modes de consommation conseillés : – frais – en conserve au naturel ou à l'huile – surgelés non cuisinés	*Pas de contre-indication* Modes de consommation déconseillés : – en conserve en sauce – préparations du commerce : poissons panés, en beignet, rillettes, mousses, pâtés, terrines… – plats cuisinés à base de poisson

Groupe d'aliments	Aliments conseillés	Aliments déconseillés
Œufs	**Œufs sous toutes leurs formes** Modes de consommation : omelettes, pochés, à la coque, au plat (poêle antiadhésive), cocotte, dur, mollets, brouillés…	*Pas de contre-indication*
Farines et dérivés	**Farines complètes, de sarrasin** **Pains complets, de seigle, au son, aux céréales, pains de mie complets** **Céréales pour petit-déjeuner type All Bran®, muesli nature, flocons d'avoine** **Biscuits riches en glucides complexes, pauvres en glucides simples, biscuits enrichis en fibres** Mode de consommation : privilégier les aliments complets (index glycémique bas)	**Farines raffinées** **Pains blancs, biscottes, cracottes, pains grillés** **Céréales pour petit-déjeuner sucrées et extrudées, barres de céréales** **Biscuits riches en glucides simples (biscuits confiturés, boudoirs, génoises, tartelettes aux fruits, biscuits roulés…)** **Biscuits extrudés (gaufrettes, meringues, crackers apéritifs…)** **Biscuits riches en beurre et/ou en matières grasses hydrogénées** **Pâtisseries, viennoiseries**
Féculents	**Pâtes, riz blanc, riz complet, semoule, blé dur précuit, quinoa, pommes de terre cuites entières, légumes secs, fruits amylacés** Mode de consommation : privilégier les féculents complets et/ou non cuisinés	**Riz cuisson rapide, pommes de terre en purée, pommes de terre en flocons** **Autres féculents cuisinés et/ou à index glycémique élevé**
Légumes	**Légumes frais** **Légumes surgelés non cuisinés** **Légumes en conserve non cuisinés**	**Légumes cuisinés du commerce** **Potages du commerce cuisinés**

Groupe d'aliments	Aliments conseillés	Aliments déconseillés
Légumes	Potages maison et du commerce non cuisinés Mode de consommation : privilégier les crudités (riches en antioxydants)	
Fruits	**Fruits frais sauf pastèque** **Fruits surgelés non sucrés** **Compotes de fruits étiquetées « 100 % pur fruits » ou « sans sucre ajouté », compotes maison sans sucre ou édulcorées** **Fruits secs** **Attention :** faire des équivalences en fonction du pourcentage glycidique de chaque type de fruits	Pastèque Fruits surgelés sucrés Compotes du commerce sucrées Fruits au sirop
Matières grasses et équivalents	Huiles d'arachide, d'olive, de colza, de noisette, de sésame, de maïs, de tournesol, de germes de blé, de pépins de raisins, de noix, de soja, huiles mélangées (variété des acides gras insaturés) Margarines végétales, margarines diététiques, matières grasses à tartiner exclusivement d'origine végétale Graisses de canard, graisse d'oie Sauces maison sans beurre ni crème fraîche En équivalence **: graines et fruits oléagineux** *sauf noix de coco*	Huiles de palme et de coprah Sauces du commerce Beurre même allégé Margarines standard (en emballage papier) Crème fraîche même allégée Noix de coco et dérivés Végétaline® Préparations industrielles contenant des graisses hydrogénées
Sucre et produits sucrés		Produits sucrés à index glycémique élevé : Sucre Confitures, gelées, marmelades, miels Confiseries Sorbets Crème de marron Fruits confits Pâtes de fruits Barres chocolatées

Groupe d'aliments	Aliments conseillés	Aliments déconseillés
Sucre et produits sucrés		**Produits sucrés à teneur en acides gras saturés élevée :** Chocolats et dérivés Pâtes à tartiner Crèmes glacées, glaces **Attention :** les produits sucrés sont autorisés mais déconseillés
Boissons	**Eaux du robinet, minérales plates ou gazeuses, de source Eaux minérales aromatisées non sucrées Thé, café, infusions, tisanes non sucrés Boissons rafraîchissantes non sucrées et/ou édulcorées Sirops édulcorés Jus de légumes**	**Eaux minérales aromatisées sucrées** **Préparations à base de thé, café sucrées** **Boissons rafraîchissantes sucrées** **Sirops sucrés** **Toutes les boissons alcoolisées**
Épices et aromates	**Toutes les épices et tous les aromates**	*Pas de contre-indication*

5. *En pratique*

Différents objectifs doivent être atteints par les patients :
– maîtrise des équivalences glucidiques (en glucides complexes et en glucides simples) ;
– maîtrise de la répartition des glucides et de la notion d'index glycémique ;
– surveillance du bilan lipidique (régime hypocholestérolémiant associé si nécessaire) ;
– surveillance des glycémies capillaires ;
– surveillance de l'hémoglobine glyquée (HbA1c) ;
– adaptation de l'insulinothérapie à la glycémie capillaire et à la ration glucidique ;
– prise en charge des différents facteurs de risques cardiovasculaires (hypertension artérielle, arrêt du tabac, lutte contre la sédentarité…).

6. Exemple de ration, de répartition et de menu

6.1. Exemple de ration d'un régime contrôlé en glucides à 8,2 MJ, 250 g de glucides

Aliments	Quantités (g ou mL)	Protéines g	Lipides g	Glucides g	Ca mg	Fer mg	Vit C mg	Fibres g
Lait demi-écrémé ou équivalent	450	16	7	22,5	540	0	0	0
Fromage	30	6	7	0	150	0	0	0
VPO maigres	150	27	7,5	0	22,5	3	0	0
Pain ou équivalent	150	12	0	75	37,5	3	0	7,5
PC crus ou équivalent	100	10	0	75	25	1	0	1,5
Légumes	450	4,5	0	22,5	180	4,5	90	13,5
Fruits	450	0	0	54	135	2,25	135	9
Huile	30	0	30	0	0	0	0	0
Margarine végétale	25	0	20,5	0	0	0	0	0
Sucre ou équivalent	0	0	0	0	0	0	0	0
Total (g)		75	71	249	1 090	14	225	32
Énergie (kJ)	8 224	1 279	2 711	4 233				
Pourcentages	100	16	33	51				

6.2. Exemple de répartition d'un régime contrôlé en glucides à 8,2 MJ, 250 g de glucides

Aliments	Quantités (g ou mL)	Petit-déjeuner g	Déjeuner g	Dîner g
Lait demi-écrémé ou équivalent	450	150	150	150
Fromage	30	0	0	30
VPO maigres	150	0	100	50
Pain ou équivalent	150	100	25	25
PC crus ou équivalent	100	0	50	50

Le régime contrôlé en glucides

Aliments	Quantités (g ou mL)	Petit-déjeuner	Déjeuner	Dîner
		g	g	g
Légumes	450	0	250	150
Fruits	450	150	150	150
Huile	30	0	20	10
Margarine	25	15	0	10
Total (kJ)	8 457	2 061	3 278	3 118
Pourcentages	100	24	39	37
Total glucides (g)	251	75	88	88
Glucides (%)	100	30	35	35

6.3. Exemple de menu d'un régime contrôlé en glucides à 8,2 MJ, 250 g de glucides

Petit-déjeuner
Thé au lait demi-écrémé édulcoré.
Pain complet et margarine végétale.
3-4 abricots.

Déjeuner
Champignons de Paris vinaigrette (10 mL d'huile de noix).
Merlan vapeur.
Tagliatelles aux légumes du soleil (dont 10 mL d'huile d'olive).
Une tranche de pain de seigle.
Une faisselle demi-écrémée édulcorée.
Deux kiwis.

Dîner
Une tranche de rôti de porc froid dégraissé.
Fondue de poireaux (dont 10 mL d'huile de tournesol)/Riz créole (avec 10 g de margarine végétale).
Pyrénées.
Une tranche de pain de campagne au levain.
Une orange sanguine.

12

Le régime contrôlé en saccharose

1. Définition et principe

Le régime contrôlé en saccharose correspond à une alimentation équilibrée au cours de laquelle l'apport total et la répartition en saccharose sont contrôlés.

2. Les indications

Les indications sont les suivantes :
1. patient à risques d'hypoglycémie réactionnelle ;
2. gastrectomie ;
3. surpoids, obésité ;
4. neurotonie.

3. Couverture des besoins et apports nutritionnels conseillés

3.1. L'énergie

Le régime est normoénergétique et le niveau énergétique est évalué selon le métabolisme de base et les activités physiques particulières de chaque individu.

3.2. Les protéines

Le régime est normoprotidique soit de 11 à 15 % de l'AET avec une répartition correcte entre les protéines animales et végétales.

3.3. Les lipides

Le régime est normolipidique avec 30 à 35 % de lipides et une répartition en acides gras réalisée selon les références (cas de l'adulte) :
- acides gras saturés : 8 % de l'AET ;
- acides gras monoinsaturés : 20 % de l'AET ;
- acides gras polyinsaturés : 5 % de l'AET avec :
  - acides gras oméga 6 : 4 % de l'AET,
  - acides gras oméga 3 : 0,8 % de l'AET,
  - acides gras polyinsaturés à longue chaîne : 0,2 % de l'AET dont 0,05 % de DHA.

3.4. Les glucides

Le régime est normoglucidique à savoir qu'en tant que compléments énergétiques de la ration, ils doivent atteindre 50 à 59 % de l'AET.

Les glucides complexes et les glucides simples doivent respectivement représenter 55 % et 45 % des glucides totaux.

Le régime étant contrôlé en saccharose, les produits sucrés sont limités à 5 % de l'apport énergétique total.

3.5. Les fibres

Les apports en fibres doivent correspondre aux besoins de chaque individu en particulier ceux en fibres solubles (évalués à 10-15 g par jour chez l'adulte) puisque celles-ci ont tendance à diminuer la glycémie postprandiale en formant des complexes avec les glucides ingérés réduisant alors l'action des enzymes digestives.

3.6. Les vitamines et les minéraux

L'alimentation étant normo-équilibrée et les produits sucrés considérés comme des calories vides (car à forte valeur énergétique et à faible densité nutritionnelle), l'ensemble des vitamines et des minéraux peuvent être correctement couverts.

3.7. L'eau

Les quantités d'eau sont déterminées selon les recommandations.

4. Le choix des aliments

Groupe d'aliments	Aliments conseillés	Aliments déconseillés
Lait	**Laits liquides nature** **Laits concentrés nature** **Laits en poudre nature**	Laits sucrés et/ou aromatisés
Laitages	**Laitages nature** **Laitages édulcorés**	Laitages sucrés et/ou aromatisés et/ou aux fruits
Desserts lactés	**Desserts lactés édulcorés** **Attention :** respecter les quantités conseillées et les fréquences de consommation recommandées	Desserts lactés sucrés
Fromages	**Fromages sous toutes leurs formes** **Attention :** respecter les quantités conseillées et les fréquences de consommation recommandées	*Pas de contre-indication*
VPO	**VPO sous toutes leurs formes** **Attention :** respecter les quantités conseillées et les fréquences de consommation recommandées	*Pas de contre-indication*
Farines et dérivés	**Farines (de blé, de sarrasin, complète), fécules, tapioca…** **Pains et dérivés nature** **Céréales pour petit-déjeuner nature, muesli nature, flocons d'avoine** **Biscuits pauvres en saccharose** **Viennoiseries, gâteaux et pâtisseries pauvres en saccharose**	Pains et dérivés avec des matières sucrantes Céréales pour petit-déjeuner sucrées et barres de céréales Biscuits riches en saccharose (biscuits confiturés, boudoirs, génoises, tartelettes aux fruits, biscuits roulés…) Pâtisseries, gâteaux et viennoiseries riches en saccharose

Groupe d'aliments	Aliments conseillés	Aliments déconseillés
Farines et dérivés	**Attention :** respecter les quantités conseillées et les fréquences de consommation recommandées **Attention :** privilégier les aliments complets	
Féculents	**Féculents sous toutes leurs formes** **Attention :** privilégier les féculents complets	*Pas de contre-indication*
Matières grasses et équivalents	**Matières grasses sous toutes leurs formes** **Attention :** respecter les quantités conseillées et les fréquences de consommation recommandées	*Pas de contre-indication*
Légumes	**Légumes sous toutes leurs formes**	*Pas de contre-indication*
Fruits	**Fruits frais** **Fruits surgelés non sucrés** **Coulis de fruits sans sucre** **Compotes de fruits étiquetées « 100 % pur fruits » ou « sans sucre ajouté », compotes maison sans sucre ou édulcorées** **Fruits secs** **Attention :** faire des équivalences en fonction du pourcentage glucidique de chaque type de fruits	**Fruits surgelés sucrés** **Coulis de fruits sucrés** **Compotes de fruits sucrées** **Fruits au sirop**
Sucre et équivalents		**Sucre** **Confitures, gelées, marmelades, miels** **Confiseries** **Sorbets** **Crème de marron** **Fruits confits**

Groupe d'aliments	Aliments conseillés	Aliments déconseillés
Sucre et équivalents		Pâtes de fruits Barres chocolatées Chocolat et dérivés Pâtes à tartiner Crèmes glacées, glaces **Attention :** les produits sucrés sont autorisés mais déconseillés
Boissons	**Eaux du robinet, minérales plates ou gazeuses, de source Eaux minérales aromatisées non sucrées Thé, café, infusions, tisanes non sucrés Boissons rafraîchissantes non sucrées et/ou édulcorées Sirops édulcorés Jus de légumes**	**Eaux minérales aromatisées sucrées Préparations à base de thé, café sucrées Boissons rafraîchissantes sucrées Sirops sucrés Toutes les boissons alcoolisées**
Épices et aromates	**Toutes les épices et tous les aromates**	*Pas de contre-indication*

5. *En pratique*

Les patients doivent :
- privilégier les aliments riches en fibres et à index glycémique bas ;
- apprendre à fractionner l'alimentation et supprimer les prises isolées d'aliments à index glycémique élevé ;
- maîtriser les signes d'une hypoglycémie réactionnelle ;
- maîtriser le ressucrage en cas de nécessité.

6. Exemple de ration, de répartition et de menu

6.1. Exemple de ration d'un régime contrôlé en saccharose à 8,9 MJ

Aliments	Quantités (g ou mL)	Protéines g	Lipides g	Glucides g	Ca mg	Fer mg	Vit C mg	Fibres g
Lait demi-écrémé ou équivalent	450	16	7	22,5	540	0	0	0
Fromage	30	6	6,5	0	150	0	0	0
VPO	150	27	15	0	22,5	3	0	0
Pain ou équivalent	200	16	0	100	50	4	0	10
PC crus ou équivalent	70	7	0	52,5	17,5	0,7	0	1,05
Légumes	450	4,5	0	22,5	180	4,5	90	13,5
Fruits	450	0	0	54	135	2,25	135	9
Huile	30	0	30	0	0	0	0	0
Beurre/Margarine	25	0	20,5	0	0	0	0	0
Sucre ou équivalent	20	0	0	20	0	0	0	0
Total (g)		76	79	271,5	1 095	14	225	34
Énergie (kJ)	8 908	1 296	2 996	4 615,5				
Pourcentages	100	15	34	52				

6.2. Exemple de répartition d'un régime contrôlé en saccharose à 8,9 MJ

Aliments	Quantités (g ou mL)	Petit-déjeuner g	Déjeuner g	Dîner g
Lait demi-écrémé ou équivalent	450	150	150	150
Fromage	30	0	0	30
VPO	150	0	100	50
Pain ou équivalent	200	100	50	50
PC crus ou équivalent	70	0	70	0
Légumes	450	0	100	350
Fruits	450	150	150	150

Aliments	Quantités (g ou mL)	Petit-déjeuner g	Déjeuner g	Dîner g
Huile	30	0	20	10
Beurre/Margarine	25	10	0	15
Sucre ou équivalent	20	20	0	0
Total (kJ)	8 907	2 245	3 660	3 002
Pourcentages	100	25	41	34

6.3. Exemple de menu d'un régime contrôlé en saccharose à 8,9 MJ

Petit-déjeuner
Thé au lait demi-écrémé édulcoré.
Pain complet et margarine végétale.
1/2 mangue.

Déjeuner
Concombres vinaigrette (10 mL d'huile de noisette).
Fricassée de colin (10 mL d'huile d'olive).
Riz basmati.
Pain au sésame.
Un fromage blanc édulcoré et morceaux d'ananas.

Dîner
Chou-fleur vinaigrette (10 mL d'huile d'arachide).
Escalope de poulet sauce moutarde (40 g de crème fraîche).
Endives au jus (250 g).
Saint Marcellin.
Deux tranches de pain aux céréales.
Melon d'eau.

Section 6

Prescriptions nécessitant une modification des apports conseillés en lipides et en glucides

13

Le régime contrôlé en glucides et en lipides

1. Définition et principe

Le régime contrôlé en glucides et en lipides correspond à une alimentation au cours de laquelle l'apport total, la répartition et la nature des glucides sont contrôlés. Ce type de prescription comprend également :
– un contrôle qualitatif des lipides en privilégiant les acides gras insaturés ;
– une limitation stricte de la quantité d'alcool ingérée ;
– souvent un contrôle de l'apport énergétique et/ou du cholestérol.

Les objectifs nutritionnels de ce régime sont les suivants :
– atteindre les objectifs glycémiques, lipidiques voire pondéraux ;
– prévenir et/ou traiter les hypoglycémies ;
– prévenir la survenue des complications micro- et macroangiopathiques ;
– prendre en charge les divers facteurs de risques cardiovasculaires (normaliser le bilan lipidique, traiter l'hypertension artérielle, arrêt du tabac…).

2. Les indications

Les indications sont les suivantes :
– diabète de type 2 (diabète non insulinodépendant) avec ou sans surpoids ;
– hypertriglycéridémies endogènes (type V, IIB et III (rare)) ;
– corticothérapie (en présence de facteur de risque de diabète).

Attention : le régime contrôlé en glucides et en lipides est fortement contre-indiqué chez les sujets âgés de plus de 75 ans et/ou en fin de vie.

3. Couverture des besoins et apports nutritionnels conseillés

3.1. L'énergie

Lorsque l'indice de masse corporelle du patient se situe dans la normalité, le régime est normoénergétique et l'apport calorique est fixé en fonction des besoins de chaque individu.

Lors des cas de surpoids ou d'obésité, un régime hypocalorique doit être associé.

3.2. Les glucides

Le régime étant contrôlé en glucides, ils représentent les nutriments de choix et doivent être généralement compris entre 50 et 55 % de l'apport énergétique total. Le taux de glucides autorisé est fixé de manière précise et exprimé en grammes par jour.

La répartition qualitative des glucides se fait de la manière suivante :
– 55 % de glucides complexes ;
– 45 % de glucides simples.

Les aliments présentant un index glycémique bas sont privilégiés car ils induisent une augmentation modérée de la glycémie et réduisent donc ainsi la résistance à l'insuline.

Les produits sucrés sont limités à 5 % maximum de l'AET car pour la plupart ils présentent un index glycémique haut et/ou sont sources d'acides gras saturés.

3.3. Les lipides

Le régime est normolipidique (30 à 35 % de l'AET) avec une répartition des acides gras réalisée selon les références (cas de l'adulte) :
– acides gras saturés : 8 % de l'AET ;
– acides gras monoinsaturés : 20 % de l'AET ;
– acides gras polyinsaturés : 5 % de l'AET avec :
  - acides gras oméga 6 : 4 % de l'AET,
  - acides gras oméga 3 : 0,8 % de l'AET,
  - acides gras polyinsaturés à longue chaîne : 0,2 % de l'AET dont 0,05 % de DHA.

Pour les patients suivant ce type de régime et présentant des risques de maladies cardiovasculaires accentués, la qualité des matières grasses est particulièrement contrôlée notamment en ce qui concerne les acides gras saturés.

Lorsqu'une hypercholestérolémie est réellement diagnostiquée, un régime hypocholestérolémiant doit être prescrit.

3.4. Les protéines

Les protéines représentent dans ce cas le complément de la ration à savoir de 10 à 20 % de l'AET.

D'un point de vue qualitatif, le rapport entre les protéines animales et végétales doit être respecté.

3.5. Les fibres

Les apports en fibres doivent correspondre aux besoins de chaque individu.

Les fibres solubles (évalués à 10-15 g par jour chez l'adulte) ont tendance à diminuer la glycémie postprandiale en formant des complexes avec les glucides ingérés réduisant alors l'action des enzymes digestives.

Quant aux fibres insolubles, celles-ci présentent la propriété de diminuer la cholestérolémie ainsi que la triglycéridémie car, tout en accélérant le transit, elles diminuent l'assimilation des lipides et augmentent l'excrétion fécale des sels biliaires.

3.6. Les vitamines et les minéraux

L'alimentation étant normo-équilibrée, l'ensemble des vitamines et des minéraux peuvent être correctement couverts.

3.7. L'eau

Les quantités d'eau sont déterminées selon les recommandations.

4. *Le choix des aliments*

Groupe d'aliments	Aliments conseillés	Aliments déconseillés
Laits	Lait liquide demi-écrémé, écrémé Lait concentré, en poudre demi-écrémé, écrémé nature reconstitué	Lait liquide entier Lait concentré entier et/ou sucré Lait en poudre entier Laits aromatisés
Laitages	Yaourts ordinaires et/ou édulcorés Yaourts 0 % MG et/ou édulcorés Fromages frais 0 % et 10 % MG nature ou édulcorés	Yaourts au lait entier et/ou sucrés Fromages frais au lait entier (20 % MG), 30 % MG et 40 % MG et/ou sucrés Laitages « crémeux »

Groupe d'aliments	Aliments conseillés	Aliments déconseillés
Desserts lactés	Desserts lactés allégés en matières grasses et sans sucre **Attention :** il convient de les décomposer en équivalences (lait, matières grasses) si nécessaire	Desserts lactés non allégés en matières grasses et/ou contenant des matières sucrantes
Fromages	**Fromages les moins riches en lipides et en acides gras saturés :** Camembert 40 %/MS Camembert 45 %/MS Camembert 25 %/MS Chèvre frais Carré de l'est Coulommiers Édam Emmental peu affiné Fromages allégés 25 % MG/MS Fromages fondus à base de pâte dure Fromages fondus 45 %/MS Fromage type Babybel® Fromage type Carré frais® Fromage type Chaource® Pont-l'évêque Raclette Reblochon Roquefort Saint Marcellin Sainte Maure Saint Nectaire Saint Paulin Selle sur Cher Tomme La quantité et les étiquetages des fromages doivent être bien contrôlés	Fromages les plus riches en lipides et en acides gras saturés : Beaufort Bleu Camembert 50 %, 60 %/MS Cantal Cheddar Chèvres mi-sec et sec Comté Emmental très affiné Fromages fondus 65 %, 70 %/MS Fromage type Boursin® Gruyère Gouda Maroilles Munster Mimolette Morbier Neuchâtel Parmesan Pyrénées Vacherin
Viandes	**Viandes de boucherie maigres** **Volailles maigres sans la peau** **Gibiers**	Viandes de boucherie grasses et demi-grasses Volailles grasses et/ou morceaux riches en peau Autres : paupiettes de viande, viandes panées, beignets, plats cuisinés à base de viandes
Charcuteries	Charcuteries maigres	Charcuteries grasses
Abats	Abats maigres	Abats riches en lipides

Le régime contrôlé en glucides et en lipides

Groupe d'aliments	Aliments conseillés	Aliments déconseillés
Produits de la pêche	**Poissons maigres, demi-gras et gras *en équivalence*** Modes de consommation conseillés : – frais – en conserve au naturel ou à l'huile – surgelés non cuisinés	*Pas de contre-indication* Modes de consommation déconseillés : – en conserve en sauce – préparations du commerce : poissons panés, en beignet, rillettes, mousses, pâtés, terrines… – plats cuisinés à base de poisson
Œufs	**Œufs sous toutes leurs formes** Modes de consommation : omelettes, pochés, à la coque, au plat (poêle antiadhésive), cocotte, durs, mollets, brouillés…	*Pas de contre-indication*
Farines et dérivés	**Farines complètes, de sarrasin** **Pains complets, de seigle, au son, aux céréales, pains de mie complets nature** **Céréales pour petit-déjeuner au son, muesli nature, flocons d'avoine nature** **Biscuits riches en glucides complexes, pauvres en glucides simples et en lipides, biscuits enrichis en fibres** Attention : les recettes doivent être avec le moins de lipides et de glucides simples possibles et ils doivent être décomposés en farine, matières grasses et sucre si nécessaire Mode de consommation : privilégier les aliments complets (index glycémique bas)	**Farines raffinées** **Pains blancs, pains fantaisies, biscottes, cracottes, pains grillés** **Céréales pour petit-déjeuner sucrées et/ou extrudées, barres de céréales** **Biscuits riches en glucides simples (biscuits confiturés, boudoirs, génoises, tartelettes aux fruits, biscuits roulés…)** **Biscuits extrudés (gaufrettes, meringues, crackers apéritifs…)** **Biscuits riches en beurre et/ou en matières grasses hydrogénées** **Pâtisseries, viennoiseries** **Autres gâteaux**

Groupe d'aliments	Aliments conseillés	Aliments déconseillés
Féculents	Pâtes, riz blanc, riz complet, semoule, blé dur précuit, quinoa, pommes de terre cuites entières, légumes secs, fruits amylacés non cuisinés Mode de consommation : privilégier les féculents complets	Riz cuisson rapide, pommes de terre en purée, pommes de terre en flocons Autres féculents cuisinés
Légumes	Légumes frais Légumes surgelés non cuisinés Légumes en conserve non cuisinés Potages maison et du commerce non cuisinés Mode de consommation : privilégier les crudités (riches en antioxydants)	Légumes cuisinés du commerce Potages du commerce cuisinés
Fruits	Fruits frais sauf pastèque Fruits surgelés non sucrés Compotes de fruits étiquetées « 100 % pur fruits » ou « sans sucre ajouté », compotes maison sans sucre ou édulcorées Fruits secs Attention : faire des équivalences en fonction du pourcentage glucidique de chaque type de fruits	Pastèque Fruits surgelés sucrés Compotes du commerce sucrées Fruits au sirop
Matières grasses et équivalents	Huiles d'arachide, d'olive, de colza, de noisette, de sésame, de maïs, de tournesol, de germes de blé, de pépins de raisins, de noix, de soja, huiles mélangées (variété des acides gras insaturés) Margarines végétales, margarines diététiques, matières grasses à tartiner exclusivement d'origine végétale Graisses de canard, graisse d'oie Sauces maison sans beurre ni crème fraîche En équivalence : **graines et fruits oléagineux** *sauf noix de coco*	Huiles de palme et de coprah Sauces du commerce Beurre même allégé Margarines standard (en emballage papier) Crème fraîche même allégée Noix de coco et dérivés Végétaline® Préparations industrielles contenant des graisses hydrogénées

Groupe d'aliments	Aliments conseillés	Aliments déconseillés
Sucre et produits sucrés	Édulcorants de synthèse Une unité ou une cuillère à soupe équivaut au pouvoir sucrant d'un morceau de sucre	**Produits sucrés à index glycémique élevé :** Sucre Confitures, gelées, marmelades, miels Confiseries Sorbets Crème de marron Fruits confits Pâtes de fruits Barres chocolatées **Produits sucrés à teneur en acides gras saturés élevée :** Chocolats et dérivés Pâtes à tartiner Crèmes glacées, glaces **Attention :** les produits sucrés sont autorisés mais déconseillés
Boissons	**Eaux du robinet, minérales plates ou gazeuses, de source Eaux minérales aromatisées non sucrées et/ou édulcorées Thé, café, infusions, tisanes non sucrés Boissons rafraîchissantes non sucrées et/ou édulcorées Sirops édulcorés Jus de légumes** **Attention : concernant les boissons édulcorées :** bien vérifier la non-présence de sucre et en contrôler les quantités ingérées	**Eaux minérales aromatisées sucrées** **Préparations à base de thé, café, sucrées Boissons rafraîchissantes sucrées** **Sirops sucrés** **Toutes les boissons alcoolisées**
Épices et aromates	**Toutes les épices et tous les aromates**	*Pas de contre-indication*

5. En pratique

Différents objectifs doivent être atteints par les patients :
- maîtrise des équivalences glucidiques (en glucides complexes et en glucides simples) ;
- maîtrise de la répartition des glucides et de la notion d'index glycémique ;
- surveillance du bilan lipidique (régime hypocholestérolémiant associé si nécessaire) ;
- surveillance des glycémies capillaires ;
- surveillance de l'hémoglobine glyquée (HbA1c) ;
- surveillance du poids ;
- maîtrise du traitement médicamenteux (antidiabétiques oraux) ;
- prise en charge des différents facteurs de risques cardiovasculaires (hypertension artérielle, arrêt du tabac, lutte contre la sédentarité…) ;
- association d'un régime hypoénergétique et/ou hypocholestérolémiant si nécessaire.

6. Exemple de ration, de répartition et de menu

6.1. Exemple de ration d'un régime contrôlé en lipides et en glucides à 8,3 MJ, 250 g de glucides

Aliments	Quantités (g ou mL)	g	Lipides		Glucides		Ca	Fer	Vitamine C	Fibres
			g/100 g	g	g/100 g	g	mg	mg	mg	g
Lait demi-écrémé ou équivalent	450	16	1,5	7	5	22,5	540	0	0	0
Fromage	30	6	22	6,5	0	0	150	0	0	0
VPO maigres	150	27	5	7,5	0	0	22,5	3	0	0
Pain ou équivalent	150	12	0	0	50	75	37,5	3	0	7,5
PC crus ou équivalent	80	8	0	0	75	60	20	0,8	0	1,2
Légumes	450	4,5	0	0	5	22,5	180	4,5	90	13,5
Fruits	450	0	0	0	12	54	135	2,25	135	9
Huile	30	0	100	30	0	0	0	0	0	0
Margarine végétale	25	0	82	20,5	0	0	0	0	0	0

Le régime contrôlé en glucides et en lipides 159

Aliments	Quantités (g ou mL)	g	Lipides		Glucides		Ca	Fer	Vitamine C	Fibres
			g/100 g	g	g/100 g	g	mg	mg	mg	g
Sucre ou équivalent	20	0	0	0	100	20	0	0	0	0
Total (g)		73		71		254	1 085	14	225	31
Énergie (kJ)	8 275	1 245		2 711		4 318				
Pourcentages	100	15		33		52				

6.2. Exemple de répartition d'un régime contrôlé en lipides et en glucides à 8,3 MJ, 250 g de glucides

Aliments	Quantités (g ou mL)	Petit-déjeuner	Déjeuner	Dîner
		g	g	g
Lait demi-écrémé ou équivalent	450	150	150	150
Fromage	30	0	0	30
VPO maigres	150	0	100	50
Pain ou équivalent	150	100	25	25
PC crus ou équivalent	80	0	40	40
Légumes	450	0	250	150
Fruits	450	150	150	150
Huile	30	0	20	10
Margarine	25	15	0	10
Sucre ou équivalent	20	10	5	5
Total (kJ)	**8 508**	**2 231**	**3 218**	**3 059**
Pourcentages	100	**26**	**38**	**36**
Total glucides (g)	**256**	85	85,5	85,5
Glucides (%)	100	**33**	**33**	**33**

6.3. Exemple de menu d'un régime contrôlé en lipides et en glucides à 8,3 MJ, 250 g de glucides

Petit-déjeuner
Thé nature.
Pain complet grillé et margarine végétale.
Deux petits suisses 10 % sucrés.
Mirabelles.

Déjeuner
Courgettes râpées vinaigrette (10 mL d'huile d'olive).
Pavé de saumon au four.
Quinoa (dont 10 mL d'huile de germe de blé) et poivrons grillés.
Une tranche de pain bis.
Un yaourt demi-écrémé édulcoré.
Deux figues fraîches.
Un café sucré (1 morceau).

Dîner
Bavette à l'échalote.
Épinards en branche (dont 10 mL de crème de soja)/pommes de terre sautées (avec 10 mL d'huile de tournesol).
Fourme d'Ambert.
Une tranche de pain au son.
Une petite banane.
Un café sucré (1 morceau).

Section 7

Prescriptions nécessitant une modification des apports conseillés en minéraux

14

Les régimes hyposodés

1. Introduction

1.1. Définition et principe

Les régimes hyposodés correspondent à une alimentation normoénergétique au cours de laquelle les apports sodés quotidiens sont limités par rapport aux apports conseillés (2 400 à 3 200 mg de sodium soit 6 à 8 g de sel/jour).

L'objectif nutritionnel de ces régimes est de faciliter le contrôle des pathologies aggravées par l'excès de chlorure de sodium qui pourrait engendrer, à plus ou moins long terme, un déséquilibre hydroélectrolytique.

On peut proposer trois types de régimes hyposodés dont le choix est réalisé en fonction de la pathologie du patient et de son évolution :
– le régime hyposodé large : 1 200 à 2 400 mg de Na/j (3 à 6 g de sel/j) ;
– le régime hyposodé standard : 600 à 1 200 mg de Na/j (1,5 à 3 g de sel/j) ;
– le régime hyposodé strict : 300 à 600 mg de Na/j (0,75 à 1,5 g de sel/j).

1.2. Les indications

D'une manière générale, les indications sont les suivantes :
– les pathologies cardiaques telles que :
  - l'athérosclérose et la thrombose,
  - l'hypertension artérielle mal contrôlée et « sensible » au sel,
  - l'insuffisance cardiaque,
  - l'infarctus et ses suites,
  - les endocardites et les péricardites,
  - les autres myocardiopathies ;

- les pathologies rénales avec :
  - l'insuffisance rénale aiguë (les patients présentent une oligurie voire une anurie générant une rétention sodée),
  - l'insuffisance rénale chronique,
  - le syndrome néphrotique ;
- les pathologies hépatiques : il s'agit de la cirrhose décompensée avec ascite ;
- au cours d'une corticothérapie : le taux de sodium journalier est à adapter en fonction de la dose de cortisone à savoir :
  - pour des doses supérieures à 1 mg/kg/j, le régime est hyposodé strict,
  - pour des doses comprises entre 0,5 et 1 mg/kg/j, le régime est hyposodé standard,
  - pour des doses comprises entre 0,1 et 0,5 mg/kg/j, le régime est hyposodé large.

1.3. Couverture des besoins et apports nutritionnels conseillés

Il s'agit d'un régime normoénergétique, normoprotidique, normolipidique et normoglucidique dont les apports sont adaptés selon les caractéristiques physiques et physiologiques de chaque patient. Il convient aussi de s'assurer d'une couverture correcte en micronutriments, en fibres ainsi qu'en eau de boisson.

1.4. En pratique

En pratique et pour ces trois types de régime, il est préconisé :
- de contrôler ou de supprimer l'apport en sel lors de la préparation des repas (sel de cuisson, sel d'assaisonnement) ;
- de contrôler ou de supprimer l'apport en sel de table ;
- d'avoir éventuellement recours (selon prescription) à du « sel de régime hyposodé » (à base de potassium) ;
- d'envisager l'achat d'aliments diététiques hyposodés (produits appauvris en sodium, voir tableau suivant) ;
- d'éviter les produits industriels qui contiennent du chlorure de sodium, du citrate de sodium, du benzoate de sodium et du glutamate de sodium ;
- de maîtriser les équivalences en sel ;
- d'utiliser des aliments sapides en substitut du sel tels que des huiles goûteuses (première pression à froid à la noix, aux olives, huiles aromatisées…), des vinaigres aromatisés (échalote, estragon, framboise, sauge…), des fines herbes, des épices, des produits céréaliers complets, des riz aromatisés, des sauces (hyposodées), du court-bouillon (hyposodé) tout en privilégiant les herbes fraîches de saison dès que possible ;
- de limiter les aliments insipides par eux-mêmes (pâtes alimentaires raffinées, fruits et légumes peu mûrs ou cultivés hors saison…) ;
- de choisir ses modes de cuisson en proscrivant les cuissons à l'eau (qui provoquent une perte de saveur importante) et en préférant les cuissons à la vapeur, à l'autocuiseur, à l'étouffée, en papillote, les braisés, les grillades…

Aliments diététiques hyposodés

Type d'aliment	Teneur en sodium moyenne ou réglementaire (mg/100 g)
Lait hyposodé liquide	**50**
Lait hyposodé en poudre	**5**
Fromages hyposodés	**< 40**
Viandes/Charcuteries/Poissons appertisés hyposodés	**< 120**
Jambon hyposodé	**< 120**
Pain hyposodé	**2**
Biscottes hyposodées	**1**
Biscuits sucrés hyposodés	**< 120**
Légumes appertisés hyposodés	**< 40**
Plats cuisinés hyposodés	**< 120**
Margarines hyposodées	**< 40**
Chips hyposodés	**< 40**
Sauces (bolognaise, aux légumes, mayonnaise, vinaigrette…), condiments (moutarde, ketchup, cornichons, oignons…) hyposodés	**< 40**
Bouillons cube hyposodés	**< 120**
Sel de régime hyposodé	**< 10**

Remarque : les emballages de tous ces produits comportent obligatoirement leur teneur précise en sodium ; ils n'en sont donc pas entièrement dépourvus et les teneurs sont variables d'une marque à l'autre. Il convient par conséquent de bien lire les étiquettes.

2. *Le régime hyposodé large*

2.1. Définition et principe

Le régime hyposodé large correspond à des apports de sodium compris entre 1 200 et 2 400 mg/j soit 3 à 6 g de sel par jour.

C'est un régime basé sur :
- une suppression des aliments extrêmement riches en sodium (plus de 1 000 mg de sodium/100 g) ;
- un évitement des aliments très riches en sodium (entre 500 et 1 000 mg/100 g de sodium) et riches en sodium (entre 100 et 500 mg/100 g de sodium) *sauf si possible concernant les fromages salés et les pains salés* ;

– un contrôle des aliments sources de sodium (entre 10 et 100 mg/100 g de sodium) et pauvres en sodium (inférieur à 10 mg/100 g) ainsi que des fromages autorisés et des pains salés.

2.2. Indications

Les indications sont les suivantes :
– cirrhose équilibrée ;
– suite d'infarctus ;
– hypertension artérielle mal équilibrée et sensible au sel ;
– insuffisance cardiaque compensée (suite de la phase aiguë) ;
– corticothérapie mineure (doses de 0,1 à 0,5 mg/kg/j).

2.3. Le choix des aliments

	Aliments à contrôler	Aliments à éviter	Aliments à supprimer
Lait	Lait liquide	Lait en poudre Lait concentré	/
Laitages	Tous les laitages	/	/
Desserts lactés	Tous les desserts lactés	/	/
Fromages	Fromages frais salés Fromages à pâte molle Fromages à pâte demi-dure Fromages à pâte dure cuite Quantités maximums : 30 g par jour	/	Fromages persillés Fromages fondus
Viandes	Viandes fraîches ou surgelées non cuisinées	Abats Plats industriels à base de viande	
Produits de la pêche	Poissons et produits de la pêche frais, surgelés, non cuisinés	Poissons panés Autres poissons fumés Mollusques/crustacés Plats industriels à base de poisson	Saumon fumé
Œufs	Œuf entier Jaune d'œuf	Blanc d'œuf	/

Les régimes hyposodés 167

	Aliments à contrôler	Aliments à éviter	Aliments à supprimer
Charcuteries	/	Andouille/Andouillette Saucisses Pâtés Rillettes Maximum : 1 fois tous les 15 jours en équivalence	Jambon blanc Jambon cru Saucissons Bacon Lard/lardons
Farines et dérivés	Flocons d'avoine Farines Pains (blanc, complet, de seigle, de campagne…) **Attention :** maximum : 150 g par jour	Céréales pour petit-déjeuner Pain de mie Viennoiseries Pains grillés Biscuits sucrés Biscottes Pâtisseries Gâteaux Muesli Biscuits apéritifs sans fromage	Biscuits apéritifs au fromage
Féculents	Féculents non cuisinés	Chips Plats industriels à base de féculents Maïs appertisé Petits pois appertisés Légumes secs appertisés	
Matières grasses ou équivalents	Beurre doux Crème fraîche Margarine Graines oléagineuses nature Noix de coco	Beurre demi-sel Sauces chaudes industrielles Graines oléagineuses salées Sauces type mayonnaise industrielles Sauces déshydratées Beurre allégé	Beurre salé Olives noires saumurées Olives vertes saumurées Sauces vinaigrette industrielles
Légumes	Légumes riches en sodium : betteraves, carottes, navets, épinards, cresson, pissenlit Légumes sources de sodium : artichaut, salades, fenouil, chou-fleur, radis, salsifis	Soupes industrielles Légumes appertisés Jus de légumes industriels Bettes Céleri	

	Aliments à contrôler	**Aliments à éviter**	**Aliments à supprimer**
Légumes	Légumes pauvres en sodium : chou rouge, brocoli, champignon, oignon, chou de Bruxelles, tomates, asperge, aubergine, concombre, courgette, haricots verts, endives, oseille, poivrons Modes de consommation : frais non cuisinés ou 4ᵉ gamme		
Fruits	Fruits frais Fruits secs Fruits au sirop Compotes Jus de fruits	/	/
Boissons	Sodas Perrier® San Pellegrino®	Rozana® Badoit® Quézac®	Vichy St-Yorre® Vichy Célestin®
Sucre et produits sucrés	Sucre blanc Sucre roux Chocolat au lait Glaces et crèmes glacées Confiseries Sorbets Chocolat noir Confiture Miel	Pâtes à tartiner Barres chocolatées Chocolat en poudre	/
Condiments	Herbes fraîches	Cornichons, câpres, oignons… saumurés	Sel Bouillons cube Levure chimique Ketchup Moutarde Curry

3. Le régime hyposodé standard

3.1. Définition et principe

Le régime hyposodé standard correspond à des apports de sodium compris entre 600 et 1 200 mg/j soit 1,5 à 3 g de sel par jour.

C'est un régime basé sur :
- une suppression des aliments extrêmement riches en sodium (plus de 1 000 mg de Na/100 g) et des aliments très riches en sodium (entre 500 et 1 000 mg/100 g de Na) *sauf concernant les fromages salés et les pains salés si possible* ;
- un évitement des aliments riches en sodium (entre 100 et 500 mg/100 g de Na) ;
- un contrôle des aliments sources de sodium (entre 10 et 100 mg/100 g de Na) et pauvres en sodium (inférieur à 10 mg/100 g) ainsi que des fromages et des pains salés si possible.

3.2. Indications

Les indications sont les suivantes :
- cirrhose déséquilibrée (ascite importante) ;
- insuffisance rénale chronique avec hyponatriurie ;
- syndrome néphrotique ;
- dialyse ;
- insuffisance cardiaque sévère ;
- corticothérapie modérée (doses de 0,5 à 1 mg/kg/j).

3.3. Le choix des aliments

	Aliments à contrôler	Aliments à éviter	Aliments à supprimer
Lait	Lait liquide	Lait en poudre Lait concentré	/
Laitages	Tous les laitages	/	/
Desserts lactés	Tous les desserts lactés	/	/
Fromages	/	Fromages frais salés Fromages à pâte molle Fromages à pâte demi-dure Fromages à pâte dure cuite Essayer avec 30 g maximum par jour	Fromages persillés Fromages fondus

	Aliments à contrôler	**Aliments à éviter**	**Aliments à supprimer**
Viandes	Viandes fraîches, surgelées non cuisinées	Abats	Plats industriels à base de viande
Produits de la pêche	Produits de la pêche frais, surgelés non cuisinés	Poissons panés Autres poissons fumés Mollusques/crustacés	Saumon fumé Plats industriels à base de poisson
Œufs	Jaune d'œuf	Blanc d'œuf Œuf entier	
Charcuteries	*Toutes contre-indiquées*		Jambon blanc Jambon cru Saucissons Bacon Lard/lardons Andouille/Andouillette Saucisses Pâtés Rillettes…
Farines et dérivés	Flocons d'avoine Farines	Pains (blanc, complet, de seigle, de campagne…) **Attention :** maximum : 80 g par jour Biscuits sucrés Biscottes Pâtisseries Gâteaux Muesli en équivalence	Biscuits apéritif au fromage Biscuits apéritifs sans fromage Céréales pour petit-déjeuner Pains de mie Viennoiseries Pains grillés
Féculents	Féculents non cuisinés	Maïs appertisé Petits pois appertisés Légumes secs appertisés	Chips Plats industriels à base de féculents
Matières grasses ou équivalents	Beurre doux Crème fraîche Margarine Graines oléagineuses nature	Sauces type mayonnaise industrielles Sauces déshydratées Beurre allégé Margarine	Beurre salé Olives noires saumurées Olives vertes saumurées Sauces vinaigrette industrielles Beurre demi-sel Sauces chaudes industrielles Graines oléagineuses salées

	Aliments à contrôler	Aliments à éviter	Aliments à supprimer
Légumes	Légumes riches en sodium : betteraves, carottes, navets, épinards, cresson, pissenlit Légumes sources de sodium : artichaut, salades, fenouil, chou-fleur, radis, salsifis Légumes pauvres en sodium : chou rouge, brocoli, champignon, oignon, chou de Bruxelles, tomates, asperge, aubergine, concombre, courgette, haricots verts, endives, oseille, poivrons Modes de consommation : frais non cuisinés ou 4e gamme	Soupes industrielles Légumes appertisés Jus de légumes industriels Bettes Céleri	/
Fruits	Fruits secs Fruits au sirop Compotes Fruits frais Jus de fruits	/	/
Boissons	Sodas Perrier® San Pellegrino®	Badoit® Quézac®	Vichy St-Yorre® Vichy Célestin® Rozana®
Produits sucrés	Chocolat au lait Glaces et crèmes glacées Confiseries Sucre roux Sorbets Chocolat noir Confiture Miel	Pâtes à tartiner Barres chocolatées Chocolat en poudre	/

	Aliments à contrôler	Aliments à éviter	Aliments à supprimer
Condiments	Herbes fraîches	/	Sel Bouillons cube Levure chimique Ketchup Cornichons, câpres, oignons… saumurés Moutarde Curry

4. Le régime hyposodé strict

4.1. Définition et principe

Le régime hyposodé strict correspond à des apports de sodium compris entre 300 et 600 mg/j soit 0,75 à 1,5 g de sel par jour.

C'est un régime basé sur :
- une suppression des aliments extrêmement riches en sodium (plus de 1 000 mg de Na/100 g), très riches en sodium (entre 500 et 1 000 mg/100 g de Na) et riches en sodium (entre 100 et 500 mg/100 g de Na) ;
- un évitement et/ou un contrôle des aliments sources de sodium (entre 10 et 100 mg/100 g de Na) voire pauvres en sodium (inférieur à 10 mg/100 g).

4.2. Indications

Les indications sont les suivantes :
- cirrhose ascitique en phase aiguë ;
- insuffisance rénale aiguë ;
- syndrome néphrotique avec œdèmes (touchant les membres inférieurs et les paupières) ;
- œdème aigu pulmonaire ;
- corticothérapie majeure (doses à plus de 1 mg/kg/j).

Attention : ce régime est fortement contre-indiqué chez les personnes âgées car il est très anorexigène à cause du choix restrictif des aliments (d'autant plus que peu sapides).

4.3. Le choix des aliments

	Aliments à contrôler	Aliments à éviter	Aliments à supprimer
Lait	Laits liquides Lait désodé	/	Laits en poudre Laits concentrés
Laitages	Tous les laitages	/	/
Desserts lactés	/	Tous les desserts lactés	/
Fromages	Fromages hyposodés	/	Tous les fromages salés
Viandes	Viandes non cuisinées fraîches ou surgelées	Viandes appertisées hyposodées	Plats industriels à base de viande Abats
Produits de la pêche	Produits de la pêche frais, surgelés non cuisinés	Poissons appertisés hyposodés	Saumon fumé Plats industriels à base de poisson Poissons panés Autres poissons fumés Mollusques/crustacés
Œufs		Jaune d'œuf	Blanc d'œuf Œuf entier
Charcuteries		Charcuteries hyposodées appertisées	Toutes les charcuteries salées
Farines et dérivés	Flocons d'avoine Farines Biscottes hyposodées Pain hyposodé	Biscuits sucrés hyposodés	Biscuits apéritif au fromage Biscuits apéritif sans fromage Céréales pour petit-déjeuner Pains de mie Viennoiseries Pains grillés Pains (blanc, complet, de seigle, de campagne…) Biscuits sucrés Biscottes Pâtisseries Gâteaux Muesli

	Aliments à contrôler	**Aliments à éviter**	**Aliments à supprimer**
Féculents	Féculents non cuisinés	Féculents cuisinés hyposodés	Chips Plats industriels à base de féculents Maïs appertisé Petits pois appertisés Légumes secs appertisés
Matières grasses ou équivalents	Beurre doux Graines oléagineuses nature	Crème fraîche Noix de coco	Beurre salé Olives noires saumurées Olives vertes saumurées Sauces vinaigrette industrielles Beurre demi-sel Sauces chaudes industrielles Graines oléagineuses salées Sauces type mayonnaise industrielles Sauces déshydratées Beurre allégé Margarines
Légumes	Légumes sources de sodium : artichaut, salades, fenouil, chou-fleur, radis, salsifis Légumes pauvres en sodium : chou rouge, brocoli, champignon, oignon, chou de Bruxelles, tomates, asperge, aubergine, concombre, courgette, haricots verts, endives, oseille, poivrons	Légumes riches en sodium : betteraves, carottes, navets, épinards, cresson, pissenlit	Soupes industrielles Légumes appertisés Jus de légumes industriels Bettes Céleri
Fruits	Fruits au sirop Compotes Fruits frais Jus de fruits	Fruits secs	/
Boissons		Sodas Perrier® San Pellegrino®	Vichy St-Yorre® Vichy Célestin® Badoit® Quézac®

	Aliments à contrôler	Aliments à éviter	Aliments à supprimer
Produits sucrés		Chocolat au lait Glaces et crèmes glacées Confiseries Sucre roux Sorbets Chocolat noir Confiture	Pâtes à tartiner Barres chocolatées Chocolat en poudre
Condiments			Sel Bouillons cube Levure chimique Ketchup Cornichons, câpres, oignons… saumurés Moutarde Curry

5. Exemple de ration, de répartition et de menu

5.1. Exemple de ration d'un régime hyposodé standard à 9 MJ/jour, 1 200 mg de sodium

Aliments	Quantités (g ou mL)	Protéines	Lipides	Glucides	Ca	Fer	Vit C	Fibres	Na
		g	g	g	mg	mg	mg	g	mg
Lait demi-écrémé ou équivalent	300	10,5	4,5	15	360	0	0	0	135
Fromage hyposodé	30	6	6,6	0	150	0	0	0	6
VP	150	27	15	0	22,5	3	0	0	150
Pain ou équivalent salé	100	8	0	50	25	2	0	5	650
Pain hyposodé	100	8	0	50	25	2	0	5	2
PC crus ou équivalent	70	7	0	52,5	17,5	0,7	0	1	3
Légumes frais	450	4,5	0	22,5	180	4,5	90	13,5	67,5
Fruits frais	450	0	0	54	135	2	135	9	13,5
Huile	25	0	25	0	0	0	0	0	0
Beurre doux	20	0	16,5	0	0	0	0	0	2,4
Sucre	40	0	0	40	0	0	0	0	0

Aliments	Quantités (g ou mL)	Protéines	Lipides	Glucides	Ca	Fer	Vit C	Fibres	Na
		g	g	g	mg	mg	mg	g	mg
Total (g)		80	77	284	1 245	14	225	34	1 179
Énergie (kJ)	9 095	1 360	2 907	4 828					
Pourcentages	100	15	32	53					

5.2. Exemple de répartition d'un régime hyposodé standard à 9 MJ/jour, 1 200 mg de sodium

Aliments	Quantités (g ou mL)	Petit-déjeuner	Déjeuner	Dîner
		g	g	g
Lait demi-écrémé ou équivalent	300	150	0	150
Fromage hyposodé	30	0	30	0
VP	150	0	100	50
Pain ou équivalent salé	100	0	100	0
Pain hyposodé	100	100	0	0
PC crus ou équivalent	70	0	0	70
Légumes frais	450	0	350	100
Fruits frais	450	150	150	150
Huile	25	0	20	5
Beurre doux	20	15	0	5
Sucre	40	0	0	40
Total (kJ)	**8 949**	**2 175**	**3 577**	**3 096**
Pourcentages	100	**25**	**40**	**35**

5.3. Exemple de menu d'un régime hyposodé standard à 9 MJ/jour, 1 200 mg de sodium

Petit-déjeuner
Une tasse de lait demi-écrémé nature.
Pain hyposodé et beurre doux.
1/2 mangue.

Déjeuner
Chou rouge vinaigrette (10 mL d'huile de colza).
Escalope de dindonneau à l'estragon.
Poêlée de légumes au thym (10 mL d'huile d'olive).
Fromage hyposodé.
Pain salé.
Reine-claude.
Dîner
Concombres à la menthe sauce au yaourt.
Sardines grillées.
Ratatouille (5 mL d'huile d'olive).
Polenta.
Pomme au four à la cannelle (30 g de sucre, 5 g de beurre doux).
Une tisane sucrée (2 morceaux).

15

Le régime pauvre en potassium

1. Définition et principe

Le régime pauvre en potassium correspond à une alimentation normo-équilibrée dont les apports en potassium sont limités par :
- une diminution des quantités de végétaux ;
- un choix quant à la consommation des végétaux crus et/ou cuits ;
- une suppression ou un évitement des aliments les plus riches en potassium.

Les apports spontanés habituels (soit 3 à 5 g/j) sont alors abaissés à 2-3 g/j en :
- supprimant les aliments extrêmement riches en potassium (plus de 800 mg/100 g) ;
- évitant les aliments très riches en potassium (300-800 mg/100 g) ;
- contrôlant les aliments riches en potassium (100-300 mg/100 g) et pauvres en potassium (moins de 10 mg/100 g).

2. Les indications

Il s'agit des cas d'hyperkaliémie ou de risque d'hyperkaliémie à savoir :
- insuffisance rénale terminale avec diminution de la kaliurèse et lorsque la clairance de la créatinine est inférieure à 15 mL/min ;
- hémodialyse ;
- dialyse péritonéale (le choix des aliments a tendance à être large) ;
- insuffisance surrénalienne ;
- hypertension artérielle avec traitement par un inhibiteur de l'enzyme de conversion.

> **Remarque**
> Lorsque la kaliémie est très élevée (supérieure à 5,5 mmol), il est possible de prescrire une résine échangeuse d'ions (*kayexalate*) au moment du repas afin d'échanger 1 mmol de potassium avec 1 mmol de calcium ou de sodium (selon le type de résine utilisé).

3. Couverture des besoins et apports nutritionnels conseillés

Il s'agit d'un régime normo-énergétique, normoprotidique, normolipidique et normoglucidique dont les apports sont adaptés selon les caractéristiques physiques et physiologiques de chaque patient. Il convient néanmoins de s'assurer d'une couverture correcte en micronutriments ainsi qu'en eau de boisson. Les apports en fibres doivent aussi être surveillés de par la réduction des quantités de légumes et de fruits et le choix des aliments qui restreint les céréales complètes.

4. Le choix des aliments

	Aliments à contrôler (5 à 300 mg de potassium)	Aliments à éviter (300 à 800 mg de potassium)	Aliments à supprimer (plus de 800 mg de potassium)
Lait	Lait liquide	Lait concentré	Lait en poudre
Laitages	Tous à contrôler	/	/
Desserts lactés	Tous à contrôler	/	/
Fromages	Tous à contrôler	/	/
VPO	Tous à contrôler	/	/
Farines et dérivés	Pains grillés Pains blancs Biscuits sucrés Pain de seigle Pains de mie Farine blanche Pain type 80 Biscottes raffinées Pâtisseries/Gâteaux Biscuits salés Viennoiseries Biscottes au son/complètes	Farine complète Flocons d'avoine Farine de seigle Muesli Farine de sarrasin	Farine de soja Céréales petit-déjeuner au son

	Aliments à contrôler (5 à 300 mg de potassium)	Aliments à éviter (300 à 800 mg de potassium)	Aliments à supprimer (plus de 800 mg de potassium)
Farines et dérivés	Farine bise Céréales pour petit-déjeuner raffinées Pains complets Fécule de maïs		
Féculents	Pommes de terre dauphines Céréales	Pommes de terre purée Pommes de terre noisette Pommes de terre à l'eau Pommes de terre au four Pommes de terre frites Légumes secs Maïs Fruits amylacés	Chips Pommes de terre flocons
Légumes	Légumes à moins de 300 mg de potassium : asperge cuite, aubergine cuite, betterave cuite, brocoli cuit, carotte crue, carotte cuite, champignons cuits, chou rouge cru, chou rouge cuit, chou vert cuit, chou-fleur cuit, cœur de palmier cuit, concombre cru, courgette crue, courgette cuite, céleri branche cuit, endive crue, endive cuite, haricots beurre, haricots vert, laitue, macédoine appertisée, navet cuit, oignon cru, oignon cuit, petits pois, poireau cuit, poivrons crus, poivrons cuits, potiron cuit, radis rose, salsifis cuite, tomate	Légumes à plus de 300 mg de potassium : Artichaut Bettes cuites Céleri rave Champignons crus Chanterelles Chicorée Chou-fleur cru Chou de Bruxelles Cresson Épinards Fenouil Frisée Mâche Oseille Pissenlit Radis noir Avocat	Légumes déshydratés/ lyophilisés

	Aliments à contrôler (5 à 300 mg de potassium)	Aliments à éviter (300 à 800 mg de potassium)	Aliments à supprimer (plus de 800 mg de potassium)
Fruits	**Fruits à moins de 300 mg de potassium :** ananas, cerise, citron, clémentine, mandarine, figue, fraise, framboise, goyave, grenade, groseille, litchi, mangue, mirabelle, myrtille, mûre, nectarine, orange, papaye, pastèque, poire, pomme, pomélo, reine-claude, pêche, raisin blanc, rhubarbe	**Fruits à plus de 300 mg de potassium :** Abricot Banane Cassis Kiwi Melon Raisin noir	**Fruits secs**
Matières grasses ou équivalents	**Mayonnaise allégée Beurre Beurre allégé Mayonnaise Margarine végétale Margarine standard Olives Crèmes Sauces du commerce Noix de coco fraîche**	Graines oléagineuses Noix de coco sèche	
Sucre et produits sucrés	**Bonbons Miel Sorbets Sirops Pâte à tartiner Pâte de fruits Confitures Glaces**	Barre noix de coco enrobée Chocolat et dérivés Sucre roux	Cacao en poudre
Boissons	**Thé Café noir**		Café moulu Café poudre soluble
Condiments	**Sel de mer Vinaigre Moutarde Cornichons**	Ail Ciboule/Ciboulette Poivre moulu Raifort frais Bouillon cube Ketchup Cerfeuil Levure de boulanger	Curry en poudre Gingembre moulu Levure alimentaire Persil

	Aliments à contrôler (5 à 300 mg de potassium)	Aliments à éviter (300 à 800 mg de potassium)	Aliments à supprimer (plus de 800 mg de potassium)
Produits diététiques			Sel de régime hyposodé Produits hyposodés industriels

5. *En pratique*

Il est nécessaire de veiller :
- au respect scrupuleux du choix des aliments ;
- à la maîtrise des équivalences en potassium ;
- à l'adaptation des modes de préparation des végétaux à savoir qu'ils doivent être :
  - épluchés avec soin,
  - découpés en très petits morceaux,
  - trempés dans l'eau pendant un certain temps (au moins 3 heures),
  - cuits à grande eau voire à l'idéal dans deux eaux différentes non salées (d'autant plus s'il s'agit de pommes de terre),
  - limités en quantité : 60 à 100 g en entrée et 150 à 200 g en accompagnement.

6. Exemple de ration, de répartition et de menu

6.1. Exemple de ration d'un régime hypopotassique à 11,1 MJ, 3 g de potassium

Aliments	Quantités (g ou mL)	Protéines	Lipides	Glucides	Ca	Fer	Vitamine C	Fibres	K
		g	g	g	mg	mg	mg	g	mg
Lait demi-écrémé ou équivalent	450	16	7	22,5	540	0	0	0	652,5
Fromage	40	8	8,8	0	200	0	0	0	56
VPO	200	36	20	0	30	4	0	0	500
Pain blanc ou équivalent	250	20	0	125	62,5	5	0	12,5	375
PC raffinés crus	100	10	0	75	25	1	0	1,5	200
Légumes crus	100	1	0	5	40	1	20	3	300
Légumes cuits	200	2	0	10	80	2	40	6	400
Fruits crus	150	0	0	18	45	0,75	45	3	375
Fruits cuits/ Jus de fruits	150	0	0	18	45	0,75	45	3	150
Huile	40	0	40	0	0	0	0	0	0
Beurre	20	0	16	0	0	0	0	0	3
Margarine	10	0	8,3	0	0	0	0	0	5
Sucre	40	0	0	40	0	0	0	0	0
Confiture	15	0	0	10	0	0	0	0	15
Miel	15	0	0	12	0	0	0	0	7,5
Total (g)		**93**	**100**	**335**	**1 068**	**15**	**150**	**29**	**3 039**
Énergie (kJ)	**11 086**	1 577	3 810	5 699					
Pourcentages	100	**14**	**34**	**51**					

6.2. Exemple de répartition d'un régime hypopotassique à 11,1 MJ, 3 g de potassium

Aliments	Quantités (g ou mL)	Petit-déjeuner	Collation		Dîner
		g	g	g	g
Lait demi-ecrémé ou équivalent	450	150	0	150	150
Fromage	40	0	40	0	0
VPO	200	0	100	0	100
Pain blanc ou équivalent	250	100	100	50	0
PC raffinés crus	100	0	0	0	100
Légumes crus	100	0	0	0	100
Légumes cuits	200	0	200	0	0
Fruits crus	150	0	150	0	0
Fruits cuits/Jus de fruits	150	0	0	0	150
Huile	40	0	20	0	20
Beurre	20	20	0	0	0
Margarine	10	0	0	10	0
Sucre	40	20	20	0	0
Confiture	15	0	0	15	0
Miel	15	15	0	0	0
Total (kJ)	11 097	2 449	3 762	1 272	3 615
Pourcentages	100	22	34	11	33

6.3. Exemple de menu d'un régime hypopotassique à 11,1 MJ, 3 g de potassium

Petit-déjeuner
Café sucré (2 morceaux).
Pain blanc grillé beurré et miel de châtaignier.
Un yaourt à l'ananas (dont 10 g de sucre).

Déjeuner
Poulet braisé (10 mL d'huile d'olive).
Carottes sautées (10 mL d'huile de colza).
Saint nectaire.
Pain de campagne.
Fraises au sucre (20 g de sucre).

Collation
Thé nature
Biscottes à la margarine.
Fromage blanc à la confiture de prunes.
Dîner
Endives vinaigrette (10 mL d'huile de noix).
Steak de thon grillé.
Tagliatelles raffinées au basilic (10 g d'huile d'olive).
Une faisselle aux fines herbes autorisées.
Une compote de poire.

16

Le régime contrôlé en phosphore

1. Définition et principe

Le régime contrôlé en phosphore correspond à une alimentation au cours de laquelle l'apport de phosphore est contrôlé à savoir qu'il ne doit pas dépasser 900 mg par jour.

2. Les indications

L'indication du régime contrôlé en phosphore est l'insuffisance rénale essentiellement lorsque la fonction rénale est inférieure à 25 mL/min.

3. Couverture des besoins et apports nutritionnels conseillés

3.1. L'énergie

Il convient d'essayer d'atteindre un niveau énergétique normal selon les besoins physiques et physiologiques de chaque patient.

3.2. Les protéines

Au vu des indications, le régime est hypoprotidique et les apports sont fixés en fonction des constantes sanguines du patient (*cf.* régime hypoprotidique).

3.3. Les lipides

Le régime peut être normolipidique et la répartition en acides gras se fait selon les recommandations.

3.4. Les glucides

Les glucides étant les compléments énergétiques de la ration, ils sont fixés selon l'apport de protéines et de lipides.

Les glucides complexes et les glucides simples doivent respectivement représenter 55 % et 45 % des glucides totaux.

Les produits sucrés sont normalement limités à 10 % maximum de l'AET.

3.5. Les fibres

Les apports en fibres doivent correspondre aux besoins de chaque individu.

3.6. Les vitamines

L'hyperphosphorémie diminuant la synthèse de *vitamine D* active, il convient d'être particulièrement vigilant quant à cet apport notamment en vitamine D endogène.

Pour ce qui est des autres vitamines, les conseils promulgués pour le régime hypoprotidique doivent être suivis.

3.7. Les minéraux

Le régime étant contrôlé en *phosphore*, l'apport doit se situer autour de 900 mg/j. À noter que la restriction protidique prescrite aide à abaisser celle du phosphore.

> **Remarque**
> Les mesures diététiques sont souvent insuffisantes pour assurer un équilibre phosphocalcique adéquat. Dans ces circonstances, la prescription d'un médicament chélateur de phosphore s'avère nécessaire.

La synthèse de vitamine D active étant diminuée, celle-ci induit une réduction de l'absorption intestinale du *calcium*. La quantité de calcium ingérée nécessite donc d'être spécialement surveillée.

De même que pour les vitamines, les apports des autres minéraux doivent être contrôlés selon les recommandations du régime hypoprotidique.

3.8. L'eau

Les quantités d'eau sont déterminées selon les recommandations. Néanmoins, dans le cas d'une pathologie rénale, les apports en eau de boisson peuvent être contrôlés.

4. Le choix des aliments

	Aliments à contrôler	Aliments à éviter	Aliments à supprimer
Lait	Lait liquide Lait concentré reconstitué Lait en poudre reconstitué	Lait concentré non reconstitué	Lait en poudre non reconstitué
Laitages	Tous les laitages	/	/
Desserts lactés	Tous les desserts lactés	/	/
Fromages	Fromages frais salés	Fromages affinés à pâte pressée *hormis beaufort, cantal et chèvres secs* Fromages affinés à pâte molle *hormis maroilles* Fromages affinés à pâte persillée Fromages fondus *hormis fromages fondus pâte dure et fromages fondus 45 %MG/MS*	Fromages affinés à pâte dure Beaufort Cantal Maroilles Fromages de chèvre secs Fromages fondus pâte dure et fromages fondus 45 %MG/MS
VPO	Viandes Produits de la pêche Œuf entier Blanc d'œuf Charcuteries	Jaune d'œuf Abats *hormis les ris*	Ris
Farines et dérives	Farines de blé raffinées Fécule de maïs Pains et dérivés à la farine blanche Céréales petit-déjeuner nature raffinées Biscuits/viennoiseries/pâtisseries/gâteaux à la farine raffinée	Farines de blé complètes Pains et dérivés à la farine complète Céréales petit-déjeuner raffinées aux graines oléagineuses Céréales petit-déjeuner aux fruits secs Flocons d'avoine Biscuits/viennoiseries/pâtisseries/gâteaux à la farine complète Biscuits salés	Farine de soja Céréales petit-déjeuner complètes

	Aliments à contrôler	Aliments à éviter	Aliments à supprimer
Féculents	Céréales raffinées et complètes Légumes secs Pommes de terre Fruits amylacés	Maïs	/
Matières grasses ou équivalents	Huiles Beurres Margarines Crèmes fraîches Fruits oléagineux	Graines oléagineuses *hormis noix de cajou, noix du Brésil, pistaches, graines de sésame, graines de tournesol*	Noix de cajou Noix du Brésil Pistaches Graines de sésame Graines de tournesol
Légumes	Légumes sous toutes leurs formes	/	/
Fruits	Fruits frais	Fruits secs	/
Boissons	Boissons sous toutes leurs formes	/	/
Sucre et produits sucrés	Sucre Confitures, gelées, marmelades Miels Produits glacées Confiseries	Chocolats et dérivés Pâtes à tartiner Pâte d'amande	Cacao en poudre non sucré
Condiments	Tous les condiments	Levure de boulanger	Levure alimentaire
Produits diététiques			Germes de blé Levure de bière

5. En pratique

Les patients doivent :
– contrôler la consommation des différents groupes ;
– maîtriser les équivalences des aliments à éviter ;
– savoir associer les autres régimes liés à l'insuffisance rénale.

6. Exemple de ration, répartition et menu

Il convient de calculer l'apport en phosphore pour le/les régime(s) associé(s) (hypoprotidique et/ou hyposodé et/ou hypopotassique) en respectant une quantité maximale de phosphore de 900 mg/jour.

Section 8

Prescriptions nécessitant une modification des apports conseillés en fibres

17

Le régime riche en fibres

1. Définition et principe

Le régime riche en fibres a pour but d'augmenter le volume fécal et d'accélérer la vitesse du transit intestinal. Il est donc prescrit lorsque les selles émises par un patient sont :
- espacées et irrégulières (moins de trois fois par semaine) ;
- de volume insuffisant car surdigérées avec disparition notamment de la cellulose et de l'amidon résistant ;
- trop peu hydratées (c'est-à-dire dures) dues à une réabsorption d'eau importante causée par un trop long séjour au sein du côlon.

Les objectifs nutritionnels du régime riche en fibres sont les suivants :
- lutter contre l'atonie intestinale en consommant des aliments péristaltiques ;
- réhydrater les selles en veillant à l'apport hydrique ;
- augmenter le volume des selles par une richesse en résidus et en eau.

2. Les indications

Les indications du régime riche en fibres sont les suivantes :
1. La constipation dont il existe deux types :
- la *constipation fonctionnelle* ou primitive (c'est-à-dire sans cause organique) qui peut être :
  - une constipation fonctionnelle passagère (suite à un voyage, un alitement prolongé, un amaigrissement…),

- une constipation fonctionnelle chronique due à : un état de stress permanent, un apport insuffisant en fibres alimentaires (diminution de la motricité du côlon), une insuffisance de musculature abdominale (fréquent chez les personnes dénutries, très sédentaires…) ;
- la *constipation organique* (c'est-à-dire secondaire à des lésions organiques) qui présente deux origines possibles à savoir :
  - une origine extradigestive qui peut être due à : une grossesse, la prise de certains médicaments agissant sur la motricité intestinale (analgésiques, antidépresseurs, opiacés, morphiniques…), certaines pathologies métaboliques et endocriniennes (hypothyroïdie…),
  - une origine digestive qui peut être due à : une obstruction du tube digestif (suite à une tumeur…), des lésions diverses de l'intestin (maladie de Crohn, diverticulose…), des lésions anales douloureuses associées à une hypotonie du sphincter anal interne, un abcès anal, des hémorroïdes, une malformation congénitale (mégacôlon).

Remarque
Le régime riche en fibres n'a pas lieu d'être appliqué lors des cas de constipation terminale, due à un problème de sphincter ou liée à un obstacle pour lesquels les fibres n'ont pas d'influence.

---

2. Les diverticules et ses complications.
3. Les diarrhées.

3. *Couverture des besoins, apports nutritionnels conseillés et choix des aliments*

3.1. Dans le cas d'une constipation primitive

3.1.1. Couverture des besoins et apports conseillés

3.1.1.1. L'énergie

Le régime prescrit peut être normo-énergétique selon le métabolisme de base et les activités physiques journalières de chaque patient.

3.1.1.2. Les protéines

Le régime est normoprotidique aussi bien quantitativement (11 à 15 % de l'AET) que qualitativement (privilégier les protéines animales de bonne qualité).

3.1.1.3. Les lipides

Là encore le régime est normolipidique (30 à 35 % de l'AET) sachant qu'il est nécessaire d'apporter suffisamment de lipides puisqu'ils stimulent la vésicule biliaire (l'insuffisance de contraction vésiculaire étant un facteur de constipation).

Il convient de plus de réaliser une bonne répartition des acides gras (8 % maximum d'acides gras saturés et le reste en acides gras insaturés) car le manque de doubles liaisons entraîne une absorption haute au niveau du côlon ce qui diminue le bol fécal.

3.1.1.4. Les glucides

Les glucides sont comme habituellement compléments énergétiques de la ration à savoir qu'ils représentent 50 à 59 % de l'AET.

La répartition entre les glucides complexes et simples se fait respectivement selon 55 % et 45 % des glucides totaux.

La quantité de produits sucrés doit être bien contrôlée et ne pas dépasser 10 % de l'apport énergétique car étant des glucides simples, ils sont absorbés à 100 % et ne laissent donc pas de résidus au sein du tube digestif. C'est pourquoi, ils n'aident pas à l'augmentation de la production de selles (à l'opposé de l'amidon qui est un sucre fermentescible favorisant le péristaltisme).

3.1.1.5. Les fibres

Les patients souffrant de constipation présentent des ingesta spontanés en fibres insuffisants. C'est pourquoi les apports sont progressivement augmentés (en se basant sur le grammage en fibres faisant suite à l'enquête alimentaire) par paliers de 5 g dans le but d'atteindre la moyenne haute des ANC soit 30 g de fibres/24 h.

Il est recommandé de privilégier les fibres insolubles (2/3 des fibres totales) à savoir les celluloses, certaines hémicelluloses et la lignine (*en petite quantité pour cette dernière car étant de consistance assez dure, elle pourrait irriter le tube digestif*) puisqu'elles s'avèrent particulièrement efficaces dans la régulation du transit intestinal en augmentant :
– le volume des selles ;
– l'hydratation des selles ;
– le poids des selles.

De plus, elles sont peu ou pas dégradées par les enzymes de la flore intestinale d'où un effet mécanique qui se prolonge tout le long de l'intestin.

Elles doivent de plus être bien réparties sur la journée en vue de potentialiser leurs effets sans agresser la muqueuse digestive.

3.1.1.6. Les vitamines

La couverture en vitamines se fait, suite aux recommandations, selon chaque individu.

3.1.1.7. Les minéraux

Normalement l'apport en minéraux peut être assuré correctement.

Il faut cependant penser à vérifier la couverture en *magnésium* celui-ci étant myorelaxant et par conséquent stimulateur du péristaltisme intestinal.

3.1.1.8. L'eau

Les apports en eau sous toutes leurs formes (eaux de boisson et eaux de constitution des aliments) doivent être particulièrement surveillés. En effet, ce constituant participe activement à la réhydratation des selles de par son action vis-à-vis des fibres. L'eau de boisson doit également être correctement répartie tout au long de la journée.

3.1.2. Le choix des aliments

> **Remarque**
> Si le patient souffre de colites, il est nécessaire d'y associer les choix du régime normal léger.

	Aliments conseillés	Aliments déconseillés
Lait	**Laits sous toutes leurs formes** **Remarques :** – La richesse en eau des laits liquides améliore l'hydratation des selles – Le lactose présente un rôle de laxatif léger en favorisant le développement de Lactobacilles dans l'intestin qui diminuent la putréfaction intestinale et la constipation	*Pas de contre-indication*
Laitages	**Laitages sous toutes leurs formes** Privilégier les laitages fermentés (yaourts) riches en bactéries lactiques qui : – produisent de l'acide lactique ayant le même rôle que le lactose – aideraient au rééquilibre de la flore bactérienne Les plus efficaces seraient ceux contenant du bifidus qui participerait activement à la régulation du transit	*Pas de contre-indication*

	Aliments conseillés	Aliments déconseillés
Fromages	Fromages sous toutes leurs formes **Remarque :** les fromages sont quand même moins riches en eau que le lait ou les laitages	*Pas de contre-indication*
VPO	Viandes de boucherie, volailles, abats, charcuteries, produits de la pêche et œufs sous toutes leurs formes	*Pas de contre-indication*
Farines et dérivés	Farine de blé complet, de sarrasin, de seigle Pains complets, de son, aux céréales, de seigle Pains aux fruits secs Pains de mie complets Biscottes complètes ou au son Pains grillés et petits pains grillés complets Cracottes complètes Céréales pour petit-déjeuner complètes, mueslis complets et/ou aux fruits secs, flocons d'avoine Biscuits riches en fibres	Farines raffinées, fécule de pomme de terre Pains blancs Pains de mie blancs Biscottes raffinées Pains grillés et petits pains grillés raffinés Cracottes au froment Céréales pour petit-déjeuner raffinées Biscuits raffinés peu hydratés
Féculents	Pâtes semi-complètes et complètes Riz semi-complet, complet, riz sauvage Semoule semi-complète, complète, Polenta complète Boulgour complet, mil ou millet complet, blé dur précuit complet Maïs et petits pois Légumes secs	Pâtes raffinées, pâtes fraîches Riz blancs Semoule raffinée, polenta raffinée Boulgour raffiné, mil ou millet raffiné, blé dur précuit raffiné
Matières grasses ou équivalents	Matières grasses sous toutes leurs formes **En équivalences : graines oléagineuses** (riches en fibres), **fruits oléagineux** Modes de consommation : les utiliser de préférence sous forme crue	*Pas de contre-indication*

	Aliments conseillés	**Aliments déconseillés**
Légumes	Légumes sous toutes leurs formes Légumes les plus riches en fibres : Topinambour Salsifis Poireau (riche en fibres insolubles) Pissenlit Fenouil Chou de Bruxelles (riche en fibres insolubles) Artichaut (riche en fibres insolubles) Asperge Petits pois (riche en fibres insolubles) Mode de consommation : le souvent plus possible sous forme crue	*Pas de contre-indication*
Fruits	Fruits sous toutes leurs formes Fruits les plus riches en fibres : Fruits secs Fruit de la passion Framboise Goyave Grenade Myrtille Rhubarbe Figue Mode de consommation : le plus souvent possible sous forme crue	**Coing** (anti-diarrhéique) **Attention :** vérifier la tolérance aux fruits suivants (de par leur richesse en fibres solubles) : Cassis Groseille Pommes Raisin
Boissons	**Eau du robinet** **Eaux minérales et de source avec de préférence celles riches en magnésium** **Thé en petite quantité, café, infusions** **Jus de fruits frais de préférence avec pulpe** **Jus de légumes frais de préférence avec pulpe** **Autres boissons rafraîchissantes sans alcool**	**Thé en grande quantité** **Toutes les boissons alcoolisées**

Le régime riche en fibres

	Aliments conseillés	Aliments déconseillés
Boissons	Modes de consommation : penser aux boissons « fraîches » qui stimulent le transit	
Produits sucrés	**Produits sucrés sous toutes leurs formes** Privilégier : Confitures avec morceaux Miels (certains auraient un effet laxatif) Chocolats enrichis en graines oléagineuses et/ou en fruits secs	*Pas de contre-indication*
Condiments	**Condiments sous toutes leurs formes**	*Pas de contre-indication*

> **Remarque**
> Même s'il n'existe pas de contre-indication, il convient néanmoins de respecter les quantités et les fréquences de consommation recommandées pour chacun des groupes d'aliments.

3.1.3. En pratique

Il peut être conseillé aux patients :
- d'avoir des repas les plus variés possibles et à heures régulières ;
- de boire au minimum 1,5 à 2 L d'eau par jour (soit l'équivalent de 8 grands verres d'eau) sachant qu'il est inutile car inefficace d'augmenter cet apport pour améliorer la constipation ;
- de limiter la consommation de thé riche en tannins à pouvoir astringent (favorise la constipation) ;
- d'exercer une activité physique régulière et de privilégier la marche lors des petits déplacements ;
- de pratiquer de la gymnastique abdominale et/ou des massages abdominaux ;
- d'aller à la selle dès que le besoin s'en fait sentir (car se retenir peut accentuer le ralentissement du transit) à heures régulières et tous les jours ;
- d'essayer, à jeun, de boire un verre d'eau glacée ou un jus de pruneaux ou de consommer 2 à 3 pruneaux (cela engendrerait une action cholagogue) ;
- de consommer le plus souvent possible des aliments sources et riches en fibres (céréales complètes, légumes secs, fruits secs, fruits et graines oléagineuses...) ;
- de bien mastiquer les aliments ;
- de privilégier les matières grasses les plus digestes et de les consommer de préférence sous forme crue (éviter les fritures, les plats en sauce, les aliments

sautés avec de grandes quantités de matières grasses…). En effet, certaines substances contenues dans les matières grasses cuites (exemple : l'acroléine) sont difficiles à digérer et diminuent l'absorption intestinale ;
- de privilégier l'huile d'olive pour ses propriétés laxatives (l'acide oléique stimule la formation de bile) ;
- de vérifier la tolérance des aliments contenant des fibres lors de leur réintroduction ;
- de consommer suffisamment de légumes : au minimum 400 g par jour (jusqu'à 800 g pour des apports énergétiques élevés) et de fruits (au minimum 2 portions par jour). En effet, la digestion de leurs fibres conduit à la formation d'acides gras volatils qui entravent la réabsorption d'eau et donc favorisent l'élimination des selles. Ils complètent ainsi les effets des fibres présentes au sein des céréales et des légumes secs (cellulose et hémicelluloses) ;
- de privilégier les végétaux :
  - crus (une voire deux crudités par repas),
  - le plus souvent entiers (c'est-à-dire non pelés) et avec les pépins (parties riches fibres),
  - les plus variés possibles et répartis tout au long de la journée (afin de potentialiser leurs effets) ;
- si l'on constate des diarrhées représentatives d'une éventuelle irritation du côlon il convient de :
  - supprimer les légumes et les fruits riches en fibres dures irritantes : radis, concombre, céleri rave, ananas, rhubarbe, poireaux…,
  - supprimer les légumes à goût fort : choux, fenouil, poireaux…,
  - supprimer les légumes secs,
  - consommer des végétaux sources de fibres douces : poire, pêche, banane (bien mûres), feuilles de salade sans côtés, tomates (sans peau ni pépins), pulpe d'aubergine, betterave, carottes jeunes…

3.2. Dans le cas d'une constipation secondaire

3.2.1. Constipation extradigestive

Le régime prescrit est le même que dans le cas d'une constipation primaire tout en associant la suppression de la cause de constipation.

3.2.2. Constipation extradigestive

Si une obstruction est constatée, un régime pauvre en résidus doit être suivi en attente de l'acte chirurgical.

Lorsque le patient présente des lésions anales douloureuses, on procède, en attente de l'acte chirurgical, à un régime riche en fibres douces et très hydratées dans le but de ramollir les selles et de limiter ainsi les douleurs. À la suite de l'opération, la réalimentation débutera avec un régime pauvre en résidus pour faciliter la cicatrisation tout en diminuant le nombre de selles.

3.3. Dans le cas de diverticules

Les fibres insolubles sont là encore à privilégier.

3.4. Dans le cas de diarrhées

À l'inverse, il faut privilégier les apports en fibres solubles (pectines, gommes, mucilages, alginates, carraghénanes, agar-agar…) de par leurs propriétés constipantes. En effet, leur ingestion entraîne, au contact de l'eau, la formation de gels visqueux ayant tendance à ralentir le transit intestinal. En absorbant l'eau en excès dans le tube digestif, elles sont ainsi particulièrement recommandées dans le traitement des diarrhées hydriques (diarrhées motrices). La quantité de fibres consommées doit néanmoins être très contrôlée et dans les cas de diarrhées importantes, un régime pauvre en fibres doit être appliqué.

4. Exemple de ration, de répartition et de menu

4.1. Exemple de ration d'un régime riche en fibres à 8,3 MJ, 30 g de fibres

Aliments	Quantités (g ou mL)	Protéines	Lipides	Glucides	Ca	Fer	Vitamine C	Fibres
		g	g	g	mg	mg	mg	g
Lait demi-écrémé ou équivalent	300	10,5	4,5	15	360	0	0	0
Fromage	40	8	8,8	0	200	0	0	0
VPO	150	27	15	0	22,5	3	0	0
Pain blanc ou équivalent	50	4	0	27,5	12,5	1	0	2
Pain complet ou équivalent	100	9	0	45	45	2	0	7
PC cru ou équivalent	70	7	0	52,5	17,5	0,7	0	1
Légumes	500	5	0	25	200	5	100	15
Fruits	300	0	0	36	90	1,5	90	6
Huile	30	0	30	0	0	0	0	0
Beurre/Margarine	15	0	12,3	0	0	0	0	0
Sucre ou équivalent	30	0	0	30	0	0	0	0
Total (g)		71	71	261	948	13	190	31
Énergie (kJ)	8 318	1 199	2 683	4 437				
Pourcentages	100	14	32	53				

4.2. Exemple de répartition d'un régime riche en fibres à 8,3 MJ, 30 g de fibres

Aliments	Quantités (g ou mL)	Petit-déjeuner	Déjeuner	Dîner
		g	g	g
Lait demi-écrémé ou équivalent	300	150	150	0
Fromage	40	0	0	40
VPO	150	0	100	50
Pain blanc ou équivalent	50	50	0	0
Pain complet ou équivalent	100	0	20	80
PC crus ou équivalent	70	0	70	0
Légumes	500	0	100	400
Fruits	300	150	0	150
Huile	30	0	20	10
Beurre/Margarine	15	15	0	0
Sucre ou équivalent	30	20	10	0
Total (kJ)	**8 300**	1 967	3 229	2 646
Pourcentages	100	25	41	34

4.3. Exemple de menu d'un régime riche en fibres à 8,3 MJ, 30 g de fibres

Petit-déjeuner
Un café sucré (1 morceau).
Un petit pain blanc individuel beurré.
Un yaourt à la myrtille (dont 15 g de sucre).
Une compote de pruneaux.

Déjeuner
Salade de fenouil au citron vert (10 mL d'huile de tournesol).
Rôti de porc aux oignons.
Blé dur précuit sauce tomate (dont 10 mL d'huile d'olive).
Un fromage blanc sucré.
Une tranche de pain de son.

Dîner
Cœur d'artichaut vinaigrette (10 mL d'huile d'arachide).
Deux tranches de jambon de Bayonne.
Salsifis au jus.
Roquefort.
Pain complet aux noix.
Une nectarine.

18

Les régimes pauvres en fibres

1. Introduction

1.1. Définition et principe

Les régimes pauvres en fibres sont basés sur une *sélection des fibres* avec une pauvreté en fibres animales et un contrôle des fibres végétales.

Ils sont donc à la base de la diététique en gastroentérologie lors des réalimentations postopératoires.

Ces régimes progressent en plusieurs stades qu'il faut adapter en fonction de l'évolution de la pathologie de chaque patient. Il existe donc une gradation de la restriction vers un élargissement progressif.

> **Remarque**
> On peut cependant aller dans le sens de la régression lorsque le patient tolère mal l'introduction de nouveaux aliments.

Les buts des régimes pauvres en fibres sont les suivants :
- *avoir une alimentation équilibrée* le plus rapidement possible et *adaptée* aux besoins des patients même si cela peut paraître parfois difficile ;
- *assurer au malade une digestion facilitée* grâce au contrôle des apports en fibres limitant ainsi l'activité sécrétoire et motrice du tube digestif. Le débit fécal est alors abaissé, engendrant une réduction du nombre de selles et de gaz ce qui permet d'assurer un confort digestif optimal par une diminution des troubles intestinaux.

1.2. Les indications

D'une manière générale, les régimes pauvres en fibres sont indiqués pour des patients présentant des troubles digestifs sévères et/ou ayant subi une opération du tube digestif.

1.2.1. Pathologies gastriques

- Dyspepsies.
- Ulcère gastrique.
- Gastrites.
- Hernie hiatale (car l'on constate une augmentation de l'acidité gastrique).
- Reflux gastro-œsophagien.
- Cancer gastrique en pré- et postopératoire.
- Gastrectomie.

1.2.2. Pathologies des voies biliaires

- Cholécystectomie.
- Dysfonctionnement vésiculaire.
- Cirrhoses[1].
- Ictères[1].

1.2.3. Pathologies du pancréas

- Pancréatectomie.
- Duodénopancréatectomie céphalique.

1.2.4. Pathologies de l'intestin grêle et du côlon

- Colopathies fonctionnelles.
- Colites (entraînant constipation et diarrhées).
- Colectomies.
- Réalimentation des gastroentérites.
- Rectocolite hémorragique.
- Maladie de Crohn.
- Diarrhées en réalimentation, diarrhées chroniques.
- Résection étendue du grêle et du côlon.
- Cancer de l'intestin grêle et du côlon.
- Anus artificiel.

---

1. Essentiellement pour le confort car le régime n'améliore pas *réellement la pathologie*.

Les régimes pauvres en fibres

1.2.5. Indications diverses

- Après une antibiothérapie prolongée.
- Après une parasitose estivale (« Tourista »).
- Après certaines pathologies graves (choléra, fièvre typhoïde).

1.3. Étude des différents types de fibres alimentaires

1.3.1. Les différentes fibres présentes dans les aliments

1.3.1.1. Les fibres alimentaires végétales (FAV)

Les fibres alimentaires végétales sont des polysaccharides c'est-à-dire des polymères glucidiques (à l'exception de la lignine qui est un polymère de phényl-propane) présents dans la paroi des cellules végétales.

Elles sont divisées en deux groupes :
- les fibres solubles avec :
  - les pectines,
  - les gommes (Guar, Caroube),
  - les mucilages,
  - les alginates,
  - les carraghénanes ;
- les fibres insolubles avec :
  - la cellulose,
  - les hémicelluloses,
  - la lignine.

1.3.1.2. Les fibres animales

Les fibres animales sont de nature protéique et sont sous forme de scléroprotéines au sein des aliments. Il s'agit du collagène, de la kératine et de l'élastine. Elles sont essentiellement présentes dans les viandes de 2e et de 3e catégories et sont indigestibles.

1.3.2. Classification des aliments en fonction de leurs teneurs en fibres

1.3.2.1. Aliments presque totalement dépourvus de fibres

Il s'agit :
- des œufs ;
- du lait et des produits laitiers (hormis les desserts lactés céréaliers et/ou avec des fruits) ;
- de la plupart des produits sucrés (sauf les confitures avec des morceaux de fruits, les gelées de fruits, certains produits chocolatés…) ;
- des corps gras ;
- des boissons (sauf les boissons à base de fruits et de légumes avec et sans pulpe).

1.3.2.2. Aliments très pauvres en fibres (moins de 0,5 % de fibres)

Il s'agit :
- des viandes de boucherie de 1re catégorie ;
- des volailles ;
- des charcuteries ;
- des abats ;
- des produits de la pêche (poissons, mollusques et crustacés) ;
- des gelées de fruits ;
- des boissons à base de fruits et de légumes sans pulpe.

*1.3.2.3. Aliments sources de fibres alimentaires végétales
   (de 0,5 à 5 % de fibres)*

Il s'agit :
- des farines raffinées :
  - farine de blé blanche,
  - maïzena,
  - farine de riz raffinée,
  - fécule de pommes de terre ;
- des pâtes raffinées ;
- des pâtes aux œufs raffinées ;
- de la semoule de blé raffinée ;
- du blé dur précuit ;
- du riz blanc ;
- du riz semi-complet ;
- du riz complet ;
- du maïs ;
- des pommes de terre cuites ;
- des pains blancs ;
- des pains de mie raffinés ;
- des pains au lait, viennois, briochés ;
- des biscottes raffinées ;
- des pains grillés et petits pains grillés raffinés ;
- des céréales pour petit-déjeuner raffinées ;
- des biscuits sucrés à la farine raffinée ;
- des biscuits apéritifs ;
- des pâtisseries et des viennoiseries à la farine raffinée ;
- de certains légumes :
  - laitue cuite, oseille cuite : 0,5 % de fibres en moyenne,
  - concombre cru, courge cuite, courgette crue, oseille crue, radis crus, tomate crue et cuite : 1 % de fibres en moyenne,
  - asperge cuite, bette cuite, betterave rouge cuite, courgette cuite, haricot beurre cuit, laitue crue, mâche crue, oignon cuit : 1,5 % de fibres en moyenne,

Les régimes pauvres en fibres 207

- aubergine cuite, céleri branche cru, navet cuit, oignon cru, poivrons crus et cuits, potiron cuit : 2 % de fibres en moyenne,
  - brocoli cuit, carotte crue et cuite, champignon cru et cuit, chicorée crue, chou rouge cuit, chou-fleur cru et cuit, cresson, céleri branche cuit, endive crue, épinard cru, poireau cuit, potimarron cru : 2,5 % de fibres en moyenne,
  - chou rouge cru, chou vert cuit, endive cuite, épinard cuit, haricot vert cuit, avocat : 3 % de fibres en moyenne,
  - fenouil cru, pissenlit cru : 3,5 % de fibres en moyenne,
  - chou de Bruxelles, céleri rave cuit, olives : 4 % de fibres en moyenne,
  - céleri rave cru : 5 % de fibres en moyenne ;
- de certains fruits :
  - citron, pastèque, pamplemousse, raisin noir : inférieur à 0,5 % de fibres en moyenne,
  - melon, raisin blanc : 1 % de fibres en moyenne,
  - ananas, cerise, clémentine, litchi, mûre : 1,5 % de fibres en moyenne,
  - abricot, banane, fraise, nectarine, orange, papaye, pomme, pêche, rhubarbe cuite : 2 % de fibres en moyenne,
  - kiwi, mangue, mirabelle, poire, reine-claude : 2,5 % de fibres en moyenne,
  - figues, myrtille : 3 % de fibres en moyenne,
  - goyave, grenade : 3,5 % de fibres en moyenne ;
- des compotes ;
- des fruits au sirop ;
- des jus de fruits et/ou de légumes avec pulpe ;
- des confitures de fruits ;
- des chocolats fourrés ;
- du cacao en poudre sucré ;
- du chocolat noir 64 %.

1.3.2.4. Aliments riches en fibres végétales (plus de 5 % de fibres)

Il s'agit :
- du son ;
- des farines complètes :
  - farine de blé complète,
  - farine bise ;
- de la farine de soja ;
- de la farine de sarrasin ;
- de la farine de seigle ;
- du germe de blé ;
- de la semoule de blé complète ;
- des pâtes semi-complètes ;
- des pâtes complètes ;
- du quinoa ;
- des châtaignes et des marrons ;

- des pains complets ;
- du pain de seigle ;
- du pain type 80 ;
- du pain au son ;
- des pains de mie complets ;
- des biscottes complètes ;
- des pains grillés et petits pains grillés complets ;
- des céréales pour petit-déjeuner riches en fibres ;
- des flocons d'avoine ;
- des mueslis ;
- des biscuits sucrés à la farine complète ;
- des pâtisseries et des viennoiseries à la farine complète ;
- de certains légumes (artichaut, petits pois, salsifis) ;
- de certains fruits (noix de coco fraîche, noix de coco sèche, cassis, coing, framboise, fruit de la passion, groseille) ;
- des légumes secs ;
- des fruits secs ;
- des graines oléagineuses ;
- du cacao en poudre non sucré ;
- du chocolat aux fruits secs ;
- du chocolat noir 70 % ;
- du chocolat noir 86 %.

1.3.2.5. Aliments riches en fibres animales

Ce sont les viandes de 2e et de 3e catégories.

1.3.3. Classification des aliments contenant des fibres végétales selon leur nature

1.3.3.1. Les aliments sources de fibres insolubles

- Les légumes : on peut proposer la classification suivante :
  - légumes riches : (3-5 %) : chou de Bruxelles, artichaut, petits pois, poireau ; (2-3 %) : aubergine, brocoli, chou vert, épinard, fenouil, potiron ;
  - légumes sources (1,5 %) : asperge, bette, betterave, carotte, céleri, champignons, chou blanc, chou rouge, chou-fleur, cœur de palmier, endives, haricots verts, oignon, navet, poivron, radis, salsifis ;
  - légumes pauvres (0,75 %) : courgette, tomate.
- Les fruits : les fruits les plus riches sont le cassis, la groseille, la mûre.
- Les légumes secs.
- Les marrons et les châtaignes.
- Les graines oléagineuses.

Les régimes pauvres en fibres

- Les céréales et leurs dérivés (les teneurs sont variables en fonction de chaque aliment mais d'une manière générale on considère qu'ils contiennent environ 2/3 de fibres insolubles).
- Les produits chocolatés (de même, ils sont composés d'en moyenne deux-tiers de fibres insolubles).

1.3.3.2. Aliments sources de fibres solubles

- Les légumes : on peut proposer la classification suivante :
  - légumes riches : 3 % : artichaut ; 1-1,5 % : aubergine, betterave, carotte,
  - légumes sources (0,7 %) : asperge, brocoli, chou blanc, chou-fleur, chou de Bruxelles, cœur de palmier, épinard, haricot vert, navet, oignon, petits pois, potiron,
  - légumes pauvres (< 0,5 %) : bette, céleri-rave, céleri-branche, champignon, chou rouge, courgette, endive, fenouil, poireau, poivron, radis, salsifis, tomate.
- Les fruits : les teneurs varient de 0,5 à 1,7 %. Les fruits les plus riches sont : cassis, coings, groseilles, pommes et raisins.

1.4. Les différents facteurs à prendre en compte lors de la prescription de régimes pauvres en fibres

1.4.1. La cuisson

Il est nécessaire :
- de limiter la sapidité des aliments afin d'éliminer les sécrétions digestives liées à une stimulation (par exemple, les viandes seront pochées, peu salées et non grillées) ;
- de limiter les modes de cuisson peu digestes : les matières grasses seront ainsi utilisées sous forme crue car leur cuisson provoque la formation de peroxydes irritants pour les muqueuses digestives.

1.4.2. La texture et la consistance

L'évolution doit se faire en fonction des capacités du patient : ainsi, au premier stade de médicamentation, l'alimentation tendra vers une texture molle afin :
- de faciliter la vidange gastrique ;
- de limiter les sécrétions gastriques ;
- de ralentir la motilité de l'estomac.

> **Remarque**
> Il est absolument nécessaire d'éviter de maintenir trop longtemps cette texture car elle devient vite anorexigène par manque d'intérêt pour les repas. C'est pourquoi l'on peut aussi essayer d'alterner entre une texture molle et normale.

1.4.3. L'acidité

Les aliments fortement acides accélèrent la vidange gastrique. Il convient donc de les déconseiller. Il s'agit des tomates, des fruits acides et/ou peu mûrs et du vinaigre.

1.4.4. Les stimulants et les irritants

Il s'agit : du thé fort, du café fort, de l'alcool, des épices et des aromates à goût fort.

1.4.5. La température

Il faut 10 à 15 minutes pour que l'estomac amène les aliments ingérés à 37 °C ce qui permet la vidange gastrique.
C'est pourquoi, en général :
– les préparations froides ralentissent la vidange gastrique ;
– les préparations chaudes accélèrent le péristaltisme ;
– les préparations glacées peuvent provoquer des diarrhées réflexes.

Les préparations doivent donc être de préférence tièdes ou peu froides mais il faudra alors faire particulièrement attention à leur qualité bactériologique.

1.4.6. Le volume des préparations

Le volume dépend du fractionnement : au début de la réalimentation, l'estomac ne supporte que de petits volumes (100 à 200 mL par repas) avec 5 à 6 repas. Par la suite, il sera possible d'atteindre jusqu'à 600 mL avec 3-4 repas.

Il faut être très vigilant quant à l'adaptation des volumes en fonction de chaque patient (âge, dénutrition, fatigue…). À titre d'exemple, les personnes âgées sont très sensibles aux diarrhées.

1.4.7. La concentration

Il faut bannir les préparations très concentrées :
– en sel car celui-ci stimule les sécrétions digestives ;
– en sucre car un excès peut entraîner des appels d'eau pouvant engendrer des diarrhées motrices. Celui-ci devra donc être correctement réparti tout au long de la journée.

1.4.8. Les différents nutriments

1.4.8.1. Les protéines

Les protéines animales augmentent la motilité et les sécrétions gastriques en augmentant la sécrétion de gastrine. Des irritations de l'estomac sont donc envisageables lors d'un excès protéique.

1.4.8.2. *Les lipides*

Ils ont la propriété de neutraliser l'acidité, la motilité ainsi que la vidange gastrique. Il faudra donc bien les répartir tout au long de la journée.

1.4.8.3. *Les glucides*

Ils ralentissent la vidange gastrique par effet hormonal et osmotique mais attention toutefois aux fortes concentrations.

Notons que par conséquent, cette alimentation est généralement fade et peu attrayante. Il faut donc absolument en tenir compte en technique culinaire lors de la réalisation des plats.

2. *Le régime pauvre en fibres végétales, à fibres animales modifiées*

2.1. Définition et principe

Le régime pauvre en fibres animales, à fibres végétales modifiées est un régime très strict à savoir qu'il est :
- pauvre en fibres végétales : les légumes et les fruits sont supprimés et les céréales sont strictement sélectionnées. Leur texture est de plus éventuellement modifiée ;
- à fibres animales modifiées : les produits animaux sont sélectionnés et leur texture est modifiée par cuisson, hachage, mixage…

La durée de la prescription peut varier de 1 à 5 jours.

2.2. Les indications

Les indications sont les suivantes :
- première étape de réalimentation après une intervention digestive. Le régime est prescrit après la diète hydrique mais il peut aussi parfois faire suite à un régime pauvre en résidus ;
- pathologies digestives les plus graves.

2.3. Couverture des besoins et apports nutritionnels conseillés

2.3.1. *L'énergie*

Étant en phase de réalimentation, on commence avec un apport énergétique très faible soit aux alentours de 2 à 3 MJ par jour (500 à 700 kcal) pour atteindre progressivement, c'est-à-dire par paliers (de 0,7 à 0,8 MJ soit 200 à 400 kcal) jusqu'à 6-7 MJ par jour (1 400 à 1 700 kcal) lorsque la durée de la prescription atteint 5 jours. À noter qu'il est difficile de dépasser ce niveau énergétique car les patients présentent souvent peu d'appétit associé à une grande fatigue.

2.3.2. Les protéines

Le régime est hyperprotidique en valeur absolue. Vu le faible niveau énergétique du départ, il est conseillé de commencer à 20-25 g de protéines par jour puis de progresser par paliers de 5 à 10 g tous les jours ou tous les deux jours.

Afin d'assurer une meilleure cicatrisation les protéines animales (riches en acides aminés indispensables) devront être privilégiées par rapport à celles d'origine végétale.

Il est de plus possible d'enrichir les préparations avec de la poudre de lait (sans oublier la vérification de la tolérance au lactose) ou de la poudre de protéines ce qui limite le volume des repas tout en améliorant leur qualité.

2.3.3. Les lipides

Ils doivent être limités à 25-30 % de l'apport énergétique total sachant que les quantités au départ avoisinent 10 à 15 g par jour. En effet, un excès de lipides pourrait engendrer voir accentuer les troubles digestifs des patients.

Au niveau qualitatif, on constate un déséquilibre en acides gras notamment en acides gras essentiels car les matières grasses pouvant être utilisées sont presque uniquement d'origine animale (beurre et crème), le choix des aliments rendant presque impossible la consommation d'huiles végétales.

2.3.4. Les glucides

Ce sont les compléments énergétiques de la ration. De par le choix des aliments, il s'avère très difficile pour le moment de respecter l'équilibre entre les glucides complexes et les glucides simples.

Les produits sucrés sont quant à eux limités à 10 % de l'apport énergétique total. En tant que calories vides et sachant que l'énergie est « précieuse » en vue du rétablissement du patient, ceux-ci présentent peu d'intérêts. Il conviendra également de bien les répartir sur la journée afin d'en limiter la concentration.

2.3.5. Les fibres

Les apports en fibres sont quasi inexistants puisque leur contrôle est à la base de ce régime. Il faudra toutefois surveiller l'apparition d'une éventuelle constipation.

2.3.6. Les vitamines

Les couvertures en vitamines sont très difficiles à assurer notamment en :
- *vitamine C* due à l'absence de légumes et de fruits sous toutes leurs formes. Or, le risque infectieux étant accentué, une supplémentation médicamenteuse peut être proposée surtout en cas de réalimentation de longue durée ;
- *vitamine E* due aux très petites quantités de matières grasses végétales. Là encore une supplémentation médicamenteuse peut être envisagée ;

Les régimes pauvres en fibres 213

— *vitamines B_1, B_3, B_5 et B_6* due à la sélection des produits céréaliers. Il est possible dans ce cas d'enrichir les préparations avec du germe de blé ou de la levure de bière.

2.3.7. Les minéraux

Pour ce qui est des minéraux, le *calcium* est bien couvert car le lait et les produits laitiers sont en quantité importante.

La restriction des viandes (notamment celles de boucherie) peut engendrer un manque de *fer* en particulier héminique. Une supplémentation médicamenteuse peut donc être recommandée.

2.3.8. L'eau

Les apports devront correspondre aux recommandations et augmentés en cas de fièvres et/ou de diarrhées.

2.4. Le choix des aliments

Groupe d'aliments	Aliments conseillés	Aliments déconseillés
Laits	**Laits écrémés, demi-écrémés de préférence (liquide, poudre, concentré)** Ils doivent être consommés en faible quantité car ils peuvent facilement entraîner des troubles digestifs. Il convient donc de bien tester la tolérance de chaque patient Le lait en poudre écrémé peut être utilisé en tant qu'enrichissant	**Laits entiers (liquide, poudre, concentré)** car les lipides qu'ils contiennent pourraient être mal digérés
Laitages	**Laitages écrémés, demi-écrémés de préférence nature ou aromatisés**	**Laitages ≥ 20 % de matières grasses et/ou aux fruits**
Desserts lactés	**Tous contre-indiqués**	**Tous déconseillés** de par leur forte concentration en sucre et/ou en graisses et/ou en céréales
Fromages	**Fromages frais salés** **Fromages peu affinés, à moins de 25 % de lipides, en petite quantité (pâtes cuites, demi-dures, molles)** **Fromages fondus** Mode de consommation : fondus dans les préparations	**Fromages persillés** (goût fort) et/ou **Fromages à plus de 25 % lipides** et/ou **Fromages très affinés (pâtes cuites, demi-dures, molles)**

Groupe d'aliments	Aliments conseillés	Aliments déconseillés
Viandes	Les morceaux de viandes choisis seront de préférence : – **maigres** car ils présentent un meilleur rapport protéines sur lipides – **de première catégorie** (c'est-à-dire à fibres musculaires courtes) car ils sont dotés d'un rapport collagène sur protéines élevé La progression de la texture se fera de la manière suivante : mixée puis moulinée puis hachée puis pochée dans un bouillon peu parfumé Modes de cuisson, recommandés : vapeur, bouillies, papillote… Les volailles seront introduites en avant-dernière étape et les viandes de boucherie à la fin (après les autres aliments d'origine animale)	Les morceaux de viandes à éviter sont : – **demi-gras et gras** – **de deuxième et de troisième catégorie** Modes de cuisson déconseillés : grillé/doré, cuisson avec de la matière grasse…
Charcuteries	**Jambon blanc non fumé découenné/dégraissé** **Filets de bacon non fumés découennés/dégraissés** **Lardons non fumés découennés/dégraissés** La progression de la texture se fait de même que pour les viandes Ils seront introduits en troisième étape (après les poissons)	**Toutes les autres charcuteries**
Abats	**Tous contre-indiqués**	**Tous déconseillés**
Poissons	**Poissons maigres et demi-gras** Ils seront introduits en second (après les œufs) mais avant les viandes car ils sont pauvres en collagène. De plus, ils peuvent facilement être mixés, moulinés, et s'effritent même entiers Modes de cuisson conseillés : sans matières grasses, court-bouillon peu parfumé et peu salé, papillote, vapeur…	**Poissons gras Poissons salés et fumés**

Groupe d'aliments	Aliments conseillés	Aliments déconseillés
Œufs	Ils sont introduits en premier et doivent être bien cuits car le blanc insuffisamment cuit est indigeste Modes de cuisson conseillés : coque bien cuit, mollet bien cuit, pochés bien cuit, au plat, au four omelette peu grillée, intégrés mixés cuits dans les préparations	*Pas de contre-indication* Modes de cuisson déconseillés : frits avec de la matière grasse
Farines et dérivés	**Farines raffinées** **Biscottes raffinées** **Pains grillés et assimilés raffinés** **Biscuits secs à la farine raffinée nature type biscuits à thé, boudoirs, génoises...** Mode de consommation : mixés et incorporés dans les préparations en vue de faciliter leur digestion ou trempés dans un liquide	**Tous les autres dérivés de la farine**
Féculents	**Semoule fine raffinée** **Riz blanc** **Pâtes raffinées de petit calibre (type coquillettes)** Mode de consommation : ils devront être bien cuits voire mixés	**Tous les autres féculents**
Légumes	**Bouillons de légumes filtrés :** bouillons clairs, passés, réalisés à partir de légumes non amylacés, peu fibreux, se digérant facilement (laitue, carottes, endives, courgettes, aubergines, blancs de poireaux...)	**Tous les autres légumes sous toute autre forme**
Fruits	**Bouillons de fruits filtrés :** bouillons clairs, passés, sucrés (à 5 % maximum) réalisés à partir de fruits peu fibreux, se digérant facilement (poires, abricots, brugnon, nectarine...)	**Tous les autres fruits sous toute autre forme**
Matières grasses et équivalents	**Corps gras émulsionnés :** Beurre de préférence allégé Margarines de préférence végétales et allégées	**Huiles végétales** **Graines oléagineuses** **Fruits oléagineux** **Graisse d'oie/de canard**

Groupe d'aliments	Aliments conseillés	Aliments déconseillés
Matières grasses et équivalents	Margarines diététiques (enrichies en acides gras essentiels, vitamines E et D) Crème fraîche de préférence allégée Modes de consommation : en petite quantité, sous forme crue, bien réparties au cours des différents repas et mélangées aux aliments	**Végétaline®**
Produits sucrés	**Sucre** **Caramel liquide** **Gelées de fruits** **Sirops de fruits dilués** Mode de consommation : peu concentrés, non pris isolément	**Tous les autres produits sucrés**
Boissons	**Eaux plates non magnésiennes** **Thé et café légers** **Tisanes, infusions** Modes de consommation : tièdes ou peu froides	**Eaux plates magnésiennes** **Eaux gazeuses** **Thé et café forts** **Boissons rafraîchissantes sans alcool (jus, nectars, sodas…)** **Alcools**
Épices et aromates	**Parfums pour desserts liquides (vanille, fleur d'oranger, café…)** **Aromates en branche** (à éliminer après cuisson) **Sel** Modes de consommation : en très petite concentration	**Aromates en poudre** **Épices**
Produits diététiques et de régime	Il est possible d'enrichir les préparations avec de la poudre de protéines et/ou d'utiliser des produits de complémentation orale voire des dextrines-maltose En cas d'intolérance au lactose, utiliser du lait sans lactose	

2.5. En pratique

Il faut veiller à :
- donner de petits volumes pour éviter de surcharger le tube digestif ;
- essayer de fractionner le plus possible les repas même si cela est difficile au départ de par le faible taux énergétique ;
- limiter le plus possible les assaisonnements.

3. Le régime pauvre en fibres végétales

3.1. Définition et principe

Le régime pauvre en fibres végétales est un régime contenant encore très peu de fibres végétales mais avec une réintroduction progressive des fruits et des légumes rendus plus digestes par la cuisson et/ou la modification de leur texture. Les fibres animales, quant à elles, sont toujours contrôlées mais les quantités sont légèrement augmentées et la texture élargie.

La durée de la prescription peut varier de 1 à 5 jours.

3.2. Les indications

Les indications sont les suivantes :
- deuxième étape de réalimentation après le régime pauvre en fibres végétales à fibres animales modifiées ;
- première étape de réalimentation pour des pathologies digestives moins graves (exemple : opération de la vésicule biliaire) ;
- gastroentérologies (colites, diarrhées peu importantes...) ;
- maladies inflammatoires en poussées.

3.3. Couverture des besoins et apports nutritionnels conseillés

3.3.1. L'énergie

En cas de première étape de réalimentation, on commence avec un apport énergétique peu élevé à savoir de 3 à 4 MJ par jour (700 à 900 kcal) et on progresse doucement par palier (de 0,7 à 0,8 MJ soit 200 à 400 kcal) pour atteindre 7-8 MJ par jour (1 700 à 1 900 kcal).

3.3.2. Les protéines

Le régime est, là aussi, hyperprotidique en valeur absolue. Le niveau énergétique du départ étant un peu plus élevé que précédemment, il est conseillé de commencer à 25-30 g de protéines par jour puis de progresser par paliers de 5 à 10 g tous les jours ou tous les deux jours.

Afin d'assurer une meilleure cicatrisation, les protéines animales (riches en acides aminés indispensables) devront être privilégiées par rapport à celles d'origine végétale.

Il est de plus possible d'enrichir les préparations avec de la poudre de lait (sans oublier la vérification de la tolérance au lactose) ou de la poudre de protéines en vue de limiter le volume des repas tout en améliorant leur qualité.

3.3.3. Les lipides

Ils doivent être limités à 25-30 % de l'apport énergétique total sachant que les quantités au départ avoisinent 15 à 20 g par jour et que les patients présentent toujours une instabilité digestive.

Au niveau qualitatif, on constate un meilleur équilibre en acides gras notamment en acides gras essentiels car les huiles végétales sont plus faciles d'utilisation.

3.3.4. Les glucides

Ce sont les compléments énergétiques de la ration. Par le choix des aliments, il s'avère plus facile de respecter l'équilibre entre les glucides complexes (50 à 55 % des glucides totaux) et les glucides simples (45 à 50 % des glucides totaux).

Les produits sucrés sont à nouveau limités à 10 % de l'apport énergétique total, bien répartis sur la journée afin d'en limiter la concentration.

3.3.5. Les fibres

On observe une augmentation des fibres non irritantes soit 10 à 15 g de fibres par jour.

3.3.6. Les vitamines

On note une augmentation des apports pour :
– *la vitamine E* car le choix des matières grasses végétales est élargi ;
– *les vitamines B_1, B_3, B_5 et B_6* car les quantités de céréales ou équivalents sont accentuées de même que leur calibre.

Cependant, une supplémentation en *vitamine C* peut toujours être envisagée due aux faibles quantités de végétaux, à leur cuisson quasi systématique et à leur sélection. De plus, les patients présentent encore un risque d'infection accentué.

3.3.7. Les minéraux

La couverture en *calcium* est à nouveau assurée et la quantité de *fer* est plus élevée car le choix des viandes est plus vaste sachant que les viandes de boucherie peuvent être proposées dès le début.

3.3.8. L'eau

Les apports doivent correspondre aux recommandations et augmentés en cas de fièvres et/ou de diarrhées.

3.4. Le choix des aliments

Groupe d'aliments	Aliments conseillés	Aliments déconseillés
Laits	**Laits écrémés, demi-écrémés de préférence (liquide, poudre, concentré)** Ils doivent être consommés en faible quantité car ils peuvent facilement entraîner des troubles digestifs. Il convient donc de bien tester la tolérance de chaque patient Le lait en poudre écrémé peut être utilisé en tant qu'enrichissant	**Laits entiers (liquide, poudre, concentré)** car les lipides qu'ils contiennent pourraient être mal digérés
Laitages	**Laitages écrémés, demi-écrémés de préférence, nature ou aromatisés ou aux fruits**	**Laitages ≥ 20 % de matières grasses**
Desserts lactés	**Tous contre-indiqués**	**Tous déconseillés** de par leur forte concentration en sucre et/ou en graisses et/ou en céréales
Fromages	**Fromages frais salés** **Fromages peu affinés, à moins de 25 % de lipides, en petite quantité (pâtes cuites, demi-dures, molles)** **Fromages fondus** Mode de consommation : fondus dans les préparations	**Fromages persillés** (*goût fort*) et/ou **Fromages à plus de 25 % lipides** et/ou **Fromages très affinés (pâtes cuites, demi-dures, molles)**
Viandes	Les morceaux de viandes choisis seront de préférence : – **maigres** car ils présentent un meilleur rapport protéines sur lipides – **de première catégorie** (c'est-à-dire à fibres musculaires courtes) car ils sont dotés d'un rapport collagène sur protéines élevé La texture est plus épaisse (hachée puis normale) et les quantités sont plus importantes Les viandes de boucherie et les volailles peuvent être servies dès le début de la réalimentation Modes de cuisson recommandés : vapeur, bouillies, papillote…	Les morceaux de viandes à éviter sont : – **demi-gras et gras** – **de deuxième et de troisième catégorie** Modes de cuisson déconseillés : grillé/doré, cuisson avec de la matière grasse…

Groupe d'aliments	Aliments conseillés	Aliments déconseillés
Charcuteries	Jambon blanc non fumé découenné/dégraissé Filets de bacon non fumés découennés/dégraissés Lardons non fumés découennés/dégraissés	Toutes les autres charcuteries
Abats	Tous contre-indiqués	Tous déconseillés
Poissons	Poissons maigres et demi-gras Ils peuvent dès le départ être servis sous forme de filets émiettés tout en surveillant qu'ils ne contiennent pas d'arêtes Modes de cuisson conseillés : sans matières grasses, court-bouillon peu parfumé et peu salé, papillote, vapeur…	Poissons gras Poissons salés et fumés
Œufs	Ils doivent être bien cuits car le blanc insuffisamment cuit est indigeste Modes de cuisson conseillés : coque bien cuit, mollet bien cuit, pochés bien cuits, au plat, au four, omelette peu grillée, intégrés mixés cuits dans les préparations	*Pas de contre-indication* Modes de cuisson déconseillés : frits avec de la matière grasse
Farines et dérivés	**Farines raffinées** **Biscottes raffinées** **Pains grillés et assimilés raffinés** **Biscuits secs à la farine raffinée nature type biscuits à thé, boudoirs, génoises…** Mode de consommation : mixés et incorporés dans les préparations en vue de faciliter leur digestion, ou bien trempés dans un liquide	Tous les autres dérivés de la farine
Féculents	**Semoule fine et moyenne raffinée** **Riz blanc** **Pâtes raffinées de petit et moyen calibre** Mode de consommation : ils doivent être bien cuits voire hachés	Tous les autres féculents

Groupe d'aliments	Aliments conseillés	Aliments déconseillés
Légumes	Légumes tendres, jeunes (car ils sont peu durs et pauvres en pépins), peu acides, peu fibreux, à goût peu prononcé : **Jeunes carottes** **Jeunes navets** **Betteraves** **Haricots verts extra-fins** **Courgettes sans pépins** **Pulpe d'aubergine tamisée** **Cœur de laitue sans côtes** **Avocat bien mûr (en petite quantité à cause de sa forte teneur en lipides)** **Cœur d'artichaut** **Endives (selon tolérance)** **Pointes d'asperges** **Potiron** **Blancs de poireau** **Champignons** **Épinards** **Cœur de fenouil…** Modes de consommation : toujours cuits, sans matières grasses (à l'eau, à la vapeur, dans leur eau de constitution), mixés, moulinés ou hachés et en morceaux le plus rapidement possible	**Tous les autres légumes sous toute autre forme**
Fruits	Fruits tendres, peu acides, peu fibreux, à goût peu prononcé : **Pommes** **Poires** **Bananes** **Coing** **Pêches** **Nectarines** **Abricots** **Cerises** Attention à bien vérifier la tolérance du patient et les supprimer en cas de diarrhées Modes de consommation : cuits réduits en purée ou écrasés à la fourchette, sans peau, sans pépins, crus si très mûrs	**Tous les autres fruits sous toute autre forme**

Groupe d'aliments	Aliments conseillés	Aliments déconseillés
Matières grasses et équivalents	**Corps gras émulsionnés :** Beurre de préférence allégé Margarines de préférence végétales et allégées Margarines diététiques (enrichies en acides gras essentiels, vitamines E et D) Crème fraîche de préférence allégée **Huiles végétales à goût peu prononcé** (tournesol, colza, soja…) Modes de consommation : en petite quantité, sous forme crue, bien réparties au cours des différents repas et mélangées aux aliments	**Huiles végétales à goût fort (olive, noix, noisettes…) Graines oléagineuses Fruits oléagineux Graisse d'oie/de canard Végétaline®**
Produits sucrés	**Sucre Caramel liquide Gelées de fruits Sirops de fruits dilués** Mode de consommation : peu concentrés, non pris isolément	**Tous les autres produits sucrés**
Boissons	**Eaux plates non magnésiennes Thé et café légers Tisanes, infusions** Modes de consommation : tièdes ou peu froides	**Eaux plates magnésiennes Eaux gazeuses Thé et café forts Boissons rafraîchissantes sans alcool (jus, nectars, sodas…) Alcools**
Épices et aromates	**Parfums pour desserts liquides (vanille, fleur d'oranger, café…) Aromates en branche** (à éliminer après cuisson) *Sel* Modes de consommation : en très petite concentration	**Aromates en poudre Épices**
Produits diététiques et de régime	Il est possible d'enrichir les préparations avec de la poudre de protéines et/ou d'utiliser des produits de complémentation orale voire des dextrines-maltose. En cas d'intolérance au lactose, utiliser du lait sans lactose	

3.5. En pratique

Les repas principaux (déjeuner et dîner) présenteront un nombre de composantes peu élevé (environ 3).

La quantité de légumes ne dépassera pas 100 à 150 g par jour. Quant à celle de fruits elle sera limitée à deux portions par jour (150 à 300 g). Il faut de plus veiller à ne pas associer les quantités maximales de fruits et de légumes lors d'une même journée.

4. *Le régime d'épargne digestive*

4.1. Définition et principe

Le régime d'épargne digestive permet toujours un travail réduit du tube digestif tout en élargissant progressivement les différents types d'aliments afin de retrouver une alimentation plus normale mais aussi tout en excluant éventuellement certains aliments qui pourraient être mal tolérés. On constate ainsi :
– une réintroduction définitive du groupe des viandes, poissons, œufs avec une quantité normale et une texture plus large mais leur choix reste identique (notamment la première catégorie pour les viandes de boucherie) ;
– une réintroduction progressive des crudités (sous forme de légumes) en petite quantité associée au maintien d'une texture modifiée.

À noter qu'il existe deux nominations possibles pour ce régime à savoir :
– régime d'épargne gastrique si la pathologie est d'origine gastrique ;
– régime d'épargne intestinale si la pathologie est d'origine intestinale.

4.2. Les indications

Les indications sont les suivantes :
– deuxième étape de réalimentation après le régime pauvre en fibres végétales ;
– troisième étape de réalimentation après le régime pauvre en fibres végétales à fibres animales modifiées.

4.3. Couverture des besoins et apports nutritionnels conseillés

4.3.1. *L'énergie*

L'apport énergétique de départ peut être plus élevé à savoir de 4-5 MJ par jour (900 à 1 200 kcal) jusqu'à presque atteindre le besoin énergétique réel du patient sachant que la prescription peut durer plusieurs semaines.

4.3.2. Les protéines

Les apports en protéines sont à adapter en fonction de l'état du patient. Ainsi, un régime normoprotidique (11 à 15 % de l'AET) ou hyperprotidique (15 à 20 % de l'AET) peut être prescrit.

Il convient encore de privilégier les protéines d'origine animale de meilleure digestibilité.

4.3.3. Les lipides

Les lipides restent compris entre 25 et 30 % de l'apport énergétique total sachant que l'équilibre entre les différents acides gras s'est nettement amélioré grâce à l'augmentation des quantités de corps gras utilisés et à leur possibilité de diversité.

4.3.4. Les glucides

Ce sont les compléments énergétiques de la ration. Au niveau qualitatif, le rapport entre les glucides complexes et les glucides simples est très proche des recommandations voire leur correspond (50 à 55 % de glucides complexes et 45 à 50 % de glucides simples). Les produits sucrés sont, quant à eux, toujours limités à 10 % de l'AET au maximum.

4.3.5. Les fibres

L'introduction des légumes sous forme de crudités augmente légèrement la quantité de fibres « irritantes ». On peut ainsi atteindre jusqu'à 15-20 g de fibres par jour ce qui améliore leur couverture tout en préservant le tube digestif.

4.3.6. Les vitamines

Les apports en *vitamine E* sont accentués (augmentation des quantités d'huiles végétales grâce à l'utilisation de vinaigrette). Il en est de même pour les *vitamines du groupe B* retrouvées au sein des céréales de par l'élargissement du choix des aliments pour ce groupe.

Quant à la *vitamine C*, une vigilance doit être maintenue car la quantité de crudités reste encore insuffisante.

4.3.7. Les minéraux

La couverture en *calcium* est assurée et la quantité de *fer* progresse et peut même correspondre aux apports conseillés puisque le groupe des viandes, poissons et œufs est servi en quantité normale.

4.3.8. L'eau

Les apports doivent correspondre aux recommandations.

4.4. Le choix des aliments

Groupe d'aliments	Aliments conseillés	Aliments déconseillés
Laits	Laits écrémés, demi-écrémés de préférence (liquide, poudre, concentré) Ils doivent être consommés en faible quantité car ils peuvent facilement entraîner des troubles digestifs. Il convient donc de bien tester la tolérance de chaque patient Le lait en poudre peut être utilisé en tant qu'enrichissant	Laits entiers (liquide, poudre, concentré) car les lipides qu'ils contiennent pourraient être mal digérés
Laitages	Laitages écrémés, demi-écrémés de préférence, nature ou aromatisés ou aux fruits	Laitages ≥ 20 % de matières grasses
Desserts lactés	Desserts lactés allégés en lipides, peu concentrés en sucre et sans céréales	Desserts lactés riches en lipides et/ou fortement concentrés en sucre et/ou contenant des céréales
Fromages	**Fromages frais salés** **Fromages peu affinés, à moins de 25 % de lipides (pâtes cuites, demi-dures, molles)** **Fromages fondus** Les quantités deviennent normales (30 à 40 g par jour) Mode de consommation : fondus dans les préparations ou tels quels	**Fromages persillés** (*goût fort*) et/ou **Fromages à plus de 25 % lipides** et/ou **Fromages très affinés (pâtes cuites, demi-dures, molles)**
Viandes	Les morceaux de viandes choisis seront de préférence : – **maigres** car ils présentent un meilleur rapport protéines sur lipides – **de première catégorie** (c'est-à-dire à fibres musculaires courtes) car ils sont dotés d'un rapport collagène sur protéines élevé La texture et les quantités sont normales Modes de cuisson recommandés : vapeur, bouillies, papillote, au four…	Les morceaux de viandes à éviter sont : – **demi-gras et gras** – **de deuxième et de troisième catégorie** Modes de cuisson déconseillés : grillé/doré, cuisson avec de la matière grasse…

Groupe d'aliments	Aliments conseillés	Aliments déconseillés
Charcuteries	Jambon blanc non fumé découenné/dégraissé Filets de bacon non fumés découennés/dégraissés Lardons non fumés découennés/dégraissés	Toutes les autres charcuteries
Abats	Tous contre-indiqués	Tous déconseillés
Poissons	Poissons maigres et demi-gras La texture et les quantités sont normales Modes de cuisson conseillés : sans matières grasses, court-bouillon peu parfumé, peu salé, papillote, vapeur, au four, poché…	Poissons gras Poissons salés et fumés
Œufs	Ils doivent être bien cuits car le blanc insuffisamment cuit est indigeste Modes de cuisson conseillés : coque bien cuit, mollet bien cuit, pochés bien cuits, brouillés bien cuits, au plat bien cuit, au four omelette peu grillée…	*Pas de contre-indication* Modes de cuisson déconseillés : frits avec de la matière grasse
Farines et dérivés	**Farines raffinées** **Biscottes raffinées** **Pains grillés et assimilés raffinés** **Biscuits secs à la farine raffinée nature type biscuits à thé, boudoirs, génoises…** **Pain blanc légèrement grillé en petite quantité et selon la tolérance** Mode de consommation : la texture est normale	Tous les autres dérivés de la farine Veiller à ce que le pain blanc ne soit pas chaud car il est très indigeste sous cette forme
Féculents	**Semoule fine et moyenne et grosse raffinée** **Riz blanc** **Pâtes raffinées de petit et moyen calibre** Mode de consommation : ils sont de texture normale et doivent être bien cuits. L'assaisonnement se fait après cuisson	Tous les autres féculents

Groupe d'aliments	Aliments conseillés	Aliments déconseillés
Légumes	Légumes tendres, jeunes (car ils sont peu durs et pauvres en pépins), peu acides, peu fibreux, à goût peu prononcé : **Jeunes carottes** **Jeunes navets** **Betteraves** **Haricots verts extra-fins** **Courgettes sans pépins** **Pulpe d'aubergine tamisée** **Cœur de laitue sans côtes** **Avocat** (en petite quantité dû à sa forte teneur en lipides) **Cœur d'artichaut** **Endives** (selon tolérance) **Pointes d'asperges** **Potiron** **Blancs de poireau** **Champignons** (selon tolérance) **Épinards** **Cœur de fenouil** Il est possible d'ajouter : **Tomate sans peau ni pépin** Modes de consommation : cuits (les quantités sont légèrement augmentées) ou crus (en petite quantité), sans ou avec peu de matières grasses ajoutée crues (à l'eau, à la vapeur, dans leur eau de constitution, au four, papillotes) en morceaux (ou hachés et en morceaux le plus rapidement possible)	**Tous les autres légumes sous toute autre forme**
Fruits	Fruits tendres, peu acides, peu fibreux, à goût peu prononcé : Pommes Poires Bananes Coing Pêches Nectarines Abricots Cerises	**Tous les autres fruits sous toute autre forme**

Groupe d'aliments	Aliments conseillés	Aliments déconseillés
Fruits	Les quantités peuvent être légèrement augmentées Attention à bien vérifier la tolérance du patient et les supprimer en cas de diarrhées Modes de consommation : cuits réduits en purée ou écrasés à la fourchette, sans peau, sans pépins, crus si très mûrs (augmentation des quantités de fruits crus)	
Matières grasses et équivalents	**Corps gras émulsionnés :** Beurre de préférence allégé Margarines de préférence végétales et allégées Margarines diététiques (enrichies en acides gras essentiels, vitamines E et D) Crème fraîche de préférence allégée **Huiles végétales à goût peu prononcé** (tournesol, colza, soja…). Introduction de petites quantités de vinaigrette peu assaisonnée Modes de consommation : en petite quantité, sous forme crue, bien réparties au cours des différents repas et mélangées aux aliments	**Huiles végétales à goût fort (olive, noix, noisettes…)** **Graines oléagineuses** **Fruits oléagineux** **Graisse d'oie/de canard** **Végétaline®**
Produits sucrés	**Sucre** **Caramel liquide** **Confitures de fruits** (*sauf prune et rhubarbe*) **Gelées de fruits** **Sirops de fruits dilués** **Crème de marron** **Confiseries** **Produits chocolatés** (*en petite quantité*) Mode de consommation : peu concentrés, non pris isolément	**Tous les autres produits sucrés**

Groupe d'aliments	Aliments conseillés	Aliments déconseillés
Boissons	**Eaux plates non magnésiennes** **Thé et café légers** **Tisanes, infusions** **Jus de fruits et nectars de fruits conseillés** (*en équivalence avec les fruits*) Modes de consommation : peu froides, tièdes voire chaudes	**Eaux plates magnésiennes** **Eaux gazeuses** **Thé et café forts** **Boissons rafraîchissantes sans alcool (boissons aux fruits, sodas…)** **Alcools**
Épices et aromates	**Parfums pour desserts liquides (vanille, fleur d'oranger, café…)** **Aromates en branche** (*à éliminer après cuisson*) **Sel** Modes de consommation : en petite concentration	**Aromates en poudre** **Épices**
Produits diététiques et de régime	Il est possible d'enrichir les préparations avec de la poudre de protéines et/ou d'utiliser des produits de complémentation orale voire des dextrines-maltose. En cas d'intolérance au lactose, utiliser du lait sans lactose	

4.5. En pratique

Il est nécessaire de toujours maintenir un fractionnement minutieux de 4 à 6 prises par jour.

Étant donné l'allongement de la durée de suivi de la prescription (plusieurs semaines parfois) les conseils généraux suivants peuvent être donnés :
- manger dans le calme et assis au moins en 20 minutes ;
- prendre des repas à heures régulières ;
- bien mastiquer ;
- ne pas boire trop glacé et de préférence entre les repas afin de ne pas surcharger l'estomac ;
- soigner sa dentition.

Pour ce qui est des modes de préparation des aliments, d'une façon générale, supprimer les graisses cuites et réaliser des cuissons, au four, à l'eau, en papillote… Réaliser des plats au goût relativement neutre pour ne pas stimuler l'appétit et entraver la digestion.

Il ne faut réintroduire qu'un seul type d'aliment par jour et tester la tolérance de chaque patient. Si l'aliment en question provoque des troubles digestifs (douleurs, diarrhées…), le supprimer à nouveau et le réintroduire dans quelques jours. En cas de nouvel échec, l'aliment pourra être définitivement exclu.

5. Exemple de ration, de répartition et de menu

5.1. Exemple de ration d'un régime pauvre en fibres à 6 MJ/jour

Aliments	Quantités (g ou mL)	Protéines	Lipides	Glucides	Ca	Fer	Vitamine C	Fibres
		g	g	g	mg	mg	mg	g
Lait demi-écrémé ou équivalent	300	10,5	4,5	15	360	0	0	0
Fromage	30	6	6,5	0	150	0	0	0
VPO 1re catégorie maigres	100	18	5	0	15	2	0	0
Biscotte/Pain grillé	80	8	3,1	56	48	1,2	0	3,5
PC crus ou équivalent	80	8	0	60	20	0,8	0	1,0
Légumes cuits	250	2,5	0	12,5	100	2,5	50	4
Fruits cuits	150	0	0	18	45	0,75	45	1,5
Huile	15	0	15	0	0	0	0	0
Beurre/Margarine	15	0	8,0	0	0	0	0	0
Sucre ou équivalent	30	0	0	30	0	0	0	0
Total (g)		53	48	191,5	738	7	95	10
Énergie (kJ)	5 962	901	1 805	3 255,5				
Pourcentages	100	15	30	55				

5.2. Exemple de répartition d'un régime pauvre en fibres à 6 MJ/jour

Aliments	Quantités (g ou mL)	Petit-déjeuner	Déjeuner	Dîner
		g	g	g
Lait demi-écrémé ou équivalent	300	150	0	150
Fromage	30	0	30	0
VPO 1re catégorie maigres	100	0	50	50
Biscotte/Pain grillé	80	40	25	15
PC crus ou équivalent	80	0	40	40
Légumes cuits	250	0	0	250

Les régimes pauvres en fibres

Aliments	Quantités (g ou mL)	Petit-déjeuner g	Déjeuner g	Dîner g
Fruits cuits	15	0	10	0
Huile	15	0	10	5
Beurre/Margarine	15	10	5	0
Sucre ou équivalent	30	15	5	10
Total (kJ)	**5 927**	1 473	2 305	2 149
Pourcentages	100	**25**	**39**	**36**

5.3. Exemple de menu d'un régime pauvre en fibres à 6 MJ/jour

Petit-déjeuner
Thé léger.
1 yaourt ordinaire à la gelée de groseille (20 g).
5 biscottes beurrées.

Déjeuner
Une tranche de jambon blanc découenné/dégraissé.
Semoule au beurre et à l'huile de germes de blé.
Comté.
3 biscottes.
Une compote de pommes.
Un café léger sucré (1 morceau).

Dîner
Potage au potiron.
Un œuf mollet.
Coquillettes à l'huile de colza.
2 biscottes.
Un fromage blanc aromatisé à la vanille (dont 10 g de sucre).

Section 9

Prescriptions nécessitant une modification qualitative globale de l'alimentation

19

Les régimes pauvres en résidus

1. Introduction : les différents résidus

1.1. Les fibres alimentaires végétales (FAV)

Les fibres alimentaires végétales sont les constituants des parois des cellules végétales. Il s'agit :
– des *fibres solubles* avec :
  - les pectines,
  - les gommes (Guar, Caroube),
  - les mucilages,
  - les alginates,
  - les carraghénanes ;
– des *fibres insolubles* avec :
  - la cellulose,
  - les hémicelluloses,
  - la lignine.

On sait que le poids des selles est corrélé à la consommation de fibres. Il paraît donc logique de limiter celles-ci dans les régimes pauvres en résidus.

1.2. Les glucides incomplètement attaquables par le tube digestif

1.2.1. *Au sein des fruits et des légumes*

On retrouve :
– **l'inuline** : dans les artichauts, les topinambours, les racines de chicorée ;

- **le raffinose** : dans les légumes secs, les choux communs, les brocolis, les choux de Bruxelles, les asperges ;
- **le stachyose** : dans les légumes secs, les haricots verts, les crosnes ;
- **le verbascose** : dans les légumes secs.

1.2.2. Au sein des féculents et de certains fruits

Depuis quelques années, de nombreuses études ont mis en évidence le fait qu'une partie de certains amidons dits *résistants* échappent à la digestion dans l'intestin grêle. Il existe ainsi trois types d'amidons résistants :
- *l'amidon cru* que l'on trouve dans la banane peu mûre ;
- *l'amidon encapsulé* comme celui des légumes secs car il est difficilement accessible aux enzymes digestives du fait d'un réseau de fibres qui l'entourent ;
- *l'amidon rétrogradé,* c'est-à-dire ayant subi des modifications qui influencent sa digestibilité en fonction des traitements qu'il reçoit. Ainsi, l'amidon des pâtes, des pommes de terre ou du riz est mieux digéré lorsque ceux-ci sont consommés immédiatement après cuisson que s'ils sont refroidis et ingérés ultérieurement. De même, les nouveaux riz précuits contiennent une quantité notable d'amidon résistant. Cet amidon se retrouve aussi dans le pain rassis (tandis que la mie de pain frais contient un amidon gélatinisé c'est-à-dire facilement accessible pour les amylases pancréatiques et salivaires et donc particulièrement bien digéré).

1.2.3. Au sein des confiseries « lights »

Il s'agit des *polyols* (sorbitol, maltitol, xylitol…) et des *fructo-oligosaccharides*.

1.2.4. Au sein des crustacés

La carapace des crustacés est composée de *chitine* qui est un polysaccharide aminé indigestible.

1.3. Le lactose

Chez les personnes intolérantes au lactose, celui-ci peut arriver au niveau du côlon incomplètement digéré et irriter alors la muqueuse digestive. Il peut aussi se transformer en acide lactique et favoriser le développement d'une flore acidophile responsable en excès d'appels d'eau et de diarrhées. Il conviendra donc d'adapter les apports en lait (essentiellement) et en produits laitiers en fonction de la tolérance de chaque patient.

1.4. Les fibres animales

Ce sont des molécules de nature protéique présentes au sein du tissu conjonctif des tissus animaux qui leur confèrent leur dureté et qui présentent la propriété

d'être peu voire pas digestibles. Il s'agit du *collagène* (essentiellement présent dans les viandes de deuxième et de troisième catégories) et de *l'élastine* (permettant de relier les muscles aux tendons).

2. *Définition et principe*

Les régimes pauvres en résidus sont des régimes, comme leur nom l'indique, *hyporésiduels* c'est-à-dire avec un choix des aliments laissant le moins possible de résidus intestinaux. Ils ont ainsi pour but de réduire et de faciliter la digestion de même que l'irritation et le péristaltisme de l'intestin. Ceci est réalisé en diminuant le débit fécal c'est-à-dire en augmentant la vacuité intestinale (par baisse du volume et du nombre de selles et de gaz). Il est donc nécessaire de limiter :
– les aliments qui accélèrent le transit intestinal ;
– les aliments qui augmentent le volume des selles.

> **Remarque**
> Ces régimes peuvent par conséquent être « constipants ».

3. *Les indications*

Les régimes pauvres en résidus sont des régimes de base en gastroentérologie. Leurs indications sont les suivantes :
– en pré- et postopératoire concernant une opération du tube digestif (colectomie, iléostomie, résections de l'intestin grêle…). Dans ce cas, ils précèdent et font suite à la diète hydrique ;
– les pathologies telles que : les subocclusions intestinales, les sténoses intestinales, les fistules basses, les colites, le grêle radique, la sigmoïdite diverticulaire ;
– les examens du côlon (scintigraphie, écho-Doppler, lavement baryté, coloscopie…) ;
– certains cas de diarrhées (le régime est associé à des aliments constipants) ;
– les pathologies inflammatoires de l'intestin en phase aiguë (maladie de Crohn, rectocolite hémorragique) ;
– les autres indications pour lesquelles le régime facilite la cicatrisation et diminue la douleur :
  - après une intervention abdominale : césarienne,
  - après une intervention proche de l'anus : épisiotomies, hémoroïdectomie, fistule anale…

4. Couverture des besoins et apports nutritionnels conseillés

4.1. L'énergie

Le niveau énergétique doit se rapprocher le plus possible des besoins réels du patient (sauf en cas de réalimentation) en fonction de son métabolisme de base et de son niveau d'activité physique.

4.2. Les protéines

Sauf en cas de cicatrisation et de réalimentation, pour lesquels le régime est hyperprotidique, les apports conseillés en protéines doivent représenter 11 à 15 % de l'apport énergétique total avec un apport protéique de sécurité compris entre 0,8 et 1 g par kilogramme de poids de forme et par jour (selon l'âge de l'individu).

4.3. Les lipides

Les lipides doivent couvrir 30 à 35 % de l'apport énergétique total avec la répartition en acides gras suivante (cas de l'adulte) :
– 8 % d'acides gras saturés ;
– 20 % d'acides gras monoinsaturés ;
– 5 % d'acides gras polyinsaturés avec :
  - 4 % d'acide gras oméga 6 (acide linoléique),
  - 0,8 % d'acide gras oméga 3 (acide alpha linolénique),
  - 0,2 % d'acides gras polyinsaturés à longue chaîne dont 0,05 % de DHA.

En cas de troubles digestifs importants, il est conseillé de réduire légèrement les lipides pour atteindre 25 à 30 % de l'apport énergétique total.

4.4. Les glucides

Les glucides représentent le complément énergétique de la ration soit 50 à 59 % de l'apport énergétique total. Néanmoins, en cas de modification des apports conseillés en protéines et en lipides, le régime peut être légèrement hyperglucidique.

Les glucides complexes et les glucides simples doivent respectivement couvrir 50 à 55 % et 45 à 50 % des glucides totaux.

Les produits sucrés sont à limiter à 10 % de l'apport énergétique total car ce sont des aliments plaisirs mais qualifiés de calories vides. Il est préconisé de bien les répartir tout au long de la journée (d'autant plus lors de troubles digestifs en vue d'éviter l'apparition de diarrhées hydriques).

4.5. Les fibres

De par la nécessité de réduire les résidus intestinaux dont les fibres font partie, les apports en ces molécules sont limités à 5-10 g par jour au maximum. Il est par conséquent recommandé de surveiller une éventuelle constipation allant à l'encontre du but recherché (à savoir la vacuité intestinale).

4.6. Les vitamines

La couverture en *vitamine C* ne peut être assurée puisque les végétaux crus sont absents du choix des aliments. En cas de suivi au long cours, une supplémentation médicamenteuse peut être envisagée.

4.7. Les minéraux

Il est conseillé de surveiller l'apport en *calcium* pour le régime pauvre en résidus strict car le lait et les produits laitiers sont peu représentés de par le choix des aliments.

4.8. L'eau

Les besoins en eau doivent correspondre à ceux recommandés en fonction de l'âge de chaque patient et accentués en cas de fièvre et/ou de diarrhées.

5. *Le choix des aliments*

Il existe actuellement deux types de régimes pauvres en résidus :
- *le régime pauvre en résidus strict* : il est basé sur la suppression de nombreux aliments d'origine différente sans tenir compte de la réelle tolérance des patients de manière individuelle. Il est par conséquent particulièrement strict et monotone même s'il est encore couramment utilisé ;
- *le régime pauvre en résidus large* : il correspond à un élargissement du régime pauvre en résidu strict suite à des expérimentations portant sur la digestibilité des aliments ce qui a permis de réintégrer :
  - le lactose (sauf si une intolérance est réellement avérée),
  - les aliments dits « irritants » tels que les graisses de constitution et les graisses cuites (en petite quantité),
  - les épices et les aromates (en contrôlant le dosage),
  - les jus de fruits (sauf ceux de pommes et de pruneau).

5.1. Le choix des aliments du régime pauvre en résidus strict

Groupe d'aliments	Aliments conseillés	Aliments déconseillés
Laits	Tous contre-indiqués	Laits sous toutes leurs formes
Laitages	Tous contre-indiqués	Tous déconseillés
Desserts lactés	Tous contre-indiqués	Tous déconseillés
Fromages	Fromages fondus Fromages à pâte dure	Tous les autres types de fromage
Viandes	Viandes de première catégorie maigres	Viandes de première catégorie demi-grasses et grasses Viandes de deuxième et de troisième catégories maigres, demi-grasses et grasses
Charcuteries	Jambon blanc découenné dégraissé non fumé Jambon cru découenné dégraissé non fumé Filet de bacon découenné dégraissé non fumé	Toutes les autres charcuteries
Abats	Tous contre-indiqués	Tous déconseillés
Produits de la pêche	Poissons maigres, demi-gras, gras Crustacés (sans la carapace et sauf les crevettes grises) Mollusques	Crevettes grises Carapace des crustacés
Œufs	Œufs durs avec le blanc bien cuit	Toutes les autres formes de cuisson des œufs
Farines et dérivés	Farines raffinées de blé, maïzena Pains blancs grillés nature Biscottes et équivalents raffinés et nature	Toutes les autres farines et leurs dérivés
Féculents	Céréales raffinées non cuisinées	Tous les autres féculents
Légumes	Bouillons de légumes filtrés : bouillons clairs, passés, réalisés à partir de légumes non amylacés, peu fibreux, se digérant facilement (laitue, carottes, endives, courgettes, aubergines, blancs de poireaux…)	Tous les autres légumes sous toute autre forme

Groupe d'aliments	Aliments conseillés	Aliments déconseillés
Fruits	**Bouillons de fruits filtrés :** bouillons clairs, passés, sucré (à 5 % maximum) réalisés à partir de fruits peu fibreux, se digérant facilement (poire, abricot, brugnon, nectarine…)	**Tous les autres fruits sous toute autre forme**
Matières grasses et équivalents	**Huiles** **Beurre** **Margarines végétales** Mode de consommation : toujours crues	**Crème fraîche** **Autres margarines** **Autres matières grasses** **Fruits oléagineux** **Graines oléagineuses**
Sucre et produits sucrés	**Sucre** **Gelées de fruits** **Miel** (*en petite quantité*) **Sirops** **Confiseries type bonbons, caramels** **Cacao en poudre** **Chocolats nature** **Sorbets nature** **Meringues**	**Tous les autres produits sucrés**
Boissons	**Eaux plates non magnésiennes** **Thé, café légers** **Tisanes, infusions** **Boissons rafraîchissantes sans alcool non gazeuses**	**Toutes les autres boissons**
Épices et aromates	**Jus de citron** **Vanille** **Fleur d'oranger** **Café soluble** **Sel** *en petite quantité*	**Toutes les autres épices et aromates**
Produits diététiques et de régime	Lait sans lactose (AL110®, Lactodiet®) Desserts lactés sans lactose Si besoin : produits de complémentation hyperprotidiques et/ou hyperénergétiques	**Confiseries « lights » à base de polyols**

5.2. Le choix des aliments du régime pauvre en résidus large

Groupe d'aliments	Aliments conseillés	Aliments déconseillés
Laits	**Laits sous toutes ses formes** Attention : il convient de bien vérifier la tolérance de chaque patient	*Pas de contre-indication*
Laitages	**Laitages nature et/ou aromatisés**	**Laitages aux fruits** **Laitages à la crème de marron**
Desserts lactés	**Desserts lactés nature et/ou aromatisés**	**Desserts lactés aux fruits cuits et/ou aux fruits secs** **Desserts lactés à la crème de marron**
Fromages	**Fromages frais salés nature** *en petite quantité* **Fromages affinés nature** *en petite quantité*	**Fromages frais salés aromatisés et/ou aux fruits secs et/ou aux graines oléagineuses** **Fromages affinés et/ou aux fruits secs et/ou aux graines oléagineuses**
Viandes	**Toutes conseillées** Attention : les viandes demi-grasses et grasses et/ou de deuxième et de troisième catégories en petite quantité	*Pas de contre-indication*
Charcuteries	**Toutes conseillées** Attention : en petite quantité, plutôt maigres et selon la fréquence recommandée	*Pas de contre-indication*
Abats	**Tous conseillés** de préférence maigres	*Pas de contre-indication*
Produits de la pêche	**Poissons maigres, demi-gras, gras** **Crustacés** (sans la carapace et sauf les crevettes grises) **Mollusques**	**Crevettes grises** **Carapace des crustacés**
Œufs	Sous toutes leurs formes : **coque, pochés, mollets, cocotte, durs, au plat, brouillés, omelettes…**	*Pas de contre-indication*
Farines et dérivés	**Farines raffinées de blé, maïzena** **Pains blancs, pains de mie raffinés et nature** Veiller à ne pas consommer de grande quantité de pain car l'amidon est rétrogradé	**Toutes les autres farines et leurs dérivés**

Les régimes pauvres en résidus

Groupe d'aliments	Aliments conseillés	Aliments déconseillés
Farines et dérivés	**Biscottes et équivalents raffinés et nature** **Viennoiseries, biscuits secs, pâtisseries à la farine raffinée nature sans fruits** **Attention** : respecter les quantités et les fréquences recommandées **Riz soufflé nature ou chocolaté**	
Féculents	**Céréales raffinées non cuisinées : pâtes, semoule, blé dur précuit, riz blanc, tapioca** **Pommes de terre en petite quantité entières non cuisinées**	Toutes les autres céréales sous toute autre forme Châtaignes, marrons Légumes secs Banane plantain Autres formes de pommes de terre
Légumes	**Bouillons de légumes filtrés** : bouillons clairs, passés, réalisés à partir de légumes non amylacés, peu fibreux, se digérant facilement (laitue, carottes, endives, courgettes, aubergines, blancs de poireaux…)	Tous les autres légumes sous toute autre forme
Fruits	**Bouillons de fruits filtrés** : bouillons clairs, passés, sucrés (à 5 % maximum) réalisés à partir de fruits peu fibreux, se digérant facilement (poire, abricot, brugnon, nectarine…) **Jus de fruits passés** (sauf pomme et pruneaux). Servir des petites quantités et les diluer éventuellement avec de l'eau lorsque tout problème digestif a été exclu	Tous les autres fruits sous toute autre forme
Matières grasses et équivalents	**Huiles** **Beurre** **Margarines** **Crème fraîche** Mode de consommation : de préférence crues	Autres matières grasses Fruits oléagineux Graines oléagineuses

Groupe d'aliments	Aliments conseillés	Aliments déconseillés
Sucre et produits sucrés	Sucre Gelées de fruits Miel (*en petite quantité*) Sirops Confiseries type bonbons, caramels Cacao en poudre Chocolats nature Sorbets nature Glaces et crèmes glacées nature	Tous les autres produits sucrés
Boissons	Toutes les autres boissons Vérifier la tolérance aux boissons gazeuses	Jus de fruits à la pomme et aux pruneaux Boissons alcoolisées
Épices et aromates	Jus de citron Vanille Fleur d'oranger Café soluble Sel en petite quantité Épices en poudre, herbes aromatiques : en petite quantité	Toutes les autres épices et aromates
Produits diététiques et de régime	Lait sans lactose (AL110®, Lactodiet®) Desserts lactés sans lactose Si besoin : produits de complémentation hyperprotidiques et/ou hyperénergétiques	Confiseries « lights » à base de polyols

6. En pratique

Proposer au moins trois repas principaux en veillant à ce que chacun soit équilibré notamment en protéines animales.

De plus, il est important de surveiller régulièrement le poids et d'observer le transit intestinal du patient.

Les modes de cuisson sont de préférence simples avec des matières grasses consommées plutôt crues (obligatoire lors du régime pauvre en résidus strict et conseillé pour le large) :
- les viandes sont grillées, bouillies, cuites à la broche, rôties… ;
- les poissons sont grillés, cuits en papillote, à la vapeur, au four, au court-bouillon peu parfumé… ;
- les œufs sont consommés bien cuits (le blanc cru étant peu digeste) ;
- les féculents sont accommodés après la cuisson avec des matières grasses crues.

Les régimes pauvres en résidus

7. Exemple de ration, de répartition et de menu

7.1. Exemple de ration d'un régime pauvre en résidus strict à 8 MJ/jour

Aliments	Quantités (g ou mL)	Protéines	Lipides	Glucides	Ca	Fer	Vitamine C	Fibres
		g	g	g	mg	mg	mg	g
Lait sans lactose	600	9	15	36	1 200	0	0	0
Fromage pâte dure	30	9	9	0	330	0	0	0
VPO maigres/1re catégorie	150	27	7,5	0	22,5	3	0	0
Œuf	50	6	5	0	0	1	0	0
Biscotte/Pain grillé raffiné	80	8	3	56	48	1,2	0	4
PC crus ou équivalent raffinés	80	8	0	60	20	0,8	0	1
Biscuits secs type petit beurre	40	2	4,8	28	8	0,4	0	1
Bouillon de légumes	400	0	0	12	0	0	0	0
Huile	20	0	20	0	0	0	0	0
Beurre/Margarine	10	0	8,2	0	0	0	0	0
Sucre ou équivalent	45	0	0	45	0	0	0	0
Total (g)		70	73	237	1 629	6	0	6
Énergie (kJ)	7 985	1 184	2 772	4 029				
Pourcentages	100	15	35	50				

7.2. Exemple de répartition d'un régime pauvre en résidus strict à 8 MJ/jour

Aliments	Quantités (g ou mL)	Petit-déjeuner	Déjeuner	Collation	Dîner
		g	g	g	g
Lait sans lactose	600	150	150	150	150
Fromage pâte dure	30	0	0	0	30
VPO	150	0	100	0	50

Aliments	Quantités (g ou mL)	Petit-déjeuner	Déjeuner	Collation	Dîner
		g	g	g	g
Œuf	50	0	0	50	0
Biscotte/Pain grillé raffiné	80	40	15	0	25
PC crus ou équivalent raffinés	80	0	55	0	25
Biscuits secs type petit beurre	40	40	0	0	0
Bouillon de légumes	400	0	200	0	200
Huile	20	0	5	0	15
Beurre/Margarine	10	0	10	0	0
Sucre ou équivalent	45	10	10	10	15
Total (kJ)		7 991	1 808	2 963	809,5	2 411
Pourcentages	100	23	37	10	30

7.3. Exemple de menu d'un régime pauvre en résidus strict à 8 MJ/jour

Petit-déjeuner
Une tasse de lait sans lactose nature.
5 biscuits secs type petit beurre.
5 biscottes à la gelée de groseille (15 g).

Déjeuner
Bouillon de légumes filtré.
Blanc de poulet poché et filet d'huile de germes de blé
Coquillettes à la béchamel.
Une tranche de pain grillé.
Semoule au lait sans lactose (15 g de semoule, 150 mL de lait sans lactose, 10 g de sucre).

Collation
Crème renversée dans lactose (150 mL de lait sans lactose, 1 œuf, 10 g de sucre).

Dîner
Bouillon de légumes filtré.
Un carré de cabillaud à l'huile d'olive.
Gruyère.
3 biscottes.
Riz au lait sans lactose (150 mL de lait sans lactose, 25 g de riz, 15 g de sucre).

20

Le régime normal léger

1. Définition et principe

Le régime normal léger est à la base de la diététique en milieu hospitalier. Il consiste à avoir une alimentation aussi proche que possible de la normale mais facile à digérer c'est-à-dire assurant une vacuité gastrique et intestinale assez rapide à la suite des repas.

Le choix des aliments doit par conséquent empêcher :
– les inconforts intestinaux et coliques (engendrant ballonnements, aérophagie, brûlures digestives, éructation, somnolence postprandiale, renvois gastriques…) ;
– le ralentissement de la digestion.

En pratique et d'une manière générale, il faut donc éviter :
– les aliments à goût fort ;
– les aliments riches en fibres ;
– les aliments riches en lipides.

Les tolérances personnelles seront particulièrement recherchées afin d'élargir le plus possible l'alimentation du patient d'autant plus que ce type de prescription peut être suivi à vie.

2. Les indications

Les indications sont les suivantes :
– dernière étape de réalimentation après une intervention digestive ;

- cas de digestion difficile quelle qu'en soit la cause (dyspepsie, gastralgie, gastrite médicamenteuse, duodénite, colopathie fonctionnelle…) ;
- cas de cardiologie en particulier en post-infarctus en vue d'assurer un meilleur confort au patient ;
- les femmes enceintes en fin de grossesse pour lesquelles on prescrit un régime normal léger large ;
- les sportifs avec là encore un régime normal léger large et particulièrement adapté ;
- les personnes âgées de par le ralentissement digestif d'origine physiologique.

3. Couverture des besoins et apports nutritionnels conseillés

3.1. L'énergie

Le régime est normoénergétique en fonction du métabolisme de base et du niveau d'activité physique de chaque patient.

3.2. Les protéines

De même que pour l'énergie, le régime est normoprotidique à savoir que les protéines doivent représenter 11 à 15 % de l'apport énergétique total.

L'apport protidique de sécurité est évalué en fonction de chaque patient.

3.3. Les lipides

Afin d'éviter les troubles digestifs pouvant être engendrés par une trop grande quantité de lipides, ceux-ci sont limités à 25-30 % de l'apport énergétique total.

La répartition en acides gras (sur la base de 28 % de l'apport énergétique total et ce, chez l'adulte) se fait alors de la manière suivante :
- acides gras saturés : 7 % de l'apport énergétique total ;
- acides gras monoinsaturés : 17 % de l'apport énergétique total ;
- acides gras polyinsaturés : 4 % de l'apport énergétique total avec :
  - acides gras oméga 6 : 3,5 % de l'apport énergétique total,
  - acides gras oméga 3 : 0,5 % de l'apport énergétique total dont 0,05 % de DHA.

3.4. Les glucides

En tant que complément énergétique, les glucides doivent représenter à 55 à 64 % de l'apport énergétique total. La répartition se fait comme habituellement soit 50 à 55 % de glucides complexes et 45 à 50 % de glucides simples.

Les produits sucrés ne doivent pas dépasser 10 % de l'apport énergétique total. En effet, ce sont des aliments plaisirs mais en tant que calories vides, ils ne doivent

pas être en quantité excessive. Il convient de plus de bien les répartir au cours des différents repas.

3.5. Les fibres, les vitamines, les minéraux et l'eau

Les apports en fibres, vitamines, minéraux et en eau doivent suivre les recommandations en fonction de l'âge et des particularités physiologiques de chaque patient.

4. *Le choix des aliments*

Groupe d'aliments	Aliments conseillés	Aliments déconseillés			Intolérances personnelles
		Goût fort	Donnent des gaz	Riches en lipides	
Lait et produits laitiers	Lait écrémé, demi-écrémé	Lait de chèvre Lait de brebis		Lait entier	
	Laitages au lait écrémé, demi-écrémé (nature, aromatisés, aux fruits)	Laitages au lait de chèvre Laitages au lait de brebis		Laitages au lait entier, à plus de 20 % de MG	
	Desserts lactés peu riches en lipides			Desserts lactés riches en lipides	
	Fromages peu affinés La quantité de fromage doit être bien adaptée et les étiquettes correctement déchiffrées	Fromages à goût fort (à croûte lavée, persillés) Fromages aromatisés	Fromages très affinés	Fromages riches en lipides	Fromages à pâte molle à croûte fleurie peu affinés
Viandes	Viandes de boucherie de première catégorie, maigres et demi-grasses Modes de cuisson : sans matières grasses, sauces dégraissées,	Viandes fumées Viande de cheval Gibier Abats	Viandes de boucherie de deuxième et de troisième catégorie	Viandes de boucherie grasses	Mouton et agneau : morceaux de première catégorie, maigres et demi-gras

Groupe d'aliments	Aliments conseillés	Aliments déconseillés			Intolérances personnelles
		Goût fort	Donnent des gaz	Riches en lipides	
Viandes	papillotes, four (rôtis), peu grillées, brochette, poêle antiadhésive, à l'eau…				
Charcuteries	Charcuteries maigres non fumées	Charcuteries fumées		Charcuteries grasses	
Produits de la pêche	Poissons maigres ou demi-gras à goût peu prononcé Mollusques Crustacés Modes de cuisson : sans matières grasses, grillés, court-bouillon peu parfumé, four, vapeur, papillote, brochette, pochés…	Poissons maigres ou demi-gras ou gras à goût prononcé et/ou fumés			Mollusques Crustacés
Œufs	Pas de contre-indication Modes de cuisson : sans matières grasses, omelette, pochés, coque, au plat, poêle antiadhésive, cocotte, durs, mollets, brouillés…				
Farines et dérivés	Farines raffinées Pains et dérivés raffinés nature Veiller à ce que le pain blanc ne soit pas chaud car il est très indigeste sous cette forme. De plus les quantités doivent être contrôlées		Farines non raffinées Pains et dérivés non raffinés et/ou aux fruits secs	Pains et dérivés aux graines oléagineuses Viennoiseries et assimilés	

Le régime normal léger

Groupe d'aliments	Aliments conseillés	Aliments déconseillés			Intolérances personnelles
		Goût fort	Donnent des gaz	Riches en lipides	
Farines et dérivés	Céréales pour petit-déjeuner raffinées et nature Biscuits secs à la farine raffinée nature		Céréales pour petit-déjeuner ou raffinées et/ou aux fruits secs Biscuits non raffinés et/ou aux fruits secs	Céréales pour petit-déjeuner aux graines oléagineuses Biscuits salés et sucrés riches en lipides Pâtisseries salées et sucrées	
Féculents	Céréales raffinées non cuisinées Pommes de terre en petite quantité entières		Céréales complètes et semi-complètes Légumes secs Maïs en grains Fruits amylacés Autres types de pommes de terre	Tous les féculents du commerce cuisinés	
Légumes	Courgettes Carottes Aubergine Laitue Batavia Romaine Frisée Chicorée Scarole Mâche Endive Feuille de chêne Betterave Pointes d'asperge Blancs de poireau Potiron Haricots verts extra-fins Haricots beurre Épinards Cœur d'artichaut Cœur de fenouil	Légumes à goût fort	Légumes riches en fibres insolubles	Avocat Sauces industrielles cuisinées	Tomates Épinards Haricots verts Navet Endive Champignons Blancs de poireaux

Groupe d'aliments	Aliments conseillés	Aliments déconseillés			Intolérances personnelles
		Goût fort	Donnent des gaz	Riches en lipides	
Légumes	Tomates Coulis de tomate non cuisiné Navet Jus de légumes (à base des légumes conseillés) Modes de cuisson : sans matières grasses, à l'eau, à la vapeur, à l'autocuiseur, au four…				
Fruits	Fruits contenant moins de 2 % de fibres	Fruits acides	Fruits riches en fibres insolubles		Pommes Prunes
Matières grasses et équivalents	Huiles à goût peu prononcé Crème fraîche Beurre Margarines Mode de consommation : sous forme crue	Autres matières grasses à goût fort	Corps gras cuits Panures/ fritures	Sauces du commerce Graines oléagineuses Fruits oléagineux	Huiles vierges Huile d'olive
Sucre et équivalents	Sucre Caramel Confitures (aux fruits conseillés) Confiseries (autres que celles déconseillées) Pâtes de fruits Fruits confits Sirops Crème de marron Sorbets nature Glaces nature Miel peu goûteux Poudre chocolatée sucrée	Marmelades Miels à goût fort Réglisse et produits à base de réglisse	Confitures de figues, de prunes, de rhubarbe Confiseries « light » à base de polyols	Sorbets et glaces non nature Crèmes glacées Nougats Dragées Cacao en poudre non sucré Chocolat et dérivés Pâtes à tartiner	Chewing-gum Cacao Chocolat et dérivés Miel

Groupe d'aliments	Aliments conseillés	Aliments déconseillés			Intolérances personnelles
		Goût fort	Donnent des gaz	Riches en lipides	
Sucre et équivalents	Mode de consommation : en petite quantité et en prise non isolée				
Boissons	Thé léger Café léger Tisanes Infusions Jus, nectars, compotes de fruits (à base des fruits conseillés)	Thé fort Café fort Boissons alcoolisées	Boissons gazeuses Boissons alcoolisées gazeuses		Jus de pomme Jus de pruneaux
Épices et aromates	Parfums pour desserts liquides Herbes aromatiques Mode de consommation : en petite quantité	Poivre Moutarde Gingembre Tabasco Vinaigre Curry Paprika Câpres Petits oignons Cornichons Harissa Piments			Herbes aromatiques

5. *En pratique*

La répartition se fait en 4 à 5 repas par jour avec :
- petit déjeuner ;
- +/- collation ;
- déjeuner « léger » ;
- collation ;
- dîner « léger ».

21

Le régime sans gluten

1. Définition et principe

Le régime sans gluten est une alimentation au cours de laquelle on supprime totalement et définitivement le gluten de l'alimentation.

2. Les indications

Les indications sont les suivantes :
– la maladie cœliaque ou entéropathie au gluten : le régime sans gluten est le seul traitement de cette pathologie. Il doit être particulièrement bien suivi en vue :
  - d'éviter les risques de cancérisation (lymphome),
  - de supprimer les signes carentiels cliniques et biologiques ainsi que les signes digestifs ;
– la dermatite herpétiforme.

3. Couverture des besoins et apports nutritionnels conseillés

3.1. L'énergie

Le régime est normoénergétique mais peut aussi être hyperénergétique lors de la découverte de la pathologie car on constate des risques possibles de dénutrition.

3.2. Les protéines

De même que pour l'énergie, le régime est normoprotidique et souvent hyperprotidique à la découverte afin de favoriser la restructuration des microvillosités de la muqueuse intestinale.

3.3. Les lipides

Là encore, le régime est normolipidique et la répartition des acides gras se fait selon les recommandations. Il convient de veiller à l'apport en acides gras essentiels pour leur implication dans la cicatrisation.

3.4. Les glucides

Les glucides sont les compléments énergétiques. À noter qu'en début de prescription, on constate souvent des diarrhées importantes chez le patient. Dans ce cas, il est possible de prescrire un régime pauvre en fibres associé à une élimination transitoire du lactose.

3.5. Les fibres

De même que pour les glucides assimilables, un régime pauvre en fibres peut être proposé à la suite ou à la place du régime pauvre en résidus selon les troubles digestifs du patient.

3.6. Les vitamines

La vitamine C doit être surveillée de par son implication dans l'absorption du fer non héminique.

La vitamine B_9 doit aussi être contrôlée car les patients présentent un risque de neuropathies.

3.7. Les minéraux

Pour ce qui est des minéraux, il convient de vérifier les apports en :
- *fer* car les patients peuvent être anémiés et présenter des troubles de la coagulation. Chez l'enfant, la carence en fer peut par ailleurs engendrer une cassure de la courbe de croissance ;
- *calcium* dû aux risques de troubles osseux (ostéopénie, ostéoporose, ostéomalacie) provoqués par la maladie ;
- *magnésium* en vue de prévenir les éventuelles tétanies et crampes musculaires souvent constatées.

3.8. L'eau

Les apports en eau doivent correspondre aux recommandations en fonction de l'âge du patient.

4. Le choix des aliments

Le principe du régime sans gluten repose sur la suppression de tous les aliments contenant du gluten à savoir :
- le blé et ses dérivés ;
- l'orge et ses dérivés ;
- le seigle et ses dérivés ;
- l'avoine et ses dérivés.

Le choix des aliments est donc très restrictif car il suppose l'élimination de nombreux produits du commerce :

Groupe d'aliments	Aliments autorisés	Aliments interdits
Laits	Laits liquides, concentrés, en poudre nature	Laits liquides, concentrés, en poudre aromatisés et/ou contenant des additifs interdits
Laitages	Laitages nature, aromatisés, aux fruits sans additifs interdits	Laitages aux céréales interdites Laitages avec des additifs interdits
Desserts lactés	Desserts lactés maison avec les aliments autorisés	Desserts lactés maison contenant les céréales interdites Desserts lactés industriels Préparations industrielles pour desserts lactés
Fromages	Fromages à pâte dure Fromages à pâte demi-dure Fromages à pâte molle non aromatisés	Fromages persillés Fromages fondus Fromages industriels à tartiner Fromages aromatisés
Viandes	Viandes fraîches, surgelées non cuisinées	Viandes du commerce cuisinées
Charcuteries	Charcuteries sans additifs interdits	Charcuteries contenant les additifs interdits
Abats	Abats frais, surgelés non cuisinés	Abats cuisinés du commerce
Produits de la pêche	Produits de la pêche frais, surgelés non cuisinés	Produits de la pêche du commerce cuisinés
Œufs	Œufs en l'état	Produits du commerce à base d'œufs
Farines et dérivés, féculents	Farines, pains et dérivés, biscottes et dérivés, céréales pour petit-déjeuner, biscuits, viennoiseries, gâteaux, pâtisseries, féculents SANS GLUTEN	Produits à base de blé (froment) et ses dérivés : farine, pains et dérivés, biscottes, pains grillés, céréales pour petit-déjeuner, chapelure, biscuits salés et sucrés,

Groupe d'aliments	Aliments autorisés	Aliments interdits
Farines et dérivés, féculents		viennoiseries, gâteaux, pâtisseries salées et sucrées, semoule et produits à base de semoule, pâtes alimentaires, blé dur précuit
	Riz non cuisiné et ses dérivés : semoule de riz, crème de riz, pétales de riz	Produits industriels à base de riz
	Maïs non cuisiné et ses dérivés : fécule de maïs (maïzena), semoule de maïs, germes de maïs, maïs égrené en conserve au naturel, maïs en épis, pétales de maïs	Produits industriels à base de maïs
	Légumes secs : frais, en conserve au naturel, farine de légumes secs (pure)	Produits industriels à base de légumes secs
	Pommes de terre fraîches, précuites, sous vide, fécule de pomme de terre	Pommes de terre industrielles cuisinées
	Fruits amylacés non cuisinés, farine de châtaigne (pure)	Produits industriels à base de fruits amylacés
	Sarrasin non cuisiné, farine de sarrasin pure	Produits industriels à base de sarrasin
	Millet non cuisiné et semoule de millet	Produits industriels à base de millet
	Quinoa non cuisiné	Produits industriels à base de quinoa
	Manioc et dérivés : tapioca, crème de tapioca Sorgho Arrow root Igname Topinambour Fruit à pain Patate douce Soja et farine de soja (pure)	Seigle et ses dérivés : farine, pains, pain d'épice… Avoine et ses dérivés : farine, flocons, riz sauvage… Orge et ses dérivés : farine, orge perlée, orge mondée Épeautre (blé ancestral) Kamut (blé ancestral) Triticale (hybride de blé et de seigle)

Le régime sans gluten

Groupe d'aliments	Aliments autorisés	Aliments interdits
Légumes	Légumes frais, surgelés, en conserve au naturel non cuisinés	Préparations industrielles à base de légumes
Fruits	Fruits frais, surgelés, en conserve, en compote sans additifs interdits Fruits secs non farinés	Fruits préparés contenant les additifs interdits Desserts industriels à base de fruits Fruits secs farinés
Matières grasses et équivalents	Toutes les autres huiles Beurres non allégés Margarines sans additifs interdits Crèmes non allégées, non transformées Fruits oléagineux Graines oléagineuses	Huile de germe de blé Beurres allégés Margarines avec les additifs interdits Crèmes allégées, transformées (chantilly industrielle, préparations industrielles à base de crème) Matières grasses industrielles à tartiner Sauces du commerce
Sucre et produits sucrés	Sucre de betterave, de canne blanc et roux, fructose, caramel liquide Miel, confiture et gelées pur fruit pur sucre Cacao pur Sorbets de fruits	Sucre glace, sucre vanillé Crème de marron Pâtes de fruits Fruits confits Confiseries (bonbons, dragées, nougats, chewing-gum…) Poudres instantanées pour petit-déjeuner Autres produits à base de chocolat Pâtes à tartiner Pâte d'amande Glaces et crème glacées Autres produits glacés
Boissons	Autres boissons	Bières, panachés Whiskies
Épices et aromates	Herbes fraîches, surgelées aromatiques nature Épices nature	Tous les autres aromates et épices Sauces industrielles Bouillons cube
Autres produits		Levure chimique Aides culinaires

5. *En pratique*

Il convient de recommander aux patients :
- de respecter strictement le choix des aliments ;
- de connaître les produits de substitution (produits sans gluten) et les adresses de distributeurs ;
- de se former à la lecture des étiquettes ;
- de contrôler et/ou d'éviter les pratiques « à risque » : repas à l'extérieur, habitudes alimentaires…

Recommandations sur les additifs

Additifs autorisés (ne contiennent pas de gluten)	Additifs interdits (contiennent du gluten)
Acidifiants	Amidon de blé, de seigle, d'orge, d'avoine
Agar-agar	Acides aminés végétaux
Antioxygènes	Gélifiants non précisés
Amidon	Malt
Amidon modifié	Matières amylacées
Arôme de malt	Polypeptides
Bétacarotène	Protéines végétales
Collagène	Gruau
Colorants	Liant protéique
Carraghénanes	
Conservateurs	
Dextrines	
Dextrose	
Exhausteurs de goût	
Émulsifiants	
Extrait de levure	
Extrait d'algues	
Extrait de malt	
Farine de Guar	
Farine de caroube	
Ferments lactiques	
Glucose et sirop de glucose	
Glutamate	
Gélatine alimentaire	
Graisse animale	
Graisse végétale	
Gomme arabique	
Gomme de Guar	
Gomme de xanthane	
Gomme d'acacia	
Inuline	
Lécithine	
Maltodextrines	
Oligofructose	
Pectine	
Polyols	
Polydextrose	
Stabilisants	

6. Exemple de ration, de répartition et de menu

6.1. Exemple de ration d'un régime sans gluten à 9,8 MJ/jour

Aliments	Quantités (g ou mL)	Protéines g	Lipides g	Glucides g	Ca mg	Fer mg	Vitamine C mg	Fibres g
Lait demi-écrémé ou équivalent	300	10,5	4,5	15	360	0	0	0
Fromage	40	8	8,8	0	200	0	0	0
VPO	200	36	20	0	30	4	0	0
Pain ou équivalent sans gluten	200	8	10	100	50	4	0	10
PC crus ou équivalent sans gluten	80	8	0	72	20	0,8	0	1,2
Légumes	450	4,5	0	22,5	180	4,5	90	13,5
Fruits	450	0	0	54	135	2,25	135	9
Huile	30	0	30	0	0	0	0	0
Beurre/Margarine sans gluten	20	0	16,4	0	0	0	0	0
Sucre ou équivalent sans gluten	40	0	0	40	0	0	0	0
Total (g)		75	90	303,5	975	16	225	34
Énergie (kJ)	9 843	1 275	3 409	5 159,5				
Pourcentages	100	13	35	52				

6.2. Exemple de répartition d'un régime sans gluten à 9,8 MJ/jour

Aliments	Quantités (g ou mL)	Petit-déjeuner g	Déjeuner g	Dîner g
Lait demi-écrémé ou équivalent	300	150	0	150
Fromage	40	0	40	0
VPO	200	0	100	100
Pain ou équivalent sans gluten	200	100	100	0

Aliments	Quantités (g ou mL)	Petit-déjeuner g	Déjeuner g	Dîner g
PC crus ou équivalents sans gluten	80	0	0	80
Légumes	450	0	350	100
Fruits	450	150	150	150
Huile	30	0	20	10
Beurre sans gluten	10	0	0	10
Margarine sans gluten	10	10	0	0
Sucre ou équivalent sans gluten	40	25	15	0
Total (kJ)	**9 847**	2 454	3 946	3 447
Pourcentages	100	**25**	**40**	**35**

6.3. Exemple de menu d'un régime sans gluten 9,8 MJ/jour

Petit-déjeuner
Thé au lait nature.
Pain sans gluten à la margarine et au miel (30 g).
Jus d'orange sanguine.

Déjeuner
Betteraves (100 g) à l'huile de noix (10 mL).
Bavette grillée à l'échalote fraîche.
Courgettes braisées (10 mL d'huile d'olive).
Comté fruité.
Pain sans gluten.
Une petite banane.
Un café sucré (3 morceaux).

Dîner
Concombres sauce yaourt à la menthe fraîche.
Fricassée de colin au citron (10 mL d'huile de tournesol).
Riz créole (10 g de beurre).
Un fromage blanc nature et morceaux de pêche.

Partie 2

Prescriptions spécifiques à une pathologie

22

Les prescriptions selon les pathologies

1. Les pathologies digestives et urinaires

Pathologie		Prescription pouvant être proposée
Troubles de la déglutition		Régimes à texture modifiée
Pathologies de l'œsophage et de l'estomac	*Œsophagites et sténoses œsophagiennes*	Régime à texture modifiée
	Chirurgie digestive haute	– Régimes à texture modifiée – Régimes pauvres en résidus – Régimes pauvres en fibres – Régime normal léger – Régime hyperénergétique – Régime hyperprotidique
	Cancers de l'œsophage, de l'intestin grêle, de l'estomac	– Régimes à texture modifiée – Régimes pauvres en fibres – Régime normal léger – Régime hyperénergétique – Régime hyperprotidique
	Reflux gastro-œsophagien/ Hernie hiatale	Régime normal léger

Pathologie		Prescription pouvant être proposée
Pathologies de l'œsophage et de l'estomac	*Ulcère gastroduodénal* ✓ *Gastrite*	– Régimes à texture modifiée – Régimes pauvres en fibres – Régime normal léger
	Gastrectomie ✓	– Régimes à texture modifiée – Régimes pauvres en fibres – Régime normal léger – Régime contrôlé en saccharose
Pathologies de l'intestin grêle, du côlon et du rectum	*Diarrhées aiguës et chroniques* ✓	– Régimes contrôlés en fibres
	Constipation ✓ *Diverticulose colique*	– Régime riche en fibres
	Diverticulites ✓	– Régimes pauvres en résidus – Régimes pauvres en fibres – Régime normal léger
	Maladie de Crohn *Rectocolite hémorragique* ✓	– Régimes pauvres en résidus – Régimes pauvres en fibres – Régime normal léger – Régime hyperénergétique – Régime hyperprotidique
	Troubles fonctionnels intestinaux ✓	– Régimes pauvres en résidus – Régimes pauvres en fibres – Régime normal léger
	Chirurgie digestive haute ✓	– Régimes pauvres en résidus – Régimes pauvres en fibres – Régime normal léger
	Cancers ✓	– Régimes pauvres en fibres – Régime normal léger – Régime hyperénergétique – Régime hyperprotidique
	Fistules digestives ✓	– Régimes pauvres en fibres – Régime normal léger
	Cirrhose ✓	– Régime liquide lacté (rupture de varices œsophagiennes) – Régimes hyposodés – Régime normal léger – Régime hyperénergétique
Pathologies hépatiques, biliaires, pancréatiques	*Hépatites* ✓ *Lithiase biliaire*	– Régime normal léger

Les prescriptions selon les pathologies 267

Pathologie		Prescription pouvant être proposée
Pathologies hépatiques, biliaires, pancréatiques	*Insuffisance hépatique (ascite)*	– Régimes pauvres en fibres – Régime normal léger – Régimes hyposodés – Régime hypolipidique
	Encéphalopathie hépatique	– Régime hypoprotidique
	Cholécystectomie ✓	– Régimes pauvres en résidus – Régimes pauvres en fibres – Régime normal léger
	Pancréatite	– Régime normal léger – Régime hypolipidique
	Pancréatectomie, DPC ✓	– Régimes pauvres en résidus – Régimes pauvres en fibres – Régime normal léger
	Cancers (pancréas, foie) ✓	– Régime normal léger – Régime hyperénergétique – Régime hyperprotidique
Lithiases urinaires oxalocalcique, phosphocalcique, urinaire		– Régimes pauvres en fibres – Régime normal léger – Régime hypoénergétique – Régime hypoprotidique

2. *Les pathologies rénales (néphropathies)*

Pathologie	Prescription pouvant être proposée
Syndrome néphrotique **Insuffisance rénale aiguë** **Insuffisance rénale chronique** **Insuffisance rénale terminale**	– Régimes hyposodés – Régime hypopotassique – Régime hyperénergétique – Régimes contrôlés en protéines – Régime contrôlé en phosphore

3. *Les pathologies respiratoires*

Pathologie	Prescription pouvant être proposée
Insuffisance respiratoire chronique ✓	– Régime hyperénergétique

4. Les pathologies de la nutrition ou métaboliques

Pathologie	Prescription pouvant être proposée
Diabète	– Régime contrôlé en glucides (type 1) – Régime contrôlé en lipides et en glucides (type 2) – Régime hypoénergétique (type 2)
Surcharge pondérale	– Régime hypoénergétique – Régime normolipidique qualitatif – Régime contrôlé en saccharose
Dyslipidémies	– Régime normolipidique qualitatif – Régime hypoénergétique – Régime hyperprotidique – Régime contrôlé en glucides et en lipides – Régime hypolipidique (hypertriglycéridémie supérieure à 10 g/L) – Régime enrichi en TCM – Régime contrôlé en saccharose – Régime contrôlé en fructose
Dénutritions	– Régimes à texture modifiée – Régime hyperénergétique – Régime hyperprotidique
Hypoglycémies réactives fonctionnelles	– Régime contrôlé en saccharose
Anémies	– Régime hyperénergétique – Régime hyperprotidique – Régime riche en fer
Galactosémie	Suppression du galactose
Fructosémie	Suppression du fructose
Intolérance aux protéines de lait de vache	Suppression des protéines de lait de vache
Phénylcétonurie	Suppression de la phénylalanine
Leucinose	Suppression de la leucine

5. Les pathologies cardiovasculaires ou MCV (maladies cardiovasculaires)

Pathologie	Prescription pouvant être proposée
Athérosclérose/Thrombose	– Régimes hyposodés – Régime hypoénergétique – Régime normolipidique qualitatif
Hypertension artérielle	– Régimes hyposodés – Régime hypoénergétique – Régime normolipidique qualitatif – Régime hypopotassique (traitement à l'enzyme de conversion)
Insuffisance cardiaque	– Régime hyperénergétique – Régime hyperprotidique – Régimes hyposodés
Post-infarctus	– Régimes hyposodés – Régime hypoénergétique – Régime normolipidique qualitatif
Chirurgie cardiaque	– Régime hyperénergétique – Régime hyperprotidique – Régimes hyposodés

6. Autres pathologies

Pathologie	Prescription pouvant être proposée
Ostéoporose/Ostéomalacie	– Régime hypoénergétique – Régime hyperprotidique
Hypercatabolisme (polytrauma)	– Régime hyperénergétique – Régime hyperprotidique
Infections aiguës	– Régime hyperénergétique – Régime hyperprotidique
Corticothérapies	– Régime hyperprotidique – Régimes hyposodés – Régime contrôlé en lipides et en glucides
Pathologies neurodégénératives/psychiatriques	– Régimes à texture modifiée – Régime hyperénergétique – Régime hyperprotidique